HEALTHCARE IN THE UK

Understanding continuity and change

Ian Greener

This edition published in Great Britain in 2009 by

The Policy Press
University of Bristol
Fourth Floor
Beacon House
Queen's Road
Bristol BS8 1QU
UK

Tel +44 (0)117 331 4054
Fax +44 (0)117 331 4093
e-mail tpp-info@bristol.ac.uk
www.policypress.org.uk

North American office:
The Policy Press
c/o International Specialized Books Services
920 NE 58th Avenue, Suite 300
Portland,
OR 97213-3786, USA
Tel +1 503 287 3093
Fax +1 503 280 8832
e-mail info@isbs.com

© The Policy Press 2009

British Library Cataloguing in Publication Data
A catalogue record for this book is available from the British Library.

Library of Congress Cataloging-in-Publication Data
A catalog record for this book has been requested.

ISBN 978 1 86134 608 7 paperback
ISBN 978 1 86134 609 4 hardcover

The right of Ian Greener to be identified as author of this work has been
asserted by him in accordance with the 1988 Copyright, Designs and Patents Act.

Cover design by Qube Design Associates, Bristol
Front cover: image kindly supplied by Science Photo Library
Printed and bound in Great Britain by MPG Books, Bodmin

For Emily, Bethany and Anna, who will probably never read what follows but were a big part of it anyway.

Contents

List of tables and boxes   viii
Acknowledgements   ix
List of abbreviations   x

one   **Introduction**   1
         Introduction   1
         Making sense of the NHS   3
         Health policy, continuity and change   4
         The book's approach   10
         Outline of the book   11

two   **The creation of the NHS and its relevance for today**   13
         Introduction   13
         Key organisational features of the NHS   13
         Healthcare before the NHS and medico–state relations   18
         Tripartism in practice   29
         The double-bed   33
         General taxation   34
         NHS principles and their inheritance   34
         Conclusion   37

three **The tripartite split**   39
         Introduction   39
         The NHS in the 1940s and 1950s   39
         The 1960s   50
         The dynamics of tripartite healthcare at the end of the 1960s   57
         The 1970s   58
         The 1980s   60
         The 1990s   63
         The 2000s   66
         Conclusion   71

four   **The double-bed**   75
         Introduction   75
         The relationship between the state and the medical   77
            profession
         The development of the double-bed relationship   81
         Developments in the 1950s   81
         The 1960s and the first organisational reform of the NHS   84

	The 1970s	88
	The 1980s	92
	The 1990s	101
	The 2000s	106
	Conclusion	111

five	**Funding the NHS**	**113**
	Introduction	113
	The 1940s	116
	The 1950s	117
	The 1960s	120
	The 1970s	124
	The 1980s	127
	Labour and health financing	131
	Conclusion	135

six	**Managing in the NHS**	**137**
	Introduction	137
	NHS administration	138
	Managerialism	140
	The Thatcher government	143
	The New Public Management in the NHS	146
	New Labour's approach to health management	152
	Conclusion	158

seven	**Nursing**	**163**
	Introduction	163
	The 1940s and 1950s	163
	The 1960s	167
	The 1970s	172
	The 1980s and further confrontations with the nurses	174
	The 1990s and 2000s	177
	Conclusion	181

eight	**The role of the public in health policy**	**183**
	Introduction	183
	Position of the public in the early years of the NHS	183
	Knights, knaves, pawns and queens	185
	Citizenship at the creation of the NHS	187
	The 1960s and 1970s	188
	The 1980s and 1990s	192
	The 2000s	197
	Conclusion	205

nine	**Health policy under Labour**	**209**
	Introduction	209
	The context of health policy in 1997	209
	The New NHS: Modern, Dependable	210
	The NHS Plan	213
	Conclusion	227
ten	**Conclusion**	**231**
	Introduction	231
	Part One: what the NHS is like today	231
	Summary of the NHS's problems	241
	Part Two: the future of the NHS. What should be done?	242
	Conclusion	255
	References	257
	Index	285

List of tables and boxes

Tables

1.1	Situational logics	11
1.2	Key events in the NHS's history and their appearance in the book	12
2.1	Key organisational features of the NHS	14
2.2	NHS principles and their description	16
2.3	Initial factors in the creation of the NHS	27
2.4	Bevan's concessions to Morrison and their implications	28
2.5	Bevan's concessions to the consultants and GPs	30
2.6	NHS principles, their logic and implication	35
3.1	The tripartite split in 1948	40
3.2	Changing relationships between consultants and GPs	44
3.3	GP problems in the late 1940s	47
3.4	Differing approaches to general practice	56
3.5	The internal market and the tripartite split	64
3.6	The tripartite split under Labour	71
4.1	The double-bed relationship	76
4.2	The logics of the double-bed relationship	79
4.3	National accountability and local paternalism	81
4.4	The 1974 reorganisation and the double-bed	89
4.5	The double-bed after the Conservative internal market reforms	101
4.6	National paternalism and local accountability	110
4.7	The double-bed relationship under Labour	111
5.1	The cost of the NHS in England and Wales, 1948-51	116
5.2	Proportional sources of NHS finance, 1948-60	119
5.3	Revenue and capital expenditure and the difficulties of cutting each	123
5.4	Arguments for and against PFI	134
6.1	Oppositions highlighted by NPM	146
6.2	NHS manager roles	161
7.1	The characteristics of nursing in the 1940s and 1950s	167
7.2	The differences between the RCN and COHSE	170
8.1	The role of the public at the creation of the NHS	188
8.2	The patient–GP relationship after the internal market reforms	195
8.3	The patient in client, consumer and customer roles in the NHS	206
10.1	The NHS's problems at the end of 2007	243

Boxes

1.1	The 'shared version' of health policy in outline	5
1.2	The book's propositions about the NHS	10
6.1	The administrative approach to running the NHS	139

Acknowledgements

This book has been a long time in preparation; consequently, there are a lot of people to thank. Jo Campling, Sue Hatt, Tom Ling and Jane Powell provided a great deal of encouragement at the beginning, without which the book may not have got started. Along the way, Alison Shaw has been incredibly patient, and Jo Campling kept providing encouragement and enthusiasm right up to her death. She was a remarkable person. I have had the pleasure of working with a number of excellent colleagues who have given me new ideas and made the analysis that follows make more sense, including Russell Mannion, Matthias Beck, Kieran Walshe, Ruth Boaden, Steve Harrison, David Hunter, Greg Marchildon and everyone at the PSA Health Politics group, including Alison Hann, Calum Paton, Rob Baggott, Stephen Peckham and Mark Exworthy. There is a massive intellectual debt to my PhD examiner Rudolf Klein, which I hope is clear in the following pages, and to Martin Powell, who was kind enough to lead work on an Economic and Social Research Council grant application to work with me under the 'Cultures of Consumption' programme, and that helped fund the generation of some of the ideas in this book. Thanks to The Policy Press's reviewers, who made me dig deeper than the first draft. Last, but by no means least, thanks to Linda Perriton for helping me to retain what remains of my sanity.

List of abbreviations

BMA   British Medical Association
CHC   Community Health Council
COHSE Confederation of Health Service Employees
EMS   Emergency Medical Service
GDP   Gross Domestic Product
GMC   General Medical Council
GNP   Gross National Product
GP   general practitioner
IMF   International Monetary Fund
MOH   Medical Officer of Health
MP   Member of Parliament
NHS   National Health Service
NICE   National Institute for Health and Clinical Excellence
NPM   New Public Management
NUPE   National Union of Public Employees
PALS   Patient Advice Liaison Services
PFI   Private Finance Initiative
RCN   Royal College of Nursing
RHB   Regional Hospital Board
TUC   Trades Union Congress

ONE

Introduction

Introduction

The National Health Service (NHS) is a remarkable institution. It represents an experiment in social engineering, an attempt to provide free healthcare to the population of the UK across a comprehensive range of services. In the US, where private medical insurance is the usual means of paying for care, over 40 million people are uninsured either because their employer does not provide it as part of its rewards package or because they cannot afford to purchase it from their own funds. Citizens of the UK, however, tend to take the NHS for granted. On the one hand, it is a national treasure, regarded by policy makers as a welfare service they must treat with extreme caution because of the disastrous electoral consequences that could result from being seen to be privatising healthcare. On the other hand, media stories run most days of sick patients not receiving the care they should have, of dirty wards and of staff shortages. The NHS seems to be the nearest thing the people of the UK have to a national religion, but also an institution portrayed as being in permanent crisis.

The NHS is also remarkable for its sheer size. It is the largest employer in Europe, with around 1.3 million employees (Secretary of State for Health, 2006). However, the name 'National Health Service' itself is misleading for a number of reasons. The NHS has not always been terribly 'nationally' organised, with significant variations in care existing from one place to another, and with increasingly different policies in place in England, Scotland, Wales and Northern Ireland. Furthermore, the NHS has not always had much of a focus on 'health', being perhaps a place where we receive treatment for illness rather than advice on how to stay healthy (Doyal, 1979). Finally, criticisms made of the NHS, especially in recent years, suggest that 'service' might be something of an anachronism because of the perception, often propagated in the media, that what it provides is often poor quality, delivered in crumbling, dirty wards with low staff morale.

The name 'National Health Service' is also a little inaccurate because it seems to refer to single entity, when in fact it represents a huge and diverse range of services from transplant surgery through to flu vaccinations, and includes organisations from large, technologically advanced hospitals to two-partner general practitioner (GP) surgeries, all of which require coordination if anything approaching a 'national' health service is to be provided. Things get more complex still because of the reforms of the past 20 years, which mean that NHS care is increasingly likely to be delivered by private or not-for-profit providers of care, possibly in private sector-built facilities. Patients in public hospitals might be offered a range of additional services such as use of televisions, telephones and private rooms by paying extra, leading many people to feel that the NHS is increasingly behaving as private organisations do in attempting to extract as much money as possible from them.

Another significant element about the NHS is that it has a prestigious and important interest group – the medical profession. This is important for a number of reasons. Any attempt at change will either have to work with, or overcome resistance from, the doctors who provide care in hospitals, GP surgeries and community health settings. The relationship doctors have with patients is private and confidential, and this raises significant challenges to those attempting to manage health services. How is it possible to manage professionals who are not only literally able to save people's lives, but are also highly regarded by the public and have such control of their day-to-day work because of the private and highly specialist nature of their work? Accounts of the history of the NHS tend to focus strongly on the relationship between the doctors and the government as being the key one for understanding the health service to the extent that one of its leading writers calls this relationship the politics of the 'double-bed' (Klein, 1990). This creates an odd situation where the largest professional group in the NHS – nurses – often tend to receive far less attention, despite them being overwhelmingly responsible for the day-to-day delivery of care (Dingwall et al, 1988). This requires an explanation.

In addition to all of the above, the NHS is exceptional because it is an extremely political organisation. Even among welfare services, about which public opinions are emotive, the NHS often arouses the strongest views. It remains extremely popular with the general public, but media coverage is often very negative, portraying a service in crisis where money is being wasted, managers are incompetent, and doctors and nurses are struggling to cope. This is certainly the television image we have come to take as normal for healthcare, not only in UK dramas such as Casualty and Holby City, but globally through US series such as ER. Health services, because of all this media attention and the fact that they are often a part of key moments of our lives, are often the subject of considerable public debate. A single tragedy involving a vulnerable patient such as a child or an older person can come to represent the failings of the health system, and raise national concerns about the care that it offers. Politicians are acutely sensitive of criticisms made of the NHS, aware that its public popularity can lead to them being vulnerable to accusations of damaging or destroying the service. This is perhaps one of the reasons why contemporary politicians seem to be unable to resist the temptation to try to reform the service with such frequency.

Making sense of the NHS

Given the complexity of the service, the range of care it offers, the difficulty of dealing with strong professional groups, the political sensitivity of the service and the long period it has been with us (nearly 60 years at the time of this book's writing), how can we make sense of the NHS?

One method would be to try to write a history of the NHS, giving a detailed account of the major events in the service's history and trying to overcome the sheer complexity the past 60 years by being as comprehensive as possible. There are already accounts of the NHS that are presented in this way, from Charles Webster's HMSO history of the NHS until 1979 (Webster, 1988, 1996) to the more medically oriented account by Geoffrey Rivett (Rivett, 1998). These sources are excellent, but this is not the approach taken here. This book aims to complement existing historical work by providing what might be termed an analytical history of the NHS rather than a detailed record of events as they occurred.

A second possible approach would be to write a political history of the NHS. Again, however, there is already an account of the development of the NHS that provides this. Rudolf Klein's *New Politics of the NHS* (Klein, 2006) is wonderfully written and a powerful account of the politics of the service since its creation. This book attempts to complement Klein's work by presenting less detail about the political arguments concerning the NHS as they have developed, and organising the account thematically instead.

Third, it would be possible to write an account of the development of the NHS that is organised by the functions that the health service provides, accounting for primary care, hospitals services and so on, and focusing on the most recent innovations in each of these areas. Two excellent books that fill this role are those of Rob Baggott (2004) and

Chris Ham (2004), with the former text especially being particularly comprehensive. This book follows this approach in organising its account thematically, rather than according to particular services, around key themes that are identified in Chapter Two as being important to understanding the development of the NHS.

The approach taken by this book, then, is to present an analytical account of the development of the NHS to explore the implications of its history to understanding the challenges it faces today. It explores the central relationships and organisational features present in the health service in England, and aims to contribute a new understanding of their importance in the development of the health service. It is neither a complete account of the history of the NHS, nor a specifically political history, nor, as already mentioned, organised around specific services.

The book presents a history of the NHS that is particularly interested in continuity and change. It is selective in what is included, and what is not. The book's success or otherwise is not about its completeness, but instead about its explanatory power in being able to account for the success or otherwise of the many attempts to reform health services in England. The choice of 'England' is deliberate, as health services in the UK are increasingly taking divergent paths. Exploring all the differences between the other countries of the UK that are part of the NHS would add little analytically to the book's account, while at the same time potentially drawing confusing elements into it.

Health policy, continuity and change

NHS policy and organisation can be thought of as representing a series of tensions between continuity and change. On the one hand, the NHS is an organisation with a considerable 'institutional memory' – whereas governments come and go, many of those who work within the health service are likely to do so for life, and many will be members of trades unions with long histories of affiliation with the NHS. There are also strong professional groups within the NHS (especially those representing doctors) that have been remarkably good at getting their members' voices heard and arguing against change. It is possible to make a case that, despite the frequent attempts at reforming healthcare in the history of the NHS, it has remained remarkably intact. In principle, the NHS has always delivered free, comprehensive care to UK citizens on the basis of need rather than ability to pay, being funded primarily from general taxation. There is a strong argument that much of the change that has taken place in the NHS, even though it seems significant to those working within it at the time, has made remarkably little difference to the overall direction of the service, or to the experience of those receiving the service's care (see, for example, Levitt, 1980). This is the 'continuity' argument.

On the other hand, however, it is equally possible to present an argument that suggests that the NHS has changed beyond recognition from the health service created in 1948. In this view, changes in society, demography, patient expectations of the care they will receive, medical technology and the organisation of health services have meant that the NHS has significantly changed. This case is usually presented with particular emphasis on the management and organisational changes coming from the Thatcher and Major governments (Taylor-Gooby and Lawson, 1993), but can equally be made in terms of the present Labour government (Greener, 2004a). Claims that the NHS is in crisis have been commonplace in the service's history (Ehrenreich, 1978; Hunter, 1994b; BBC News, 2004) – surely an organisation that has experienced so many difficulties and so much reform must have also undergone significant change?

The 'standard account' of the development of health policy and its critique

In a book published nearly 20 years ago that can be regarded very much as a precursor to this one, Harrison et al (1990) suggest that much scholarship on the NHS at that time could be summarised in terms of presenting the 'shared version' of the development of health policy. This is summarised in Box 1.1.

Box 1.1: The 'shared version' of health policy in outline
- Health politics is incremental.
- The policy process is one of partisan mutual adjustment.
- The medical profession is hugely influential, at least in defensive terms.
- The position of lay health authority members is weak in relation to that of both clinicians and senior managers.
- The position of consumer health organisations is even weaker.
- The centre has little direct operational control over the implementation of most of its national policies, but does control funding.
- The role of health authority manager has been reactive and consensus seeking.
- The policy inertia resulting from the distribution of power between health authorities, health departments and the medical profession is made worse by complexity of service as a whole.

> • The whole complex and slow-moving edifice has been underpinned by an extremely durable political consensus, as no government has directly challenged the basic deal struck between the then Labour government and the medical profession during the founding period of 1946-48, and because of the high and continuing popularity of the NHS (Harrison et al, 1990, pp 7-8).

The NHS at the beginning of the 1990s was therefore characterised as an organisation that was slow to change, and where policy was the result of a number of significant interests negotiating with one another in a slow and time-consuming process where it was difficult to achieve radical change. The position of the medical profession was clearly important because any government will effectively depend on the doctors to run health services for it – healthcare requires skilled professionals to deliver it and this means that they will have at least some ability to block changes they regard as unwelcome. The shared version's suggestion of doctors' defensive ability was about health professionals being able to block or ignore central policy because of their strong local control over health services, and so, even if radical policy was put in place by the government, it did not necessarily mean it would be implemented in quite the way policy makers envisaged. Because of the strength of the medical profession, both health authorities (organisational bodies overseeing the running of local health services) and patients had had little say with regard to what went on in health services for much of their history.

The government was weak in the shared version in terms of its ability to influence local health organisation directly, but did control finance from the centre, and so had some influence over health services. Health authority managers, given their lack of control over medics especially, had to negotiate and achieve consensus for decisions rather than leading their organisations through active decision making. This tended to result in inertia because whereas doctors controlled local health services, they were unable to determine policy or funding, and central government, which could control both policy and funding, was weak in terms of its ability to influence the running of health services locally. All of this was in a political environment, according to the shared version, in which government did not want to confront the doctors, and feared the political consequences of attempting significant reform.

It is important to say that Harrison et al did not claim that the NHS was actually like the shared version, but instead that this was how it was, how the literature overwhelmingly portrayed it. It is an account of policy that confirms the continuity approach described above – healthcare is portrayed as producer-dominated, conservative, with consensus-seeking managers and a government not able to really control things. The NHS is subject to considerable inertia, as its organisational plan is based on a deal between the medical profession and the government back at the creation of the service, and it remains in place because managers have not overturned medical dominance and because politicians are afraid of reforming health services for fear of being accused of attacking an institution that has been described as the closest thing the English have to national religion (Klein, 1993).

The main problem with the shared version is that it makes no attempt to explain the dynamics between the elements it identifies, or to tell us why they are there. From the perspective of the 2000s, it also needs bringing up to date as the pace of reform has gathered considerably since the 1990s.

Other accounts of the development of the NHS

In addition to the standard account, there are a number of alternative narratives explaining the development of the NHS in the UK welfare state.

First, there is a debate around the extent to which the UK welfare state was part of a 'golden age' or 'consensus' (Kavanagh and Morris, 1991) between the main political parties from the 1950s to the beginning of the 1970s, which meant that remarkable continuities in policy and organisational form occurred in those years, even when there was a change in government. This apparent continuity ran alongside a period of sustained British economic growth during a time in which the government felt entirely comfortable, in contrast to today, in running the economy substantially through fiscal policy (adjustments to the government's tax and spend plans). Fiscal policy was a central instrument of Keynesian economic thought, an approach to managing the economy based on attempting to 'smooth' the path of economic growth through increasing taxation and reducing government expenditure in times of boom, and vice versa in times of recession. Big, interventionist government was fashionable and entirely philosophically in keeping with the NHS, created by nationalising hospitals to create a virtual monopoly provider of healthcare in the UK. On the surface of it, there appears to be at least some kind of case arguing that a 'golden age' of the NHS occurred in its first two decades, in which it was generally supported by politicians and the public, and relatively free from challenge or significant reform (Hill, 1993).

The 'golden age' of welfare is usually dated as ending in the 1970s as a result of 'fiscal crisis' in which the government, faced by slowing economic growth on the one hand, and a public sector that was continuing to grow year on year on the other, was forced to engage in 'cuts' to budgets (Lowe, 1993). These cuts meant, at the operational level, the introduction of a range of managerial technologies into the NHS, significantly changing its organisational form. As well as this, there was something of an intellectual crisis of welfare more generally, in which Keynesian economic thought was effectively discarded by a New Right monetarist solution that was intrinsically hostile to big government and believed that there ought to be a far stronger role for the private sector in providing welfare services (Pierson, 1998). No longer was the state to be a monopoly provider of care but instead seemed to be recasting itself as a funder of services only, and one that was particularly difficult to satisfy. It was to demand that public and private providers of care compete with one another to secure the best possible deal through the creation of public sector markets ('quasi-markets'). There are clear tendencies in the NHS towards the greater use of management techniques developed in the private sector, and of market mechanisms based on economic thought, so these elements must clearly form part of the account here.

This book is concerned with linking its analysis of the NHS with wider influences in society, and, as such, specific elements demand special attention in terms of the development of healthcare in the UK. The term 'health' is not at all unproblematic, and has seen its meaning and context considerably changed during the history of the NHS. In the 1940s, it would have been unusual for a patient to challenge medical expertise, and to some extent that remains the case, but today there is considerably greater scope for questioning diagnoses and far greater awareness of complementary medicines, leading to greater expectations of clinicians. Today it is possible to argue that we do not simply 'have' health, but that we 'consume' it, we purchase it and subject it to far greater scrutiny than has been the case before (Newman and Vidler, 2006). Health is not only something to be promoted through campaigns to get people to eat healthily and take more exercise, but is also a means of challenging the NHS to provide a wider range of services through a consumerist agenda. Patients have gone from being presented as passive figures receiving medical care from doctors who 'know best', to instead being portrayed as 'co-producers' of care, demanding improvements in services and the right to choose their own healthcare provision (Greener, 2005b). Equally, the government is increasingly making it clear that healthcare is not only the state's problem, but that the public must play a role in looking after itself and not just rely on the NHS to pick up the pieces when people fall ill (Secretary of State for Health, 2006).

There appears in existing accounts of the development of the NHS a particular focus on the shifting balance of power between the medical profession on one hand and the state on the other (Klein, 1979; Day and Klein, 1992; see especially Klein, 2001). This work usually talks about an accommodation, implicit at the time of creation of the NHS, that the state would fund the health service, but leave the operational control of it largely to the medical profession. This suited both parties. The state could put into place a national health service to meet the recommendations of the inter-war Beveridge Report (Beveridge, 1942), which made an explicit assumption that in the postwar period a national, comprehensive health service would exist in the UK to defeat the 'giant' of disease blocking the path to a civilised society. In turn, the medical profession was to be given an almost free hand in running health services, so long as it allowed the state to set the overall budget for health services. Over time, however, the 'concordat' between state and medicine appears to have progressively broken down; the state has felt the need to interfere in the running of health services, and the medical profession is increasingly free to criticise publicly the allocations of money given to the NHS. The relationship between state and medical profession is clearly, then, one that must be a central part in the telling of the story of the development of the NHS.

An additional element necessary to an account of the development of the NHS is often significant in its absence. As academics have become more sensitive in their analyses of the development of welfare services, they have increasingly come to the conclusion that they must also pay special attention to the role of gender in the provision of services (Daly and Rake, 2003). Many existing accounts of the development of the NHS have something of a tendency to play down gender in health services, or even to not mention it at all. However, of the total sum spent on the NHS, around three quarters is expenditure on salaries and wages, and around three quarters of those employed in the NHS are women. To ignore gender as an analytical category, not only in terms of the delivery of healthcare, but also of its impact on the population, would appear to be an oversight (Doyal, 1979).

The book's approach

> Out of ignorance, and a misguided faith in a conception of rationality that is at odds with practice, reformers have failed to recognise the NHS's power structure, the capacities of groups to bargain and influence, and the importance of historical legacy for the shape and character of organisational arrangements. (Hunter, 1986, p 9)

The book suggests that, in order to understand the tensions present in health policy and organisation today, it is first necessary to have an understanding of the creation of the NHS, and of the inheritance this presented to subsequent policy makers and those working within the health service itself. Understanding the NHS in terms of a series of inheritances is useful because it forces an explanation of exactly how they come to limit the choices of policy makers and those working in health services. This means that the book focuses on dynamics that either reproduce the past or challenge and change it.

The propositions around which the book is organised are summarised in Box 1.2.

Box 1.2: The book's propositions about the NHS

- To understand the problems of NHS reform today, it is necessary to understand its earlier organisational forms and the inheritances they bring to policy today.
- Policy makers inherit health services that are the result of previous decisions, and are underpinned by ideas and structures that the present government may find outdated or even wholly objectionable. It is by exploring how they deal with these inheritances that health reform can be explored from a new perspective, explaining why some reforms tend to work and others do not.
- Understanding the NHS in terms of a series of inheritances is useful because it forces an explanation of exactly how they come to limit the choices of policy makers and those working in health services.

The book therefore suggests that governments have to deal with inheritances in terms of both institutions and resources, and have to try and work out how to make policy that either works with the grain of those inheritances, or reforms them so that they become different. If inheritances limit the scope for reform, an important job is working out exactly how this happens – what mechanisms exist for the reproduction of the past in the present and into the future?

The second characteristic of the book is that it explores the dynamics of the NHS. A useful framework within which to achieve this, which the book returns to frequently, is that of Archer (Archer, 1995, 1996, 2000; Archer et al, 1998), who suggests that relationships comprise relations between interest groups, and that specific logics are created through the nature of their interactions.

The logics within which interests work are characterised as being either necessary, where interests require the support of others to attain or retain dominance, or contingent, where interest groups are not related or do not require such support from others. As well as exploring how interests are related to one another in terms of being necessary or contingent, they must also be examined to see if they are compatible or not. The combinations of necessary and contingent, and compatible and incompatible relations, create logics that are outlined in Table 1.1.

Table 1.1: Situational logics

Emergent property	Situational logic
Necessary compatibilities	Protection
Necessary incompatibilities	Compromise
Contingent incompatibilities	Elimination
Contingent compatibilities	Opportunism

Source: Derived from Archer (1995, p 218)

Situational logics, it must be stressed, condition behaviour; they do not determine it. They do, however, create substantial opportunity costs for actors trying to work against them (Greener, 2005a). They vary from each interest having an incentive to protect their relationship (protection) through to one where they may be forced to compete to destruction (elimination). Utilising Archer's framework allows the book to explore the basis of relationships, and how they have changed during the history of the NHS.

Outline of the book

The book proceeds as follows. First, the creation of the NHS will be explored, emphasising the importance of how it can inform debates around health services 60 years ago, the organisational structures that were put in place to address them, and their relevance for today. As such, the creation of the NHS will be explored in terms of putting in place inheritances that future policy makers will have to work with and try to understand.

Next, the book explores the split within the medical profession created by the NHS – the 'tripartite' split between hospital consultants, GPs and local authority health services. The relationship between the state and the medical profession is then explored – the 'double-bed' (in Klein's terms). This relationship has dominated the political science literature on the NHS, and clearly deserves close consideration. The book then considers the history of funding health services in the NHS, and asks why it is that, 60 years after the creation of the NHS, it is still funded primarily from general taxation.

The book then moves on to explore other key professionals working within the NHS: its managers, who have grown in influence and importance in recent years, and nurses, who remain remarkably absent from accounts of the development of the NHS despite their importance in terms of delivering care. It then explores how the role of the public in health services has changed, particularly over the past 20 years.

The book then moves towards its conclusion by tying together the accounts of policy since 1997 presented in previous chapters into a unified exploration of Labour's health reforms, and concludes by presenting both a critique of the state of health policy at the end of 2007 and a look to the future to consider what might be done to rectify the problems of health policy and organisation.

First, then, it is necessary to consider the creation of the NHS, and its continuing relevance today. The reader will find, as they progress through the book, that certain aspects of the NHS's history appear in several of the chapters. This is a necessary evil coming from the decision to present an analytical rather than chronological history of the NHS. It is hoped that the explanatory power offered by arranging the material in this way outweighs the repetition it leads to, as those events are covered from different perspectives. Table 1.2 gives an indication of particular key events and their most significant coverage throughout the book, and important links will be signalled in the chapters themselves.

Table 1.2: Key events in the NHS's history and their appearance in the book

Event	Chapters
The Hospital Plan	Three, Five
NHS Management Inquiry	Four, Six, Seven
Conservative internal market	Three, Four, Six, Eight
NHS Plan	Three, Four, Five, Nine
Performance management	Four, Five, Six, Nine
Private Finance Initiative (PFI)	Three, Five, Nine

TWO

The creation of the NHS and its relevance for today

Introduction

When the NHS began to provide care in 1948 it comprised of a number of organisational features that were the result of its infrastructural inheritances, of compromises and innovations in the process of designing the new service and of ideas about the role of the medicine within it.

This chapter suggests that three key organisational features are central to understanding the NHS of 1948, and alongside them, three key principles that were, to varying extents, embedded in its organisational form. It aims to answer the questions of where these organisational features and principles came from, and what their implications were. It will do this by outlining the process through which the three organisational features and principles emerged, before going on to examine the logics that each created. Every organisational choice creates tensions between the interests that are promoted or excluded as a result. Organisational choices create inheritances that shape the institutions within which those providing health services have to work, choices that favour some courses of actions over others. By examining the logics of these organisational choices, insights into the dynamics of the NHS can be gained.

Key organisational features of the NHS

Rather than presenting the debates and arguments that led to the creation of the NHS, and then show how key organisational features and principles emerged, it perhaps makes more sense to make clear what these features and principles are, and then to show the debates that led to their appearance. The danger of this approach is that 'Whig history' gets presented that only includes the elements that the author deems relevant for the argument at hand. However, in the case of the NHS, there is a strong consensus within the literature as to what the most important organisational elements found in its creation were, so exploring their development will hopefully give the reader additional clarity as well as forming a basis for subsequent chapters that will discuss their development in the period after the NHS's creation.

Three key organisational features dominate discussions over the NHS. They are tripartism (Ruggie, 1996); the 'double-bed' relationship between the state and the medical profession (Klein, 1990); and the general taxation funding mechanism chosen for the NHS (Moran, 1999) (see Table 2.1).

Table 2.1: Key organisational features of the NHS

Organisational element	Description
Tripartism	The split between hospital, GP and local authority or community health services
The double-bed	The relationship between the state and the medical profession
General taxation funding	Funding the NHS from general taxation as a whole rather than from an insurance or hypothecated tax system

Tripartism refers to the split in health services between hospital (acute) medicine, general practice medicine and community (personal) health services. This split was put in place by the health service's creators as a result of a series of political compromises during its creation (Honigsbaum, 1989). Hospital medicine was dominated by the prestigious consultant grouping of doctors, represented largely by the Royal Colleges, where specialist medicine was practised (Mohan, 2002). General practice medicine was the first port of call for most patients entering health services, but was less prestigious than specialist hospital medicine, and run by doctors often practising alone or in small groups in poor conditions (Webster, 1998b). Finally, personal health services were run by local government and included what were often regarded as 'Cinderella' areas of the NHS, including mental healthcare, which attracted less attention and status than hospital medicine and where the most vulnerable groups of society often received support (Means et al, 2002, 2003). Tripartism refers to the organisational split that resulted between these three services: hospitals were nationalised and so owned and (theoretically) run by the government; general practice services were within the scope of NHS, but were to be independently contracted for; and personal health services were run by local government, so were organised in a different way. The NHS might have been a 'national' health service, but it was split three ways in terms of its service provision. An account of the creation and subsequent development of the NHS must explain the reasons why this split occurred, and explore why the division has remained significant throughout the service's 60-year history. It must also explore how the relationships between the three parts of the health service have affected its subsequent history.

The 'double-bed' relationship between the state and the medical profession is based on analysis by Rudolf Klein (1990) that provides a powerful interpretation of the way the government and its institutions interact with doctors and their representatives. Doctors are clearly central to the ability of the NHS to treat and care for people, but are not the only professional group working in healthcare – they are not even the largest. However, it is almost impossible to write about the history of health organisation in England without considering the status and importance of doctors, and their ability for much of the NHS's history to have a considerable influence on both policy making and implementation.

The term 'double-bed' refers to the relationship of mutual dependence between the state and the medical profession. This mutual dependence was based on the state requiring the services of the doctors for the NHS to function, and the doctors needing to work for the state as the NHS was becoming the effective monopoly purchaser of health services in the UK. In the theoretical terms developed in Chapter One, the relationship between the state and the medical profession is therefore a necessary one. A relationship of mutual dependence, however, is not automatically a harmonious one, and a considerable part of the NHS's history is taken up with either the state or the doctors arguing for greater control or autonomy. The relationship can be characterised as necessary, but to varying degrees compatible or incompatible in the service's history.

The importance of the system of financing healthcare chosen by the NHS, funding services predominantly through general taxation, is that it favours redistribution and fairness, but carries with it a series of problems, including a tendency towards resource poverty. Funding services from general taxation is redistributionary in that those with higher incomes, because they pay more tax both relatively and absolutely, pay more for them than those on lower incomes. However, everyone receives the same level of service, regardless of how much tax they pay. Access to NHS services is based on need rather than ability to pay, and even if the better-off are able to receive healthcare more quickly through the use of the private sector, they still have to pay taxation that contributes towards the NHS. This principle, through which all taxpayers in the UK contribute towards the cost of the NHS, but at different rates according to their incomes, means that the NHS scores highly in international league tables for fairness and equity (World Health Organization, 2000).

The NHS's funding mechanism, based on general taxation, comes with a cost; health services have to compete with other public services for resources. This means that health services, in a year when public finances are tight or when other priorities are deemed more important, risk receiving less funding than they might receive through a health insurance system. A health insurance system would be demand-led rather than, with a general taxation system based on the taxation resources available, supply-led. Equally, there is often a tendency for governments not to invest in NHS infrastructure at the level required because of the difficulty in securing increases in funding year after year to pay for them. Healthcare in the UK is only now coming up to the level of investment enjoyed by other European countries for years – although the NHS still has a reputation as a place where inefficiency is rife, in international terms it has cost the British people far less than just about every other healthcare system in the developed world.

Tripartism, the double-bed and the general taxation means of paying for the NHS are key parts of the organisational settlement of 1948 that have significantly informed healthcare debates since that time. It is therefore important to explain how they came into being, as well as being clear about their implications for later policy. However, the NHS, as well as having organisational features, has a series of key principles that informed its creation, and again, that influence policy today (not least by policy makers often citing their importance; see the introduction of Secretary of State for Health, 2000). These are summarised in Table 2.2.

First, the NHS provides care that is free at the point of delivery. This means that citizens do not first have to consider whether they

Table 2.2: NHS principles and their description

Principle	Description
Care is provided free at the point of delivery	Care is provided free when needed, rather than being provided on the basis of ability to pay, or being insured for the care needed
Care is universal	Care is provided to everyone within a population, regardless of gender, ethnicity, age or disability
Care is comprehensive	Regardless of the condition a patient has, the NHS should be able to provide some kind of care

can afford healthcare, but instead can expect to receive it regardless of their ability to pay. This is important because of the peace of mind it gives to economically vulnerable groups – giving them an assumption that should they fall ill, they will not have to worry about finding potentially large sums of money to pay for healthcare. The situation in the UK has therefore been contrasted with that of the US, where a lack of health insurance coverage for a large number of Americans (estimates vary, but a figure around 40 million is typical) means that considerable uncertainty is attached to the future for those who are unable to pay for their own healthcare.

Second, the NHS offers universal care. This means that all citizens have a right to receive its care, based on need, rather than on ability to pay. Health insurance systems, in contrast, may only offer care based on the insurance coverage of the particular individual rather than how sick they are. In the UK we often take for granted the fact that we will receive care free (principle one) regardless of who we are (principle two), but in other countries, particularly the US, this is far from the case.

Third, the NHS provides comprehensive care. This means that citizens are entitled to receive the full range of care that the NHS offers. This is a more contentious principle as it is not always clear what it means, or how far comprehensiveness is meant to extend (Powell, 1997). It is certainly the case that care is often different from city to city within England, and so it does not mean that everyone, even if diagnosed with exactly the same illness, will receive the same care, or even the same level of care. However, it does mean that the NHS should provide treatment of some kind for the injured or for those diagnosed as sick.

Having explained in outline the organisational features and principles on which the NHS was founded, it is now important to try to explain how they came into being in order to provide an insight into the reasons why they were a part of the NHS in 1948. In each case, this will give us an idea of the implications of these organisational choices for subsequent policy because of the logics they created for subsequent health organisation.

The NHS of 1948 was the result of a series of institutional inheritances from the pre-war and inter-war healthcare services in the UK, the choices by policy makers (particularly Aneurin Bevan) in attempting to design the new health services, and the compromises that resulted from the subsequent debates between interest groups almost right up to the day the NHS came into being.

Healthcare before the NHS and medico–state relations

For much of the 19th century, the predominant notion of the state's relation to the economy and its people was based on the principles of laissez-faire and balanced budgeting. This meant that the state only interfered in the marketplace where there was a dire need, and did not spend more than it received in taxation in any given year. Local authorities led the way in terms of health improvement through programmes of improved sanitation, with relatively little role for the central state in welfare services. By the end of the 19th century, however, there was a definite trend towards a more collectivist approach. The percentage of the population employed in agriculture had declined significantly since 1850, with a sharp decline in agricultural prices causing real poverty for those working in that section of the economy, but increasing affluence for those in urban areas who could now afford food more cheaply. Although standards of living were improving in urban areas, an increased awareness of working-class poverty was appearing through surveys from the likes of Charles Booth in Liverpool and Seebohm Rowntree in York.

The Conservatives had extended voting rights to the male working classes in the late 1860s, with further reforms in the 1880s rebalancing constituencies between urban and rural areas. Even though many adult men (and all women) were unable to vote, there was a growing momentum for change, which was combined with the working classes finding ways of mobilising their own supporters and having their own representation. The first Labour Members of Parliament (MPs) were elected in 1900.

The Liberals and Conservatives responded to this challenge by attempting to head off socialism, with Balfour, Churchill and Lloyd-George joining to offer what appeared to combine a genuine commitment to social justice with political pragmatism, and which introduced welfare change into the political agenda. This led to a programme of reform that resulted in the National Insurance Act of 1911, with Part 1 putting in place a general scheme of insurance against ill-health and its consequences for manual workers, which was financed through the contribution of employees, their employers and the state. Manual workers gained free access to GPs and access to sanataria for tuberculosis, but not access to hospitals, with financial compensation for ill-health provided instead.

As such, the pre-First-World-War story represents the state progressively becoming involved in healthcare provision. This was then gradually extended in the inter-war period through the expansion of benefits and cover for health insurance, but often with concerns from the medical profession that their private practice might become eroded with increased state intervention, or that increased state intervention would lead to reductions in clinical freedom.

The origins of the tripartite split can be traced back to the history of medicine, in the differences between physicians, surgeons and apothecaries. The 1858 Medical Act required state registration of qualified doctors, and the 1911 National Insurance Act the panel system through which poorer patients could gain access to a family doctor (Digby, 1999). The Act gave primarily manual workers (but not their spouses or dependants) the right to access doctor services, but often on the terms specified by the numerous local and national societies that administered the system. The number of societies administering the systems meant that considerable differences in coverage and access existed depending on whom a worker registered with (see particularly Harris, 2004, p 226). National Health Insurance (NHI) was gradually extended in terms of its coverage and payment rate until the Second World War, but with still considerable differences between societies persisting, and growing calls for a unified system with universal coverage.

The hospital sector was split between voluntary and municipal hospitals. Voluntary hospitals developed as charitable institutions for the poor during the 19th century, but gradually found themselves increasingly dependent on patients who could pay for their services through contributionary schemes until concerns grew that they were losing their original mission of treating the poor.

Municipal hospitals were part of the increasingly wide range of health services provided by local government during the 19th and early 20th century. Infant welfare was central to local authority provision in the period after the First World War, with health visitors undergoing a considerable expansion in the inter-war period. The main problem with municipal health services was that they were largely dependent on taxation from local rates systems, so the most deprived areas also had the least to spend on health services. Even after 'block grant' systems were introduced to try to increase the role of central government in funding local services in 1929, this appeared to make little difference to the problem.

Hospitals were often equipped with apparatus that members of staff were not qualified to use and staff carrying out surgical treatment often lacked the necessary training, experience and qualifications (Cohen, 1943). Hospitals were fragmentary in organisation, and often in a deplorable state. Little or no cooperation between different types of hospital existed, with possibly even local rivalries existing between the voluntary and public hospitals. The 1,000 or so voluntary hospitals were self-governing institutions proud of their independence and only loosely associated with each other (Honigsbaum, 1989) and the 3,000 public hospitals were distributed between hundreds of separate local authorities that were only vaguely concerned with their regulation (Webster, 1998a). The majority of voluntary hospitals faced financial crises of one kind or another, with only 8% of income coming from the government, and most money therefore having to come from patients themselves or from subscription schemes (Eckstein, 1958).

General practitioners acted as the gateway to health services, performing not only routine medical work, but also surgical work, at least some of which they were unqualified to deal with (Webster, 1998b). Morale among GPs was low because of overwork and an inability to keep up with medical advances (Lowe, 1993). Most GPs worked alone, and after a long training had to take out a substantial loan to purchase the goodwill of a practice, which then had to be financed from a fairly fixed salary as fees were often low. Many GPs therefore had a real need to work in areas that offered the possibility of private income, and these better-off areas, by definition, were probably those that needed GP surgeries least (Powell, 1996).

To be admitted to hospitals, patients had to be referred by GPs. This created a particular dynamic between hospital consultants and GPs. Consultants required GP referrals in order to be able to retain their honorary posts, and therefore their access to private, paying clients. The relationship between consultants and GPs was a necessary one; consultants needed GPs for referrals, and GPs needed consultants to be able to refer patients. It was a system not without its flaws, but it suited both sets of doctor groups and meant that they had a largely compatible relationship.

By 1939, NHI covered nearly half the population, but that left children, those not covered by health insurance and their spouses, many women not in employment, the self-employed, higher-paid employees and many older people outside the system (Leathard, 1990). Those who were insured faced considerable variations in uncertainty with regard to the extent of provision in terms of additional benefits, including dental and ophthalmic care and hospital and specialist treatment, depending on healthcare history and geographic location. Leathard summarises the drawbacks of the pre-war system under five headings:

(1) shortage of facilities and trained manpower;
(2) inequitably distributed services, both geographically and functionally;
(3) uneconomic use of services arising from irrational organisation;
(4) lack of adequate funds making any significant expansion impossible;
(5) the persistence of certain unsatisfactory clinical conditions (Leathard, 1990, p 23).

Wartime

It was the Second World War that created the impetus for change (Webster, 1988). The think-tank Political and Economic Planning feared that air-raid casualties could be as high as 300,000 and, with remarkable speed and efficiency, an Emergency Medical Service (EMS) was put in place (Glennerster, 1995). This outburst of planning activity during wartime has been expressed as a paradox by Titmuss (1950) because 'where human lives are cheapest, the desire to preserve life and health is at its highest'. The energy and organisation of the EMS was so impressive that calls quickly appeared for the immediate conversion of the hospital scheme into a National Hospital Service (Honigsbaum, 1989).

The NHS went through its formative process during the time of creation of what has been called the 'classic welfare state' (Lowe, 1990) or the 'Keynesian welfare state', and formed a central plank in the effort to slay the disease giant Beveridge (1942) identified as blocking the path to civilised postwar society. Beveridge's plan of centrally planned welfare dovetailed with the emergent economic thought of the time, as Keynes' General Theory (Keynes, 1997) found favour with those in power as a means of redistribution and economic planning (Kavanagh, 1985; Kavanagh and Morris, 1991). Three main elements dominated the approach: the recasting of social problems away from being the result of individual blame to recognition of them as societal in nature; the recognition that the state had a legitimate role to play in providing public services; and the proposal that where the state did not provide public services itself, it would enter into partnership with the charitable and private sectors for their provision (Osborne and McLaughlin, 2002). The NHS of 1948 was closely bound up with the rationalistic flavour of the times, and the faith in health professionals to solve the problems of society through the application of scientific knowledge.

The inter-war discussions of what the NHS trailed in the 1942 Beveridge Report might look like in practice, resemble a torturous process of bluff and counter-bluff between the numerous parties involved, with attempts by coalition government figures to consult as many interested parties as possible. The first attempt to summarise the results of these discussions publicly came in the 1944 White Paper (Ministry of Health, 1944), largely written by Sir John Hawton, who emerged later to become a significant figure in the negotiations between the medical profession and Aneurin Bevan after 1946.

The 1944 proposals were based on two principles: first, that the new service should be comprehensive: and second, that it should be free. These two principles were enshrined in legislation two years later, but by then in a completely different organisational form. Quite what was meant by 'comprehensive' and 'free' was not entirely clear; the status of industrial and school medical services, mental health services, and dental and ophthalmic services for non-priority cases was a source of considerable discussion (Webster, 1988, pp 55-6); and the door was left open for direct or indirect charges for appliances and hospital treatments, especially through 'hotel' charges for hospitals (Ministry of Health, 1944, p 12).

The decision over whether or not health services should be universal in scope was even more complicated. It appears that it became linked in GP's minds with services being administered at the municipal level and so held the potential, in their view, to impinge on clinical freedom, as it held the potential for civil servants to have line management authority over doctors. Even so, by June 1942, the medical profession looked set to approve a healthcare system based on universal access, with the British Medical Association (BMA) approving the move by a small majority (Honigsbaum, 1989, pp 204-5). But the BMA then quickly reversed its decision after further negotiations in March 1943 in protest against plans for a salaried, municipally controlled GP service. It seems likely that had plans for municipality been dropped, universality would have been established as the third principle on which health services in the UK were based by 1944. There was, then, considerable progress toward the principles, if not the eventual organisational form, of the NHS (Allsop, 1995, pp 27-30).

In 1944, a White Paper presented an outline of what a national heath service might look like (Ministry of Health, 1944). The preferred organisational solution was to put hospital planning in the hands of 'joint boards' that were to represent local authorities in the larger areas thought necessary to run a hospital service, and that would secure hospital services from both municipal and voluntary hospitals in those areas. Payment for services would come from both local and central government funds. General practitioner services in health centres would be run by local authorities, and be largely accountable to them. Those GPs in 'individual practice' would be contracted instead to a Central Medical Board, and free to undertake private practice. Local authorities would also run clinics along with their domiciliary and environmental health services, giving them substantially more involvement than in the health service of today.

Presenting the White Paper as being the end of a political process, however, conceals as much as it reveals. There was no consensus over the 1944 White Paper; 'for many Labour members it represented a minimum on which to build for the future, while for many Conservatives it represented the limit to which they were prepared to go' (Powell, 1994, p 337). The 1944 White Paper does present the dominant view of the inter-war Ministry of Health of a service administered predominantly at the local level. But with this came several tensions; the advent of the EMS during the war demonstrated that it was possible to organise on a national level, and it was also clear that many of the voluntary hospitals across the country could not afford to return to their pre-war state, as they were verging on bankruptcy. The earlier 1941 Brown proposals committed the government to the same 'joint boards' as the 1944 White Paper, but did not commit to a free service. It appears therefore that there was commitment to the health service being free before there was support for it being comprehensive, but even that was a contested issue within the medical profession (Honigsbaum, 1979, p 196).

After the publication of the 1944 White Paper, Health Minister Henry Willink continued to negotiate with the medical profession until the end of the war, making concessions over medical representation on health organisation bodies, limiting the Central Medical Board's powers to intervene in the distribution of GPs, introducing health centres for GPs on an experimental basis first, removing financial links between local authorities and voluntary hospitals, and making joint boards primary planning rather than executive bodies (Powell, 1994, p 335).

As such, it is hard to consider the 1944 White Paper as being a particularly consensual document, representing too little for Labour's 'New Jerusalemers', too much state interference for the Conservatives, and too much medical interference for the doctors. Its movement towards the twin goals of comprehensiveness and providing a free service were not considered and obvious, but rather contingent and faltering. The BMA was no longer in favour of universalism, but wanted instead to introduce the new health service by extending NHI (Pater, 1981, pp 170-3). The Ministry of Health favoured a local organisation system. The medical profession appeared rather more interested in testing the limits of what they might negotiate than in agreeing a coherent plan for the future of the health service (Klein, 2006). By the end of the war, there was enough momentum to assume that a health service of some kind was to be established, but a number of additional contingencies dictated the exact nature of the final organisational form of the NHS.

Discussions over healthcare principles also appeared to have reached a consensus, with the state to offer a free, comprehensive and universal healthcare system. Socialism clearly played a large part in the decision to nationalise hospitals, but another key element was the influence of Keynes in economic thought. If the 19th century was dominated by laissez-faire and balanced budgets, Keynes suggested instead that economies could become stuck in a position of 'demand-deficiency' where the government needed to intervene in the economy in order to avoid the waste and loss of unemployment. Keynes provided an intellectual reason for government increasing its role in welfare services such as healthcare, suggesting that doing so might actually help the economy avoid the extremes of boom and bust. Public expenditure, as well as being justified in terms of social cohesion in the Liberal reform programme, might also offer greater economic efficiency. This was an idea of great appeal to socialists, who wished to nationalise the production of key areas of the economy, providing a neat fit between their ideas and those of Keynes. In healthcare, the faith in experts that socialists tend to hold (Clarke et al, 1992) was invested in its archetypal professional group – the doctors.

Medical knowledge, in retrospect, was at the beginning of a wave of progress at the end of the Second World War (Le Fanu, 1999). Medical practice was, however, very different from anything we would recognise today. Doctors seldom examined their clinical practice in a systematic way, with the concept of the randomised controlled trial being a new one and only really taken up in the *British Medical Journal* as representing a gold standard for scientific papers from 1947 onwards. In general practice settings, there were few drugs of any efficacy, with what amounted to placebo prescribing common (Rivett, 1998, p 55).

Wartime had seen the widespread use of antibiotics, which were the new wonder drugs, but were primarily available only by injection until the mid-1950s. Cortisone was not available on a widespread basis until about the same time because of the difficulty of its extraction. New drugs for psychiatric illnesses that could calm agitated patients were synthesised, and were gradually to have a profound impact on practice for mental illness from the 1960s onwards. Cardiac surgery, buoyed by improvements in sterilisation and operating room procedure, saw improvements in cardiac catheterisation, pacemaking and, eventually, the possibility of surgery inside the chest. Wartime provided the opportunity for surgeons to acquire experience of operating on the heart, removing the taboo of cardiac surgery, and led to work on repairing damaged hearts, particularly in young people (Rivett, 1998; Le Fanu, 1999). Wartime had given orthopaedic surgery increased impetus, with systems of rigid internal fixation and rehabilitation allowing patients with severe fractures to be able to get up and move about, and an understanding of fracture healing improving. Joint replacement was first carried out in the 1950s and substantial improvements in technology came about through further innovations after that time.

The end of the war and the Labour government

Labour achieved its first majority government at the end of the Second World War. Despite its considerable parliamentary majority, the result was regarded as uncertain even on polling day (Morgan, 1990). Had the Conservatives been elected, it is likely that the NHS would have been administered far more at the local authority level, that hospitals would not have been nationalised and that Willink, the Conservative Health Minister Elect, would have negotiated a far different settlement from the one achieved by Aneurin Bevan (Powell, 1994, p 337; Harris, 2004).

If the election of Labour was not entirely predictable, and had profound implications of the creation of the NHS, the appointment of Bevan as Minister for Health and Housing was both brave and, at least to some degree, unexpected; Webster (1988) described it as 'audacious'. Bevan took over perhaps the most politically sensitive portfolio in the government, being responsible for rebuilding houses as well as honouring the wartime promise to create a national health service – all for a figure that played no part in the coalition government and with a reputation as something of a loose cannon. The appointment of Bevan accounts significantly for the course of events leading up to the creation of the NHS.

Bevan favoured an approach to health reform that was based on the nationalisation of the inheritance of voluntary and municipal hospitals. Bevan viewed this as the best way of dealing with the problems of the local hospitals, with the voluntary hospitals sometimes in a difficult financial situation, and with competition and duplication between the two types of services in some areas, and underprovision in others. Nationalisation was bold in that even Beveridge, who had been instrumental in making it possible for a national health service to come into being, rejected this way of organising health services, preferring instead that the system of society financing and local provision remained (Webster, 1988). However, proposals for nationalisation predated Bevan in the plan put together by the Chief Medical Officer Sir Arthur MacNalty in 1939, so were not entirely original (Klein, 2006, pp 5-6), even if they did represent a discontinuity with wartime proposals. Nationalisation also dealt with the claim expressed by President of the Royal College of Physicians Lord Moran, that doctors would only enter the NHS if all the hospitals in the country were taken out of the hands of the municipal government (Titmuss, 1958, p 142). As such, it was a 'vehicle for giving the consultants what they wanted as well as what Bevan wanted' (Glennerster, 1995, p 51).

If nationalisation of the hospitals was bold, Bevan wanted to go further still, nationalising personal health services as well in the name of administrative unity (Honigsbaum, 1989). This second proposal, however, was to be a casualty of the concessions required to create a politically viable service (see below).

Bevan also made the decision not to consult with the medical profession, but that his proposals, to preserve sovereignty, would go to the Houses of Parliament before the doctors got to see them (Eckstein, 1958; Rintala, 2003). This resulted in Bevan appearing disengaged and uncompromising to at least the BMA, and made subsequent negotiations with that group rather more difficult. Table 2.3 shows Labour's election, Bevan's appointment and his subsequent refusal to initially negotiate with the medical profession. Each of the events on the left is considered in terms of its consequences and its organisational implications.

After coming up with his proposals, Bevan then had the job of getting internal political support within the government for his ideas. The debate in Cabinet between Bevan and Local Government Minister Herbert Morrison resulted in a compromise; Bevan wanted a national health service, a full nationalisation of the disparate hospital service in the UK and, for administrative clarity, the unification of many of the personal health services that were run by local authorities. Morrison, however, wanted a locally run health system (Eckstein, 1958). There was some irony in this conflict, as Morrison was instrumental in Bevan being appointed to his post as Minister of Health and Housing in the first place. Morrison regarded a nationalisation of hospital services as potentially hugely damaging to local government because of the loss of resources and influence that it would suffer as a result. Bevan appeared to win support from the Prime Minister, however, who summed up the Cabinet debate in his favour. Bevan's attempt to bring community

Table 2.3: Initial factors in the creation of the NHS

Contingent event/ feature	Consequences	Implications
Labour's election to power in 1945	Large majority made radical policy possible. Put socialist government in power with commitment to nationalise means of production	Nationalisation a possible approach to welfare reform because of socialist principles and the large government majority
Bevan's appointment as Minister of Health and Housing	Favouring of the nationalisation option for hospitals	Created national network of publicly owned hospitals resistant to privatisation
Bevan not negotiating with medical profession prior to NHS Act	Eventual granting of concessions (below) to GPs through BMA	Bevan required to give GPs independent status in NHS

health services under national control was a casualty of him winning the debate over nationalisation of the hospitals (Klein, 2006).

Bevan was allowed to nationalise the hospitals, but had to leave personal health services (community and social services) in the control of local authorities. The result was the product of political compromise rather than administrative or ideological logic. Bevan gained unity for his hospital service at the expense of administrative unity for the service as a whole. The result of this compromise is that health and social services staff have worked with different pay and conditions (even where they effectively do the same job), and that divisions in working practices and methods of care exist. The compromise with Morrison is summarised in Table 2.4.

Bevan's second compromise came in his dilemma over how he was to gain the support of the medical profession. Bevan sought to preserve the sovereignty of Parliament by refusing to discuss the contents of his proposals for the NHS with the doctors before they were released there. However, Bevan did talk about the principles of his organisation with several leaders of the medical profession with whom he tried to work out his ideas for the health service (Rintala, 2003). Despite the relative secrecy of his proposals, Bevan had therefore met with many of the most important doctors with whom he would have to deal later

Table 2.4: Bevan's concessions to Morrison and their implications

Contingent factor	Consequences	Implications
Nationalisation of the hospitals achieved at the expense of administrative unity between hospital and personal or community health services	Separation between hospital and community health services. Other health organisations have little incentive to take over 'Cinderella' services. Social services organised separately from health services	Creation of administratively distinct services. Isolation of low-prestige community health services with few resources. Separate pay, conditions, coding systems, performance systems, administration

on. Bevan appeared to have favoured the consultants in his proposals because the Royal Colleges were able to take decisions on behalf of their members without recourse to consultation, whereas the BMA, largely representing the GPs, required full consultation and often a vote (Honigsbaum, 1989).

Bevan's negotiations with the 'medical Lords' prior to the release of his proposals suited a style of consultation that was informal, and that suited the consultants more than the GPs. Bevan was able to secure participation in the new health service of at least one key doctors' grouping quickly and efficiently (from his perspective) through the means of the consultant contract in which he 'stuffed their mouths with gold'. To achieve this, Bevan allowed consultants flexible working conditions, special status in teaching hospitals in the new NHS (Jones, 1994) and private practice in NHS hospitals. General practitioners, however, appeared to have received relatively few concessions by the time the NHS Act was published in 1946, and had considerable concerns that the state might be attempting to make them employees of the NHS rather than independent contractors. They were also worried, under proposed plans for the establishment of surgeries, that the government might be able to compel them to move to work in areas where few GPs worked at the time, and that they might lose built-up rights to receive payments for the 'goodwill' embodied in their practices that new partners or GPs wishing to take over practices of retiring GPs would have to pay for.

Bevan then had to make compromises to ensure the cooperation of the GPs, a more difficult body to negotiate with than the consultants because of their system of representation and their need for the democratic approval of decisions, which took a considerable amount of time. Bevan had to guarantee that he was not planning to erode the autonomy of the GPs and that he was planning to effectively allow them to administer themselves within health services (Pater, 1981), and he had to offer reassurances over their freedom to work where they wished, despite initial proposals to prohibit the sale and purchase of practices. Amending legislation was issued to make it clear that the Labour government was not attempting to create a salaried GP service and that they would continue to be paid according to the numbers of patients on their books (on a 'capitation' basis). The end result of these negotiations was that the NHS acquired a third administrative dimension, with a tripartite structure between hospital, GP and community services being created. Bevan's concessions to the consultants and GPs are summarised in Table 2.5.

Tripartism in practice

The founding of the NHS, then, created a very specific organisational form, and one that has proven to be remarkably resilient to attempts to change it.

Community health services

Community health or personal health services are often regarded as the 'Cinderella' element of the health service, underfunded from being under local authority control, and occupying the less visible aspect of medicine. Chronic care services, especially where they do not cure, but simply manage conditions, do not command the attention or resources that acute, or hospital, care does. Mental illness is particularly representative of this, where a long-term condition that may or may not be curable requires the support of health professionals in often trying and difficult conditions. Rather than being able to offer dramatic solutions, care is about helping to manage conditions, and there is little of the innate glamour of high-technology medicine such as transplantation. As such, community health services do not offer spectacular cures or cutting-edge medicine; they often appear on the edges of accounts of the development of the NHS and they are positioned only contingently to the other services of the NHS – the hospitals and GPs.

In many respects, it would be more rational for health services to be run by local authorities than by a central department at the national

Table 2.5: Bevan's concessions to the consultants and GPs

Concession	Constraining factor	Logic
Concessions to the consultants		
Private practice allowed in contracts	Consultants prepared to battle to retain privileges	Continuity through consultant contract
Teaching hospitals given 'special' status	Creation of 'fiefdoms'	Research funding and prestige conferred on consultants
'Acute' medicine funded as a priority	Relative resource richness	Hospitals attractive to new doctors – rewards, prestige
Consultants afforded 'special' status in negotiations	Consultant 'infiltration' of committees and decision-making processes in the NHS. 'Concordat' over funding and control	Ability to exert negative power over decision making
Concessions to the GPs		
GPs remain independent contractors	'Family doctors' remain independent	Regulation of GPs is independent of state
GPs positioned as 'gatekeepers' to service	State needs GPs so is reluctant to challenge their position. Relative shortage of doctors means state cannot challenge their position. GPs predominant in decision making at 'community' level	State dependent on GPs to act as gatekeepers. Negative power over decision making

level, but this clashes with the idea of a 'national' health service. Central government tends to be suspicious of giving greater control of public services to locally administered bodies, and attempts at 'co-terminosity', or combined administrative arrangements, have yet to prove successful. This is because health and social service staff are employed on a different basis, with different pay and conditions (even for remarkably similar jobs), they record information about their activities in a different way (Greener, 2003b) and have different systems of performance measurement. There can be considerable suspicion between staff in the two areas, and teamworking is not always present.

Hospital services

Before the NHS, hospital consultants theoretically relied on GPs for their referrals, putting in place a dependency of sorts. But the creation of the NHS meant that consultants were no longer dependent on GPs for their positions or for their ability to access private patients – consultants were now employed in the NHS on a salaried basis. As such, the relationship was no longer a necessary one, as it was no longer based on mutual dependence. It was now contingent. Status disparities between the two groups now had free reign. It was the consultants who were the practitioners of specialist medicine; in the hierarchy of medicine, there was little doubt in most consultants' minds that they were higher up the 'ladder' than GPs. Consultants had the ability to treat private patients, thus supplementing their income, were more likely to be conducting research than GPs and, in a hospital attached to a university, may have had students, or at least junior doctors, who would be expected to hang on their every word. As well as this, specialist medicine undoubtedly occupies a more prestigious position than general medicine, displaying the full force of the curative model of healthcare in all its miraculous glare. The resource networks around consultants stretched rather wider than those of GPs, and the financial rewards available were potentially much greater.

State funding for acute medicine has supported the consultants' position through its emphasis on acute care (at the expense of public health, for example), embedding consultants further into their networks of superior resource advantage. Equally, the Royal College representatives of the consultants have demanded, and often received, privileged access to the policy process, effectively vetoing reforms in the late 1960s because of their managerial content. But the very advantage that their representation system gave them in the negotiations with Bevan became more contested as the profession became more socially disparate. As a consequence of this, the Royal Colleges, especially in the face of the internal market reforms of the 1980s, became less able to represent their members, and the government rightly determined that it was better able to resist the demands of the consultants, forcing through the reforms against their wishes.

But the consultants and the prestigious Royal Colleges also represent the cutting edge of medicine, with several of their number occupying elite social as well as occupational positions. Prominent doctors present television programmes, and are asked by the media for their opinions on plans to reform health services. It is remarkably difficult to drive through change in the face of determined opposition from this group and, even if reforms are legislated that appear to remove power from them, implementation often flounders. Consultants, secure in their local professional fiefdoms, are strongly positioned to simply ignore attempts from above to reform their practices; the difficulty of measuring their performance, and the notion of 'clinical autonomy', means that it is remarkably difficult to challenge doctors' behaviour.

GP medicine

The tripartite organisational split in the UK also carries with it a specific dynamic, at the centre of which is the GP. In the UK, the GP is effectively the gatekeeper for the NHS. If the public require care (outside of an emergency case), and want to see a doctor (rather than utilising NHS direct services), then they must consult first with a GP. The GP then provides (or not) access to additional networks of care. This may involve an endorsement to access drugs, or the booking of an appointment for further care with other practitioners, including hospital consultants and community health services. Patients therefore have necessary relationships with their GPs, but GPs have the right to refuse to refer or prescribe for their patients – a relationship asymmetry because it may be more work or effort for the GP to refer the patient than to send them away empty-handed. As such, GP and patient interest may not always be compatible.

General practitioners have jealously guarded the independence granted by Bevan in the creation of the NHS. The GP is the family doctor, the representative of the NHS with whom patients have most contact and it is a brave government that attempts to reform the relationship between doctors and patients. It is also significant that, in times of contentious health reform, leaflets appear in surgery waiting rooms outlining the case against them. General practitioners are most able to mobilise support for the cause of the NHS against government reform; little wonder that health reform tends not to antagonise this group.

Equally, GPs, in the same way as consultants, carry considerable negative power. Because of their organisational independence, clinical autonomy and the confidentiality of the doctor–patient relationship, they are able to hold a remarkable degree of control over their own destiny, vetoing or simply ignoring organisational change they do not wish to cooperate with. Occupying an elevated social standing in local communities, they are a highly entrenched professional grouping able to resist change and command the respect and sympathy of the communities they serve; they are family doctors. As such, governmental attempts to reform this group without their consent are remarkably fraught with political danger because of their potential to create adverse publicity. It was an independent GP who was elected as an MP in the 2001 General Election with the sole motive of preventing the closure of a local hospital. The dark face of GP power was shown by the hold that serial killer (and GP) Harold Shipman seemed to have over his local community, with several of his patients apparently unwilling to accept his guilt, and the considerable time over which he was able to perpetrate his crimes (Smith, 2002).

The double-bed

The remarkable growth in medical knowledge coming from wartime and the concerted medical and surgical research prior to it brought a belief that medicine as a profession was coming of age. Most of the dramatic change occurred in the context of hospital medicine, where it seemed there were no limits in what might be achieved by brilliant young doctors challenging medical orthodoxies and finding new treatments that bordered on the miraculous. Medical practice, at the cutting edge, was being transformed beyond imagination. There was a groundswell of support for improved access to healthcare from the public in return for the sacrifices made during wartime. Investment in healthcare, especially that of the hospitals (Jones, 1994), appeared to offer the state substantial potential for excellent returns in the nation's health. There seemed to be a wonderful marriage of political and medical interest.

This marriage of interest between the state and the doctors was only apparent, however, outside of the cut and thrust of the debate over the formation of the NHS, and would come into play only if the NHS got off the ground, giving both parties a clear need for one another. If the Labour government had not been set on creating a nationalised health service, the problem of securing medical cooperation in a health service would have been for local authorities to deal with, even if failure would have had significant implications for the national government. Equally, had the medical profession not found itself working for a monopoly employer of their services, doctors would have retained considerable autonomy from the state, albeit with far less guarantees in terms of the security of their future employment given the precariousness of the postwar health system. If the relationship under the NHS can be characterised as being a necessary one, there was no guarantee it would remain a compatible one, however, with plenty of scope for the needs of both state and doctors to diverge.

General taxation

Funding the NHS from general taxation created a system whereby the NHS was redistributionary between rich and poor, and therefore carried with it a strong egalitarian element. However, it also put in place a means of controlling healthcare expenditure that future Chancellors of the Exchequer were to be grateful for. As the sum allocated to healthcare in the government public expenditure round was supply-led, based on available taxation, the NHS had to work within a specified budget set centrally by the state. The alternative to this, utilising an insurance-based system, would mean that health expenditure would instead be demand-led, as the sums paid to the NHS would instead be following treatment decisions by doctors and nurses.

As such, the use of general taxation to fund health services is paradoxical in that it is redistributionary, but may result in everyone receiving less healthcare than they would under an insurance-based system. Arguments against a change in the way the NHS is funded have always run up against the problem that virtually any alternative system of funding healthcare services is likely to result in an increase in the service's budget that central policy makers, particularly those in the Treasury, cannot entirely predict. Funding health services from an insurance system is not an open-ended commitment, as there will always be rules concerning the qualification for treatment, for example. However, funding healthcare from general taxation is a remarkably efficient means of imposing a limit on the total amount of healthcare expenditure that will be allowed, and so is understandably popular with the government of the day. Even economically radical Chancellors of the Exchequer have come to the conclusion that general taxation funding should remain (Lawson, 1991).

NHS principles and their inheritance

The principles that the organisational form of the NHS rests on were largely decided during wartime, but have proven to be remarkably durable. Their logics are outlined in Table 2.6.

The decision to make the NHS free at the point of care meant that health services were to be provided on the basis of need rather than the ability to pay, and has a strong socialist element to it. It also created

Table 2.6: NHS principles, their logic and implication

Principle	Logic	Implication
NHS is free	Free healthcare expected by the public as a right. Political danger from charging for health services	Popularity of free healthcare with population makes it difficult to withdraw
NHS is universal	Implicit rationing – waiting lists. Danger of reallocation of waiting lists	Universal service but not necessarily the same – tension between universal/national and differentiated/local
NHS is comprehensive	Political expediency and fear of resource commitment	Commitment to provide NHS services, but not same in each locality. Aspirational as much as actual

a sense of expectation of receiving healthcare as a right for the British public, especially for those who did not carry the memory of having to pay for it themselves. This makes it politically extremely dangerous for any politician challenging the right to free care. It is far easier to grant the citizenry new rights than to remove old ones, and it would be a brave Prime Minister who endorsed the introduction of a more directly contributionary means of funding health services because of the political outrage opposition parties and the media would be able to generate.

Making the NHS universal (providing care to all citizens) brings with it particular problems. A universal service may also mean a standardised service, with no scope for local differences in care delivery. Does the 'National' in NHS mean that services must be the same everywhere, laid out in national standards, and with clear policies on what care is, or is not, provided? Providing care for everyone can often seem like a commitment to provide the same care for everyone, when the two are not at all the same. One version of universalism is for the NHS to provide a health service that is locally differentiated, where everyone has guaranteed access to care, but where the actual care may differ from locality to locality. This option, however, carries with it the risk of what has become known as the 'postcode lottery', in which some services or treatments are provided in some areas but not others. A universal commitment to provide care is not the same thing as a universal commitment to provide the same care to everyone.

The NHS's universalism also carries with it an implicit assumption that it may be necessary to wait for treatment. If everyone in the country has the theoretical right to treatment, some treatments are going to be oversubscribed unless local providers are to be continually reconfigured to try to exactly meet the needs of their local populations (which leads back to tensions between responsibility at the national and local and local levels). Once waiting lists appear, it is left to either doctors or managers or some other group to try to decide who should be treated first, and on what basis. Doctors, as well as being a key professional group, also become gatekeepers to care, making decisions about access to care. An implicit rationing system appears in which doctors must work within budgetary and infrastructural limits rather than being led by patient need.

Universal care, as with free care, is a popular policy. However, the NHS has found it very difficult to be transparent about the order in which patients are treated on waiting lists because it brings to light a number of difficult questions about who should be treated, and who should be treated first. It also means that policy makers (and in the NHS of the 2000s, local managers) can be blamed by local people who believe they are not being treated quickly enough or who do not appear to qualify for the treatment they believe they should receive. Universal care would be difficult to remove, even if it is being challenged by government exhortations to look after ourselves better and the prioritising of care in some very specific areas for those who have led healthier lives over others. The public do not often link universalism with the need to wait for treatment, but the two are inextricably bound up with one another.

Finally, there is the NHS's comprehensiveness, perhaps the most difficult of the NHS principles to operationalise. NHS care is not comprehensive in providing every kind of treatment imaginable, but the NHS will offer some kind of treatment to citizens who require it. There is a difference between being treated immediately with the latest available technologies, and being treated with adequate but not cutting-edge medicine after a period of waiting. Often the NHS has managed the latter but not the former. Because NHS infrastructure has been substantially underfunded for much of its history, it has often lacked the resources to be able to provide the most up-to-date treatments, although it has always offered some kind of alternative, usually after a wait in the case of popular services.

The NHS is comprehensive in that it will typically offer some kind of care, but not necessarily the particular care envisaged by the patient, or that which the GP or consultant believes the patient should receive.

So expectant mothers might want a water birth and personal midwife attention, but find this service unavailable and are cared for instead by a midwife who is also trying to look after several other mothers in labour. Patients therefore cannot really be viewed as consumers; within the NHS they do not pay directly for their own treatment, and they do not have a free choice of the type of treatment they receive. Policy makers could not afford to provide a universal, free healthcare system that also allowed patients to be prescribed any kind of medical treatment. Where new treatments appear increasingly costly (Le Fanu, 1999) and where cheaper alternatives exist for most of the services required by patients, comprehensiveness is in place in the NHS, but is not an open-ended commitment for care.

Conclusion

The purpose of this chapter was to show how the NHS of 1948 created a number of institutional legacies that strongly influenced its future, and that are shaping the policy discussions of the service nearly 60 years later. It claims that the legacies described above suggest that the double-bed and tripartite relationships at the heart of the NHS are crucial in understanding debates in the service today.

The following chapters take up the organisational elements described above, showing how the tripartite and double-bed relationships developed in subsequent years, as well as providing a history of how the system of general taxation funding has survived within the NHS. As well as this, it is necessary to explore how health services have been administered and managed, especially considering the increased focus on the importance of management since the 1980s. It is also crucial to ask the question of why it is that accounts of the NHS (this one included) spend so much time exploring the medical profession when it is not its largest professional group. What about the nurses? Finally, recent policy has placed the role of the health service user under greater scrutiny, and it is therefore important to understand the role of patients in the organisation and delivery of healthcare organisations within the very particular organisational characteristics of the NHS.

Once the book has dealt with these questions by presenting their history, it will bring the account together around a discussion of health policy under Labour in the decade 1997-2007, before presenting a critique of the direction of health policy and an attempt to bring the book to a close by looking to the future, and working out what an historical account of the NHS might suggest for how health services could be better run.

THREE

The tripartite split

Introduction

The story of the tripartite split in the NHS is one of policy makers' and doctors' attempts to overcome, or use to their advantage, the organisational separation between health services resulting from the organisational compromises present in the founding of the NHS in 1948. This chapter considers the development of the tripartite split one service at a time, but also in terms of the boundaries of the services in relation to one another.

The NHS in the 1940s and 1950s

The creation of the NHS split health services into three largely separately administered services. First, there were the hospitals. Hospitals were nationalised under Bevan's plan, brought into the public sector because of the often precarious state of voluntary hospitals in many locations, but also because this created the possibility of a service with unified planning and delivery of care within the public sector. Second, there were independent contractors, such as doctors and dentists, who managed in the lead-up to the creation of the NHS to secure sufficient assurances that their services would remain independently contracted. This book deals with GPs for the most part when considering independent contractors because of their significance as gatekeepers for access to care within the NHS. Third, there were local authority health services, consisting of health visitors, home nurses, domiciliary midwives and ambulance services, with Medical Officers of Health (MOHs) responsible for coordinating services and often taking a lead on public health. Local government health services were also supposed to develop health centres in order to establish multidisciplinary teams of those working in local health services. Local government had lost control of its municipal hospitals in the nationalisation of the hospitals in 1948, and so had lost its most significant health asset.

If hospital medicine carried the greatest status, GPs could at least console themselves with their independence, but local government health services were hugely variable from location to location, and ranked a clear third in terms of public profile and funding. These three parts of the NHS are summarised in Table 3.1

Table 3.1: The tripartite split in 1948

Hospitals	Nationalised into the public sector
GP services	Remained independent contractors
Local authority health services	Coordinated by MOHS – services including health visitors, home nurses, ambulance services

Hospitals

In 1948, the NHS took over around 2,600 hospitals, with experienced local authority managers mostly taking over the Regional Hospital Boards (RHBs). Consultants entered hospitals not as independent contractors but as employees, in a clearly defined career structure progressing from house officer eventually through to consultant. Distinction awards were on offer for those of above-average ability, and were decided on by other consultants.

Hospitals were divided up into 'natural' districts, which were overseen by Hospital Management Committees, which in turn reported to RHBs, which were meant to be responsible for the application of government policy, the development of strategy and budgetary control, as well as the development of specialities. Hospital areas were organised around hubs of local teaching hospitals, which as a concession to the consultants had their own Boards of Governors, and so were outside the control of the RHBs. General practitioners were part of the independent contractor services that were placed outside the control of either regional boards or local authorities. There was a clear element of inheritance, as the 140 or so Executive Councils overseeing these services were effectively renamed insurance committees from the pre-NHS that were responsible for GP, dentist, optician and pharmacist services. The nationalisation of the hospitals led to local health services coming under local authority control under the auspices of the new local health authorities, largely under the control of the MOHs.

Hospital medicine has been the dominant force in the NHS since its creation. It is where most specialist medicine is carried out, and therefore has tended to attract doctors with the highest qualifications and abilities seeking the chance to work at the cutting edge of their discipline. Hospital medicine tends to be mostly concerned with acute conditions, dealing with the worst illnesses and injuries, and can therefore make a claim for resources that can be seen to be literally saving people's lives, unlike investment in GP practices or public health, which may take time to generate a return. This sounds a little cynical, but it is always harder for those in charge to invest in an area where returns may come years from the commitment of funds as they may be creating a legacy for their successor rather than popularity for themselves. Acute medicine is therefore a politically good area for politicians to be seen to be spending money. However, there are other reasons why hospital medicine has dominated the NHS.

First, the increase in medical knowledge in the late 19th and early 20th century made clear the importance of sterile practice in surgery, leading to a significant rise in patient survival. Improvements in technique, often coming from doctors' wartime experiences, meant that surgery underwent a transformation from being something only to be resorted to when facing imminent danger of death, to a more everyday occurrence, albeit one with still significant risks attached to it (Le Fanu, 1999). General practitioners carried out minor surgeries in their practices (some GPs still refer to their practices as 'surgeries' today), but the site where practice was most common was the hospital. Surgical and medical specialties began to grow up in the 20th century based around the hospital where technologies unimagined 50 years earlier were the embodiment of the 'new' medicine sought out by the public: 'The exigencies of the machine increasingly dictated the organisation and structure of the hospital' (Brandt and Gardner, 2003, p 28).

A second reason for hospitals being dominant in medicine came from the UK's wartime experience. Fearing extensive bombing from an early date, the EMS was set up in the early days of the war, effectively passing the pre-war mix of voluntary and municipal hospitals into public hands in order to deal with the anticipated casualties (Honigsbaum, 1989). Thankfully, bombing never occurred on the scale feared by the government, but the EMS showed that nationalising hospitals was a possibility. It also showed that public services could be planned on a large scale in order to achieve greater efficiency and organisation than was the case under the old system, which suffered from duplication and waste in some areas, and a lack of provision in others (Addison, 1975). This is an important point because it shows how radically ideas about health organisation can change from one period to another. In the 1940s, state-controlled monopolies were regarded as providing an efficient means of planning services, and the socialist government (Labour in the 1940s) believed that services such as healthcare, but also industries that were key to the national economy, such as steel and coal, were too important to leave to the private sector. The best solution, the government believed, was to nationalise them and bring them under state control where they could be most efficiently managed without the waste and disruption of the market. The argument in relation to the organisation of public (and other) services today would be almost exactly the opposite, that public control of services is bureaucratic, wasteful and unresponsive, and that only the dynamism of the market can make services efficient (Forbes, 1986).

Ideas about health organisation are very much a function of their time, and can change dramatically from one era to the next. In the 1940s, the increased role of the state during wartime fitted well with the belief of the postwar Labour government that the state should control vital public services, and so the nationalisation of the hospitals, with all the opportunities for planning and efficiency this appeared to create, created an attractive proposition for socialist policy makers. In Webster's (1998b, p 22) words, 'The constructive energies of the Department of Health were dedicated to the hospital sector'.

The dominance of the hospitals was therefore due to the nature of the medicine practised in them (acute and specialist), the breakthroughs in acute medicine in the late 19th and early 20th century demonstrating that it was an area of rapid improvement, and the wartime experience of nationalising the hospitals and the opportunity this offered socialist policy makers for planning healthcare on a much larger scale after the war by taking greater control of the network of hospitals in the country.

In terms of their relationship to other areas of the NHS, hospitals were in something of a vulnerable position before the creation of the NHS. Patients, as today, would receive referrals from their GPs if they required hospital care, but faced the significant problem that, unless their health insurance covered them for hospital care, they would have to find the funds for care themselves. This was a significant problem. Hospital care is expensive not only because of the treatments it provides, but also because if patients are required to stay in hospital while being treated, additional 'hotel' costs for staying can quickly accrue. General practitioners were therefore necessary partners for hospital doctors in the pre-war health system, with consultants often not receiving a salary from hospitals, instead depending on the fees of patients referred to them. If GPs did not refer patients, consultants would struggle to justify their appointments in hospitals; even though they received no salary, a hospital appointment carried with it both prestige and the potential to generate a considerable private income. Referrals were therefore hugely important; without them, both hospitals and consultants would struggle financially.

The relationship between consultants and GPs before the NHS, although consultants may have looked down on their colleagues because of the generalist rather than specialist medicine they practised, was therefore one that can be characterised as being necessary. It was a relationship that both GPs and consultants needed, a mutually dependent one, with GPs needing consultants to refer specialist cases on to, and consultants needing GPs for their appointment at the local hospital, and so for access to private fees. The creation of the NHS, however, changed this because consultants became salaried employees of hospitals, and hospitals were no longer financially dependent on receiving referrals for patients as they were separately funded by the Department of Health. Hospitals and consultants were no longer dependent on GP referrals. The relationship between GPs and consultants no longer carried with it a two-way dependency, and was far more one-sided than before. General practitioners still needed to make referrals for patients requiring specialist care, but consultants no longer had to foster their relationships with GPs with great care in order to preserve their hospital appointments. Consultants could begin to regard themselves almost as doing favours for GPs in seeing their patients. The relationship moved from a demand-led basis in which fee-paying patients and their GP referrers held power, to one that was supply-led, where salaried consultants and hospitals, secure in their receipt of funds from the NHS, decided the terms on which patients would be referred. These changes are summarised in Table 3.2.

The founding of the NHS effectively left two groups as 'othered', or having to define their roles in the healthcare system in relation to hospital medicine, struggling to find a coherent identity as a result: GPs and those working in local authority health services.

GPs

The plebiscite of GPs taken by the BMA in January 1948, just six months before the launch of the proposed NHS, saw 84% voting against its introduction (Morrell, 1998). By the introduction of the NHS, GPs were relieved of administrative roles such as bad-debt chasing, but faced increased demands from patients because of greater access to their services than had been the case prior to the NHS, as well as concerns about increased demands for out-of-hours care and the need to provide an increasing number of certificates and prescriptions within the new NHS system.

Table 3.2: Changing relationships between consultants and GPs

Pre-NHS	NHS in 1948
Consultants depend on GP referrals to secure their posts, and so access to private medicine	Consultants are salaried and hold posts independent of GP referrals
Consultants are required to foster good relationships with GPs in order to maintain referrals	Consultants are no longer dependent on GP referrals and there is no incentive to preserve relationships with GPs
The consultant–GP relationship is necessary – based on mutual dependence	The consultant–GP relationship is weighted on consultant's side, and GPs still need consultants in order to be able to refer patients – a power imbalance

At the founding of the NHS, there were around 18,000 GPs, the vast majority of whom were male, and 50% of whom worked in single-handed practices, often working from their own homes. The NHS brought greater security of income than had been the case for GPs prior to the NHS as they no longer had to collect fees from insurance companies and individual patients. Urban GPs with large lists of registered patients often became affluent, but had problems serving all their patients. In contrast, GPs in rural areas, who might have depended significantly on private practice, which was no longer available, and where there were small patient lists, suddenly became rather worse off. In his early survey of the NHS, Eckstein (1958) examined variations in practice size in the North of England and found huge variations, with affluent areas such as Harrogate having large numbers of GPs, but poorer areas such as Leeds and Bradford having a relative scarcity (Eckstein, 1958).

It quickly became fairly clear that GPs, despite their agitation between the announcement of Bevan's plans and the final NHS legislation, were on the worse end of the deal that created the NHS; 'the rate of remuneration of general practitioners … was seen to be unfair and almost certainly led to the slow level of recruitment in the first four years of the service' (Godber, 1975, p 22). The problem was not just one of pay; Calnan and Gabe (1991, p 144) argue that GPs had become an 'isolated and defensive group who had lost interest in challenging the dominance of hospital specialists'. General practitioners were contracted to provide 24–hour care, but remained independent practitioners, were self-employed and organised their own professional lives. Pay was entirely based on capitation – the number of patients registered on their list, and with expenses based on an average figure. This system had a built-in bias to try to enrol as many patients as possible on to doctors' lists, but with little incentive to improve services once they were enrolled. Many GPs reported that little had changed with the creation of the NHS, with the changes that did occur being financial rather than clinical:'Nothing changed very much except we didn't have to send out monthly bills, and didn't have 20 percent bad debts' (Payer, 1996, p 107). In a survey of the literature in 1958, Titmuss concluded that GPs appeared to have lost no clinical freedom or autonomy as a result of joining the NHS (Titmuss, 1958).

General practitioners acted as gatekeepers to the NHS, sanctioning referrals to other health services and writing prescriptions (Dowling, 2000). The gatekeeper role is hugely important because it provides a first barrier to accessing health services, so limiting the flow of patients into secondary care. The gatekeeper role also, for the vast majority of the history of the NHS, has created a system by which, through delay and implicit rationing, costs are kept down. International comparative figures show the relatively low rates of referral and prescription in the NHS compared with other health systems. Patients in the UK see their doctor more (5.4 times a year on average) than the French (5.2) or Americans (4.7), but GP consultations are far shorter (about six minutes, compared with 15–20 minutes). Doctors in the UK prescribe fewer drugs (6.53 per capita) compared with French (10.04) or West German (11.18) doctors (Payer, 1996, p 106).

Pemberton (1949) examined GP practices in Sheffield in 1947 and found high workloads, with doctors typically seeing 350 patients per week in the winter and 260 in the summer, with, remarkably, around a third of consultations taking place in patients' homes. The quality of care offered by GPs is hard to establish, but seems to have been hugely variable. Collings (1950, p 563) suggested that the state of general practice was 'bad and still deteriorating' and that inner-city practice was 'at the best unsatisfactory and at the worst a source of public danger'. Hadfield (1953), however, was not so pessimistic, suggesting that nearly 60% of GPs were in good or adequate premises, although 24% still lacked essential facilities and 10% were totally unsuitable or inadequate. Taylor (1954) suggested that around a quarter of GPs (particularly in industrial areas) lacked essential items of equipment, had poor case notes and did not see patients when necessary. Within that last quarter was a final 'twentieth for whom it is difficult to find any excuse.... No doubt a similar inefficient sediment can be found in any profession; but in medicine it matters more to the public' (Taylor, 1954, pp 8–9).

General practitioners also actively campaigned in the early years of the NHS to make it more difficult for patients to change their registered doctor, resulting in rule changes in 1950 to prevent what they called the 'abuse' that might result from people changing doctors.

The driver for the reform of local health services, the formation of health centres within which teams of professionals would work, largely disappeared with the creation of the NHS through responsibility for their development being passed to the local authorities, and its priority being lowered to avoid antagonising already-angry interest groups in general practice (Eckstein, 1958, pp 247-52).

Consultants often regarded GPs as second-rate doctors, non-specialists not deserving of their respect. Because of the lack of resources attached to referrals, consultants had a vested interest in defining their specialism as narrowly as possible to try to prevent what Payer (1996, p 106) pithily calls 'GP rubbish' referrals and so keep their workloads down. General practitioners still wished to refer patients, but consultants who wished to minimise their NHS work were now in an incompatible relationship with their GP colleagues; they had no financial incentives to see their patients and carry out the extra work.

In the early years of the NHS, there were few financial incentives to redevelop GP practices and the profession appeared gripped in something of a malaise, treating as much as 90% of all NHS patients (Rivett, 1998, p 162), but often in cramped conditions. Health centres, where GPs could share facilities and ancillary support, had not taken off in the way envisaged by the architects of the NHS (see Eckstein, 1958), and there appeared to be a need for local authorities to invest considerably in GP services to get initiatives that provided more integrated care off the ground. The problem was that improved facilities and the employment of more staff invariably meant higher costs for GPs, who were paid from a global sum of money (the 'pool') that was divided among them. There was an incentive to run a GP practice as cheaply as possible, not investing in facilities, because this could make the GP better off. Many GPs provided excellent care despite this, but there was clearly always a built-in incentive to be as cost-conscious as possible – in contrast to much of the activity of hospital consultants.

Morale among GPs was low. As they saw hospital services improve and consultants achieve greater status (and income), GPs found that their referrals no longer carried the same importance as before the NHS. From there being a necessary relationship between GPs and consultants, it was now entirely contingent – the tripartite arrangement had effectively removed the mutual dependence between the two doctor groupings.

The GPs also faced a problem in that their representative body – the BMA – had done little to endear itself to the Department of Health in the period leading up to the creation of the NHS, and this provoked among policy makers an attitude of what might be viewed as benign indifference towards the state of general practice where improvements were not actively sought, especially as hospital medicine in contrast appeared so dynamic (Webster, 1998b). At the local level, GPs were often suspicious of MOHs, who effectively organised local authority health services, because of the administrative boundary between them, but also because of possible conflicts between the two groups over boundaries involving the management of groups such as nurse visitors. These nurses were now technically employed by local authorities, but needed to work closely with GPs, especially because GPs often utilised them as a resource of their own surgeries.

The problems of the GP service in the 1940s are summarised in Table 3.3.

In 1952, the Danckwerts pay award went some way to addressing the problem of GP pay, and 1952 was also the year that saw the founding of the College of General Practitioners. Danckwerts suggested a pay rise for GPs of around 25%, and the government, despite not anticipating such a large award, paid it on condition that there were incentives built in to improve general practice. The flat-rate capitation system was

Table 3.3: GP problems in the late 1940s

Problem	Concern
Referrals no longer carry status for consultants	GPs suffer a reduction in status and ability to refer patients in a timely fashion
GPs are required to provide 24-hour care	GPs are required to perform out-of-hours work from both their own homes and patients' homes
Pay is based on capitation	There is an incentive to have large 'lists' of patients, but heavy workloads come with this
GP services are hugely variable	Heavy workloads often mean that GPs are using outdated medicine and working in poor conditions
Gatekeeper role for general practice	GPs are required to see patients with a variety of illnesses but to refer on 'specialist' cases, so work is often relatively mundane

changed to give a higher relative return to practices with medium-sized lists, and it was made easier for new doctors to enter practices through an initial practice allowance. There were also financial encouragements to form partnerships and group practices. This, however, eroded the differential between consultant and GP pay. In 1955, the BMA put forward a proposal for an increase of around 25% for the period 1951 to 1954, leading eventually, after several years of rather public argument between the state and the consultants, to the establishment of a Royal Commission on medical pay.

The gulf between hospital and general medicine was made most explicit in the Royal Commission on Doctors' and Dentists' Remuneration (in 1958), where Lord Moran, then president of the Royal College of Physicians, had a famous exchange with the Chair of the committee:

> The Chairman: It has been put to us by a good many people that the two branches of the profession, general practitioners and consultants, are not senior or junior to one another, but they are level. Do you agree with that?
>
> Lord Moran: I say emphatically No. Could anything be more absurd? I was Dean at St. Mary's Hospital Medical School for 25 years, and all the people of outstanding merit, with few exceptions, aimed to get on the staff. It was a ladder off which they fell. How can you say that the people who fall off the ladder are the same as those who do not?... I do not think you will find a single Dean of any medical school who will give contrary evidence.
>
> The Chairman: I think you are the first person who has suggested to us that general practitioners are a somewhat inferior bunch. (Rivett, 1998, p 163)

General practitioner groups, despite later retractions from Moran, were understandably furious. Moran probably reflected the views of his peers in a frank, if somewhat incautious, manner, but he had made explicit the unsayable – the gulf between specialist and generalist medicine was wide and growing.

Local authority health services

If GP services appeared to be struggling in the NHS, local authority health services may have been in an even worse state. Section 28 of the 1946 NHS Act gave local authorities responsibilities for the 'prevention of illness, the care of persons suffering from illness or mental defectiveness, or the after-care of such persons'. However, these responsibilities were often enacted in an uneven and inconsistent manner. In some areas, for example, patients discharged from hospitals found themselves resettled by active local authority healthcare teams, but in others such care appeared almost non-existent (Jones, 1954). The Ministry of Health conceded by the mid-1950s that there was a lack of expertise, with trained staff scarce, and that progress in dealing with 'mental deficiency' had been 'slow and uneven' (Ministry of Health, 1953). In addition, local authorities were responsible for the provision of Occupation Centres (to try to provide skills to those with learning difficulties), hostels, social clubs and after-care, but once again, provision varied considerably from one location to the next (Welshman, 2006b).

The role of the MOH changed with the creation of the NHS from the development of services to assisting in service provision by others. From 1948, local authorities were responsible for nursing in the community and the development of preventative and social support services, including home-help services. Local authorities began to bring nursing services in-house from voluntary nursing organisations, with visiting nurses becoming increasingly important as hospitals began to discharge patients increasingly rapidly. In London, home helps were crucial because of the shortage of hospital beds, and were used to keep the chronically sick cared for in the community rather than in hospitals (Land, 1991). The role of the health visitor came under challenge as GP services became free, as patients increasingly wished to consult with doctors instead, and because of the organisational boundary between the two groups.

Putting the development of health centres under the control of local authorities was largely stifled by GP concerns that it would increase their links with local authorities (which were responsible for their development), but also because of the lack of a template demonstrating what such centres would look like. Health centres were few and far between, and where they did appear, GPs often used the centres only as branches of their own practices. It was hard, at the end of the 1950s, to consider local authority health services as being an area of innovation or dynamism, despite the huge importance of the care offered there.

The 1960s

The Porritt Report of 1962 (General Medical Services Committee, 1962) recommended that the three parts of the NHS be brought under the control of a single area board, with a doctor being chief officer, and professionals being well represented in making decisions about healthcare in their localities. The report fed into the discussions leading to the first organisational reform of the NHS between 1968 and 1974. However, the process of negotiation and consultation with the many interest groups involved in the NHS meant that the goal of reuniting health services at either national or local level became lost. Plans for 'co-terminosity' of boundaries between local authorities and health authorities were meant to begin to address the problems of working between those two areas, but difficulties in the setting of the new local areas and the negative reaction of the Department of Health for plans to give local authorities greater powers, meant that the opportunity to bring services closer together was lost (Glennerster, 1995). The 1960s were not notable for the reunification of health services, but for the continued dominance of the hospitals.

The Hospital Plan

The peak of the faith in hospital medicine came in the 1960s with the Hospital Plan (Minister of Health, 1962). Capital building in the NHS was at a derisory level, with figures of around £9-10 million per year in the 1940s, rising slowly in the 1950s to around £20 million a year by 1960. It had been three times the 1950s level in the pre-war period (Glennerster, 1995, p 87), and the Guillebaud Committee (Ministry of Health, 1956) had suggested that a figure of £30 million a year was necessary simply to account for the annual depreciation of buildings. The money had been used chiefly to patch up existing infrastructure rather than to replace outright many of the crumbling buildings the NHS had inherited (Watkin, 1978, p 59).

Health Minister Enoch Powell asked the RHBs to put together a proposal for increased capital expenditure, and in January 1962 the Hospital Plan was published. The Hospital Plan attempted to replace outdated infrastructure, and put in place a generic blueprint for the size and scale of what hospitals were needed in the NHS according to the template of the District General Hospital. It was a remarkable document; the development of 90 new hospitals was proposed, and the upgrading of an additional 134. It aimed to create a network of District

General Hospitals, which would each serve a population of 100,000 to 150,000 people, and which would each have 600 to 800 beds.

Powell then asked for plans from local authorities for community health services. Local authorities, because of the tripartite split, were not under Powell's direct control, but he reasoned that creating hospitals without the community health services to support them was ridiculous – an example of what we would today call 'joined-up' thinking. The Hospital Plan also reflected one of the high points of the use of rationalistic planning in government, and occurred at a time when the Treasury was attempting to model the economy in evermore sophisticated ways.

The building of District General Hospitals meant that to keep pace with medical technology and changing medical practice, increasingly large sums of money would need to be invested in healthcare. The changing structure of the population, with increasing numbers of people reaching old age, meant that increased resources from the NHS were required. The buildings themselves were physical manifestations of the faith in planning in the 1960s, embodying this approach to medicine and health organisation. They were designed according to the very latest ideas about efficiency, and were in direct contrast to the smaller 'cottage hospitals' they were designed to replace. They were sites where the best in medical expertise (the consultants) could work together for the furtherance of medical knowledge and the improvement of patient care. Faith in medical expertise was at its greatest – breakthroughs in medical technology could be incorporated into the new hospitals and the very best treatment delivered on the largest possible scale. This was paternalism on a massive scale. The financial aspects and implications of the Hospital Plan are covered in greater depth in Chapter Five.

Mental health services and the birth of community care

All was not entirely well in the hospitals, however. The mental health services were a case study of a specialism at the bottom of the medical hierarchy, where patients were often vulnerable because of their inability to voice their views. If local authority health services were under-resourced because of their lack of visibility, this also applied to mental health services. The lack of visibility of mental health services seems to have led to conditions within some of them becoming scandalously bad (see Robb, 1967). Documentary evidence for the period shows patients ignored and, as there was often little hope of cure or sometimes even treatment, mental health services came low down the list of both public and political priorities. The mental health services also illustrated the powerlessness of the NHS administrative structure. For example, faced by compelling evidence of the terrible state of mental health services at Ely Hospital, Secretary of State Crossman was forced to publish an uncensored report by Geoffrey Howe, later an important figure in the Thatcher governments of the 1980s, damning the conditions there, and subsidise the mental health charity MIND to complain to the government so that a scandal was created on which he could act. This convoluted way of securing policy change illustrated the extent to which institutional inertia dominated.

The area of mental health, as well as being one of often appalling conditions, was also one of remarkable innovation. The increasing availability of psychotropic drugs had a significant implication for GPs and local authority health services and hospitals as the 1960s wore on. The new drugs meant that for many patients with mild or moderate degrees of mental illness, easy and effective treatment could now be managed by GPs rather than by institutionalising patients. However, to simply close down the mental institutions and move treatment to the community was not practical because of the lack of resources available there. This did not stop Enoch Powell in 1961 from making dramatic statements about the closure of the old institutions (National Association for Mental Health, 1961). Throughout the 1960s, the goal of policy was to return patients to ordinary life as much as possible, with health services providing necessary support. The number of beds available in mental hospitals was to be reduced from 160,000 to 80,000 within 16 years. The movement towards this new conception of 'community care' was driven not only by the availability of psychotropic drugs, but also by the claims of libertarians claiming that mental institutions deprived patients of their civil liberties (Welshman, 2006a). This was, in turn, allied with a practical eye from the Department of Health that treatment in the community may well produce cost savings, although it was unclear to anyone in the field at that time exactly what the costs of the new policy would be. It was equally unclear whether patients could be released to care for themselves adequately. Moving patients from mental hospitals into the community meant a transfer of patients from the hospital sector (albeit its least glamorous part) and required a concurrent movement in resources, and for new community health services to be able to take up the challenge to deal with it. Sadly, it does not seem that either of these conditions was fulfilled.

Criticisms of the hospital status quo also began to appear from elsewhere. The 1960s were the decade in which second-wave feminism came to the fore. One of its recurring topics was the concern that much of medicine appeared to be organised according to the convenience of the medical profession rather than the women who were on the receiving end of its treatment. Childbirth was an area of particular concern, with criticism that it was becoming over-medicalised, not to make it safer, but because it suited male doctors, and that midwives' roles under the NHS had been largely reduced by making them junior to male consultants (Dingwall et al, 1988). Practices such as episiotomy were still widespread when they were, in the majority of cases, unnecessary and were performed not on the basis of clinical need but of convenience. Any radical critique will tend to over-reach itself, but there is certainly evidence that the medical profession was not doing all it could for its patients – feminism can therefore be seen as a radical precursor of the consumerism movement that was to follow.

GP services

With respect to GP services, the College of General Practitioners continued to try to drive improvements, claiming that family medicine had its own skills and knowledge, and that it was as important as anything the hospital services could offer. However, GP services still faced the problem that, within a certain practice size range, they received the same remuneration regardless of the quality of care offered. Writing in the 1960s, Enoch Powell (Powell, 1966) suggested that although GPs continued to regard themselves as independent contractors and dynamic entrepreneurs, the reality of the situation was some way from this – with competition between doctors no longer relevant, there was very little of the private enterprise system evident. If GP services were to be based on a different logic to private enterprise, it was not yet clear what that logic was to be.

General practitioners' frustration with pay and conditions grew. General practitioner groups believed that the gap between their pay and that of the consultants was too wide, but the BMA struggled to represent them because of its aspirations to speak as a unified voice for the medical profession as a whole, and it was by no means clear that consultants felt strongly about the plight of their professional colleagues. A General Practitioners' Association was created to attempt to represent GPs and put forward their case more forcefully, and the membership of the Medical Practitioners' Union rose dramatically. The NHS had been in existence for little over 15 years with relatively little in terms of industrial action, but the increase in competition between representative groups for GPs led to the potential for a more conflictual future.

General practitioners and consultants also appeared to be moving down very different professional lines. In 1961, the Standing Medical

Advisory Committee put in place a group to try to work out the role of family doctors over the next 10-15 years. The subsequent Gillie Report (Central Health Services Council Standing Medical Advisory Committee, 1963) saw the future of GPs in a role that coordinated resources between hospitals and care in the community setting, mobilising care on behalf of patients as it was needed. However, this role appeared to anger both older GPs, who felt that it bore no resemblance to their current practice, and younger GPs, who felt that it underplayed their status as medical professionals. The outgoing Conservative Minister of Health, the BMA and the College of General Practitioners met to discuss the report, finding little agreement among the GPs in terms of pay, but a need for help over the provision of premises and access to hospital facilities (Rivett, 1998).

General practitioner numbers actually fell in 1964, and then again over the subsequent two years. The medical pay review body then gave largely unsympathetic awards to the GPs, creating a new mood of militancy, and eventually the Charter for the Family Doctor Service was submitted by James Cameron (Cameron, 1965). The charter aimed to reduce patient lists to 2,000, reduce bureaucracy, shorten the working day, create better access to hospital facilities for GPs and increase the ability of practices to choose how they would be paid. The BMA adopted it, giving it wide publicity, and Cameron called for undated resignations to be sent to BMA House until a new deal was met.

At the end of the discussions, GPs received a pay rise of about one third, and despite an economic crisis, the government went reluctantly along with the deal, not least because Minister of Health Robinson threatened to resign if it did not. Despite the increase in pay, however, there was still very little idea of how a career structure in general practice might work, or what the characteristics of the 'better' GP might look like.

There was, as a result of changes stemming from the GP charter, an upsurge in interest from GPs in health centres. Rental charges were no longer a charge against personal income. Doctors even began to build their own premises, employing receptionists and incorporating nurses and midwives who needed to be given space and resources of their own. As a consequence of this and the improvement in GP pay, Rivett (1998) argues that something of a renaissance of GP medicine took place in the 1960s. Conditions certainly improved, but whether much ground was gained on the consultants is less certain.

One of the significant problems facing general practice has been the difficulty of defining the role of GPs without reference to the dominant form of medicine in hospitals. A generic initial model was that of the family doctor, who often worked alone in premises that may have been a part or extension of their house. The family doctor was an extension of the panel doctoring system present before the NHS, in which GPs were set up to provide their services to either those covered by national insurance or those who could pay fees through private means. Patients were often seen in the parlour of the house of the GP, with it not being unusual for private patients to have a separate entry point (the front door) compared with those receiving their care through the national insurance system (who might enter through the back door instead). The range of treatments the GP could offer was remarkably limited compared with the modern cornucopia of drugs, with few effective, tested drugs on offer. Antibiotics, for example, only became available on a widespread basis during the 1950s. Taylor's accounts of general practice in 1954 (Taylor, 1954) give an indication of what family doctoring meant, based on intimacy and domesticity, but also the considerable social distance between doctor and patient (Marinker, 1998). Taylor gave clear categories of illness that paid little or no attention to psychological conditions, and were based clearly on biomedical categories used by hospitals and learned by doctors during their medical training.

Balint's (1957) ideas about general practice, published only three years after Taylor's report, presented a very different view. Balint had worked with the Tavistock Institute, and was instrumental in popularising psychotherapeutic techniques with general practice being based on the development of human relationships rather than the biomedical model of diagnosis (Balint and Norell, 1973). Although his ideas never spread as widely among GPs as he had hoped, those Balint worked with were instrumental in shaping the *The Future General Practitioner* (Royal College of General Practitioners, 1972), which attempted to shape a new understanding of GP practice from the 1970s onwards (Calnan and Gabe, 1991). Balint was immediately influential in trying to get GPs to think beyond drugs, and to try to achieve continuity of care with personal lists of patients as practices grew (Marinker, 1998). Even if doctors did not agree with Balint's psychotherapeutic evangelising, they often agreed with the good sense of seeing their own patients regularly and its fit with the traditional notion of family doctoring. Bowling (1981), for example, suggested that GPs were happy to continue with ear syringing rather than delegate it to nurses within their surgeries because it helped to cement the doctor–patient relationship.

A third model of general practice was developed by Tudor-Hart (1988) and is based on a synthesis between epidemiology and primary care. Tudor-Hart first became widely known for his critique of the disparity between the need for care and the availability of care – care in several urban areas with greater health support needs appeared lacking because of the unwillingness of doctors to live in those areas, whereas areas that were more attractive to live in, already well served by doctors, tended to attract more doctors. This 'inverse care law' (Tudor–Hart, 1971) presented a view of the patient as being part of a community (Marinker, 1998), with an emphasis on the results of experimental scientists dominating practice rather than the case-by-case constructions favoured by Balint's approach. Tudor–Hart contrasted his approach to that of Balint because of his emphasis on the social context of medicine (Berridge, 1999). Table 3.4 summarises the different approaches to general practice.

Table 3.4: Differing approaches to general practice

GP role	Description
Family doctor	GP as centre of community, but distant from it. Biomedical categories of diagnosis and treatment
Personal/biographical (Balint)	Psychotherapeutic, personal, relationship-based. Non-biomedical diagnosis and treatment
Epidemiological/primary care-driven (Tudor-Hart)	Patient is part of a community with large-scale experiments appropriate to examine local areas. Emphasis on the social context of medicine

Local authority care – from control to care?

Local authority care for those with learning difficulties in the 1960s was characterised by Welshman (2006b) as representing a movement from 'control' to 'care'. Welshman suggests that, at the creation of the NHS, eugenics was the dominant ideology, provision was based on the separation of people with learning difficulties from the rest of society and physical restraint was often necessary. As the 1960s developed, however, a new language of care and integration began to appear, based on the beginnings of an idea of community care in which facilities would be provided in local settings for adult and child training in basic skills. This was allied with social changes that recast those with learning difficulties in a more favourable light, making it easier for politicians to fund new facilities. Progress, however, was slow, and a combination of economic difficulties and the low priority afforded those in need of this type of care (Ham, 1980) meant that, as with local authority services at the creation of NHS, provision was geographically uneven.

Local authority services represented neither the glamorous, high-technology medicine of the hospitals nor the everyday medicine of the GPs, but instead provided a range of local health services, which made a considerable difference to their recipients in terms of preserving their independence and offering respite for informal carers. As well as this, societal changes characterised by Lewis (1992) as the 'deregulation of personal life', such as the advent of the contraceptive pill, led to family planning services becoming more widely available, with legislation in 1967 enabling local authorities to provide services on a general basis. From a mixed start, the MOHs appeared to have become more organised, and at least begun to provide some level of consistency.

The dynamics of tripartite healthcare at the end of the 1960s

By the end of the 1960s, then, a clear dynamic was in place between the three areas of healthcare in England. Hospital medicine was dominant and apparently unassailable in the minds of planners, although criticisms were mounting from elsewhere. The Hospital Plan had invested significant sums in high technology, and consultant medicine that no longer had any significant dependence on referrals from GPs. Hospitals had survived changes in government between Labour and Conservative and back again, apparently being able to show an equal fit with either political party. If it was a Labour government that gave the consultants a privileged position within the NHS through the concessions Bevan was prepared to give them, it was the Conservatives who reinforced it through the Hospital Plan. The only dissenting voice appeared to come from the feminist movement, and was directed at medical practice more generally. Other criticisms, however, were soon to follow.

General practice had been in a poor state at the creation of the NHS, and had struggled in the following decade to find a clear identity and role within the health service. The removal of the importance of the referral link meant that consultants no longer had to court GPs in order to retain their living, and disdain for their generalist colleagues appeared to surface quickly. Newly qualified GPs yearned to be something more than the community or family doctor, and imagined alternatives that positioned them in a more therapeutic role, or as the leaders of teams engaged in community-oriented medicine. What they often found, however, was that they were required to act as gatekeepers for the NHS, dealing with everyday conditions while referring on any specialist cases. From the low point in the early 1960s when GP numbers actually fell, an improvement in morale had come from the implementation of the GP Charter and from the increased interest in setting up health centres. But this improvement came from a low base, and the lack of good working relationships with consultants often led to GPs continuing to be poorly regarded by their hospital specialist colleagues.

Local authority healthcare had lost most as a result of the creation of the NHS. The nationalisation of hospitals meant that it had lost its most significant stake in local healthcare provision, and it was left with a range of services that, in the early years of the NHS, it struggled to coordinate. This led to hugely variable local authority services being in place, with much depending on the individual abilities of the local MOH. By the end of the 1960s, however, things appeared to be settling down, even if hospital medicine continued to dominate.

The 1970s

If the high point of the District General Hospital and of the faith in the combination of state planning and medical expertise came in the 1960s, critiques of hospital medicine began to appear more widely by the 1970s. Thomas McKeown suggested that there had been unjustified concentration on acute medicine and hospital services, while much of the improvement in healthcare was due instead to the environment, better food, cleaner water and general improvements in the standard of living (McKeown, 1962, 1976). McKeown's conclusion was that society was misdirecting its health investment, and was later radicalised further in the development of the critique that acute medical care might be responsible for making its recipients more ill through a process of 'iatrogenesis' (Illich, 1977).

Medical research had resulted in a period of dramatic development in the postwar period, but was beginning to become a victim of that success, as subsequent improvements were never going to be as impressive (Le Fanu, 1999). Hospitals began to be seen as expensive in an era of increased public financial stringency, and impersonal and alienating for patients because of their increased size (Turner, 1987). As early as 1958, Titmuss had suggested that there was a danger that 'the hospitals may tend increasingly to be run in the interests of those working in and for the hospital rather than in the interests of the patient' (Titmuss, 1958, p 122). There was certainly discursive space developing for a greater critique of hospital–dominated health services.

The criticisms of the status quo in medicine created greater space for local authority health services to develop, based on new agendas in public health and greater care in the community. Public health still had a strong environmental element, with a notable success being the actions of the National Society for Smoke Abatement, made up of MOHs and a cross-party group of MPs, which resulted in the 1956 Clean Air Act. The MOHs had smoothly running empires of the limited range of health services under their control by the end of the 1960s (Rivett, 1998), overseeing community nursing, social work and after-care, ambulances and school health. However, the recommendations of the Seebohm Report (DHSS, 1968) led to the separation of social work from medicine, and directors of social services were appointed, so the MOHs lost a significant part of their work. Community nursing was then organised into a new hierarchy, so MOHs lost control of this area as well. Finally, ambulance services were placed under the control of the new regional health authorities and the health centre programme began to wind down. The new area of 'community medicine' began under the reformed NHS in 1974.

Community medicine addressed concerns that health services needed to address groups rather than individuals, and the perceived need to create a new specialty that included public health doctors, medical administrators and epidemiologists. Some areas of community medicine stressed health promotion, while others emphasised planning and management and the need for the evaluation of services. Community health services have always been ambiguous; they can be a generic term for care that addresses population groups rather than focusing on individual patients, but are also a rallying point for those involved in non-hospital services, including general practice (Lewis, 1999). In either case, new discourses of care were emerging to challenge the pre-eminent hospitals. Equally, new ideas about treatment were moving care from hospitals to the community. This was most present in the case of the old mental illness hospitals, where as far back as the early 1950s new drug-based therapies were becoming available that created possibilities for the release of patients. The closure of the old mental illness hospitals, however, proceeded rather slowly. Wright et al (1994) suggest they had experienced a fall of only around 7,000 places during the 1970s to about 51,500.

Community care, born most formally after the 1974 reforms but present in theory and practice before then, was the mainstay of care until its transformation in the late 1990s into 'social care'. Community care, as with many other areas of care outside of hospitals, has many meanings; it can be the alternative to the institutions where mentally ill patients were located in the 1940s and 1950s (care in the community) but also a cheaper alternative to hospital care, being mobilised in a similar way to primary care, but across perhaps a wider range of services and involving lay carers as well (care by the community, which makes clear the overlap with the modern social care agenda of direct payments and individual budgets). There is a sense that community care has been shorthand for trying to move patients away from expensive hospital care settings into something cheaper, with this also carrying with it a positive discourse of allowing people to stay in their homes for as long as possible.

The 1970s also mark the beginning of the emergence of the idea of the primary healthcare team. In the early part of the decade, Lewis (1999) suggests that a model that can be characterised as 'GP-centred and negative' was in place, in which GPs were positioned at the centre of the team, and other members, such as practice nurses, were there to protect them from 'trivia'. However, this gradually gave way to one that was 'GP-centred and positive', in that it gave more recognition to the contribution that other members of the team might make. This was still a long way from suggesting that those working in primary healthcare teams were doctors' equals, but showed that some progress was being made.

The 1970s were dominated by the economic problems most industrial nations suffered from, and by the NHS reorganisation of 1974. The former did not have as significant an impact on the tripartite split in medicine as might have been expected, while the latter was important in removing most of the remaining NHS services from local authority control, putting the focus instead on the ideas of community care and primary care to fill the gap left behind. Both were to be significant in the following decade.

The 1980s

Hospital-based medicine was explicitly challenged in the 1980s by the appointment of general managers in posts explicitly created to make the NHS more business-like by giving clearly designated individuals the responsibility for running services (DHSS, 1983). These individuals could be doctors (in fact, the NHS Management Inquiry even suggested that they were the 'natural' managers of the NHS), but in the future, health services had to be more accountable and to take greater responsibility for improving services to both patients and to the community in the wider sense. In Alford's (1972) terms, the dominant interest of the consultants was being challenged by the corporate rationalisers from the new managers. Hospitals were no longer to be regarded as churches, where the sacred practice of consultant specialist medicine was to be carried out (Klein, 1993), and were criticised for being expensive and producer- rather than patient-focused. Policy makers began a search in earnest for ways of making them more accountable. The creation of the 'internal market' later in the decade gave managers increased legitimacy to challenge medics, and so represented a continuation of the corporate rationaliser theme (Ham, 2000). They also reinstated the importance of GP referrals for consultants, a topic that will be picked up again below. The state, while still continuing to fund hospitals in a privileged way, was beginning to demand greater control of its investment in them.

General practitioners found themselves challenged by the Conservative administration to find savings when 'limited list prescribing' was introduced to decrease the range of prescriptions GPs could make, as well as beginning the process of standardising the drugs available within the NHS. The limited list produced a bizarre alliance of opposition between the medical profession, the pharmaceutical industry and the Labour Party, but the government refused to back down, and it was introduced in November 1984. The notion that the NHS could be 'primary care–driven' also began to appear, with the government appealing to GPs to drive improvements in healthcare as the doctors closest to the patient (Peckham and Exworthy, 2003). This fitted well with ideas about introducing markets into healthcare as patients were encouraged to choose their GP, and GPs encouraged to be responsive to patient wishes in the way that they referred patients needing further care. Doctors in both hospitals and GP surgeries found themselves criticised for providing a poor service to their patients, with the Acheson Report on inner-London GPs in 1981 (Acheson, 1981) particularly critical of the care available.

In community care, the 1981 Community Care Act was designed to try to address an incentive within the health system that rewarded health organisations for closure and penalised social services. Savings from hospital closures accrued to health authorities, while the cost of looking after the patients fell to local authorities (Walmsley, 2006). A rule change in 1983 allowed board and lodging allowances in voluntary or privately run accommodation to be funded from social security payments if a person could show financial need (Johnson, 2005). This, apparently by accident (Klein, 2006), created a mixed economy of care, with the number of beds in voluntary organisation-run homes increasing by 271% between 1980 and 1990 (Walmsley, 2006), and public expenditure on private residential care increasing from £10 million in 1979 to £1,872 million in 1991 (Means and Smith, 1994). The government had created an almost perfect voucher system that maximised consumer choice and power in the new market (Glennerster, 1995), the upshot of which was the creation of a market for residential care, paid for by the social security budget rather than by health or social services.

The growth in community-based services was ideological as well as the result of hospital closures and accident, with the incoming government having an attachment to a trinity of 'family, private market and voluntary sector' (Berridge, 1999), and the idea that care in the community should also mean care by the community (Hunter, 1993a). At the end of the 1970s, Graham (1979) suggested that the burden of informal care within the family fell on women, but by the mid-1980s an equalising appeared to have taken place, with some 3.5 million women carers and 2.5 million men looking after an older or disabled person (Berridge, 1999). The 1989 White Paper on Community Care (DH, 1989) acknowledged that informal carers' total contribution to care was greater than that funded by central government or local authorities (Hunter, 1993a).

Public health's role within the NHS remained as ambiguous as ever. After the 1974 reforms, public health posts were created at all organisational levels of the reformed NHS, but after the removal of the area tier of organisation in 1982, a division between management and specialist roles appeared to take place, and 20% of all public health doctors sought early retirement (Berridge, 1999). Griffiths' (DH, 1989) focus on the management of individual health organisations carried with it the concern that analysing health problems that went across health communities, such as public health, could get lost. Concerns about AIDS added urgency to the public health agenda, however, and the Acheson Report of 1988 (Acheson, 1988) made a concerted argument to upgrade the status of public health professionals in the NHS, leading to the appointments of Directors of Public Health, and, aided by breakthroughs in information technology, an increased role particularly for epidemiology. This was allied with a greater focus on health promotion and national campaigns to warn against smoking and stress the importance of vaccination and better nutrition. AIDS appeared to represent a watershed in which health promotion gathered in importance, and after which government ministers wondered whether an increased emphasis on prevention might lead to a reduction in health expenditures later on.

The 1990 NHS and Community Care Act attempted to address the increase in expenditure for community-based services, ending funding from an open-ended social security budget and replacing it by a cash-limited, locally administered budget that supported only those users who were individually assessed as requiring its support (Walmsley, 2006). Services were to be tendered for on a competitive basis (under the same process that ancillary services were subject to in hospitals). Local authorities were tasked with drawing up plans for community care, giving them a new role, and emphasising the need for the joint planning and commissioning of health and social services, but which was something that very few local areas achieved in practice in the following decade. The architect of the reform, Roy Griffiths (who was also responsible for the NHS Management Inquiry at the beginning of the decade), managed to persuade Margaret Thatcher to give local authorities a bigger role in organising community care on the grounds that they become 'enabling authorities' (Glennerster, 1995), and that the funds would probably be spent on the private sector rather than on local authority care itself. Discussion about local authority care during the 1980s had become centred on the use of the social security budget, and the 1990 Act moved local authorities closer still to a role within the mixed economy of care where they would regulate and purchase care within the market, but increasingly supply very little of it.

The 1990s

The 1989 internal market reforms (Secretary of State for Health, 1989) recast the relationships between the three areas of the NHS again. The importance of the reforms was that they sought to attempt to increase the status and importance of GP referrals within the NHS. The internal market of the 1990s, by creating GP 'fundholders', attempted to make GPs purchasers of care, receiving a budget to this end, and with patient referrals having funding attached to them (following the mantra that money should 'follow the patient'). General practitioners could purchase care from a wide range of providers, including complementary and alternative therapies, and nearly half of fundholders did so (Baggott, 2004, p 38). They were also given the incentive to prescribe and refer economically because they were allowed to reinvest any surpluses on the budgets they were given for their activities back into their practices. The fundholder model created what economists call a 'principal–agent' relationship between patients and their GPs, in which patients (principals) effectively made doctors their expert agents who made healthcare decisions on their behalf (Mooney, 2003). In some respects, this was a direct continuation of the past – GPs have always referred and made prescription decisions on behalf of their patients. What was different now was that, by making patients principals, GPs were meant to be accountable to their patients for the decisions they had made. Funds were given GPs to provide services on behalf of their patients, and patients had the right to ask how decisions had been made (Clarke and Newman, 1997). The government also appeared to be trying to re-establish the necessary relationship between the GPs and consultants that had existed before the NHS in order to try to drive improvements in the NHS. The changes to tripartite relationships stemming from the internal market reforms are summarised in Table 3.5.

Table 3.5: The internal market and the tripartite split

Change	Importance
GP fundholders	GPs given budgets and are able to purchase care from consultants – referrals carry resources with them again. GPs get to reinvest budget surpluses in their own practices – incentive to prescribe and refer less. GPs able to commission care from a wider range of providers – including complementary and alternative therapies
Principal–agent relationship between GP and patient	GPs meant to work for best interests of patients – to act as their agent – referring and prescribing as necessary. Patient meant to be in charge
Consultants work in NHS Trusts	Consultants still salaried, but some managerial pressure to receive GP contracts. Block contracts mean that they have a number of spaces to fill, but no incentive to work beyond that point

However, the lack of a working information system made it extremely difficult to keep track of patient referrals, and 'block' contracting was commonplace, in which GPs did not so much refer individual patients to the best possible providers as fill spaces on pre-booked contracts that might have become contested only if the hospital provider was manifestly failing to provide adequate care (Le Grand et al, 1998b). Equally, GPs varied tremendously in how dynamically they took up their contracting role, with some attempting to drive up standards through it, but others apparently more content to try to save money by both referring and prescribing less (Coulter, 1995). Oddly, given its potential for driving up standards, patient satisfaction as a whole appeared to fall for patients of fundholding GPs, suggesting that they may have experienced the economies made through reduced referrals and prescribing as a reduction in service (Dusheiko et al, 2004b). Another concern was that it was extremely difficult for a relatively small GP surgery to influence the care practices of a very large hospital – even a large GP practice threatening to remove contracts from a hospital would only have a very limited effect because of the uneven bargaining power of the two, and the fact that most hospitals, because of a capacity shortage, had waiting lists for most treatments. The Conservative internal market reforms are explored in terms of their financial implications in Chapter Five, with their implications for managers and nurses discussed in Chapters Six and Seven, respectively.

The GP contract negotiated in 1990 moved more of the work for individual preventative services, such as vaccination, higher on the agenda for GPs. Increased numbers of practice nurses were employed to deal with this work, which many GPs found mundane, and practices changed to accommodate offices for nurses, where cervical smears, injections and health promotion clinics were run, all of which attracted extra fees into the practice.

This shows an emphasis on GP surgeries taking a greater role in public health, which was located predominantly in local government prior to 1974, but also crossed over into local university departments where Chairs of Public Health were sometimes found. Public health appeared to have lost status as a discipline with the rise of the hospital and the sense that public health itself was associated with the improvement of local sanitation during the 19th and early 20th century, which was now largely a job completed. However, it established a new identity as the 20th century drew on, becoming more associated with lifestyle issues. The government increased its interest in a range of comparative health indicators and took increasing responsibility for them from 1992 with the publication of *The Health of the Nation* (Secretary of State for Health, 1992), which Klein (Klein, 2006) sees as a hugely important turning point in health policy. From that time, a commitment was made to allocate resources to attempt to demonstrate gains in a range of areas from smoking cessation to the improved monitoring of cholesterol. This shift has led to massive television campaigns of increasing sophistication and impact, and has clear links with the notion of the 'risk society' (Beck, 1992), in which individuals find themselves taking greater responsibility for their lives, perceiving issues previously ignored as inevitable risks to be countered and either insured against or proactively prevented (Peterson and Lupton, 1996). The government appeared to be acknowledging that it had responsibilities for the provision of healthcare that went beyond the healthcare system itself; this was a more collectivist, societal definition of health.

On coming to power in 1997, Labour abolished fundholding on the grounds that it was bureaucratic (involving the monitoring of large numbers of contracts) and inequitable (as not all GPs were fundholders) (Secretary of State for Health, 1997). Labour also claimed to have abolished the internal market, although this is not really the case (Powell, 1998). Instead, it recast relationships within it on to a longer-term basis through contracts of increased duration, and combined GP practices into Primary Care Groups, which eventually became Primary Care Trusts, and which took over from the district health authority as the purchaser of care within the health service.

The 2000s

By 2000, Labour set about creating a new internal market, known, as the market for community health services was, as the 'mixed economy of care' (Secretary of State for Health, 2002). Addressing the problem of the lack of capacity to treat patients quickly, the private and not-for-profit sectors were invited to provide more care to the NHS (initiatives to shorten waiting lists since the 1980s had seen NHS patients referred to private hospitals and clinics) on the grounds that this would not only increase the capacity of the NHS, but would also drive up standards by creating competition.

Patients were no longer restricted by their GPs making decisions about where they should receive care, but instead were to be offered choices of where and when they could receive any required secondary referral (DH, 2001a, 2006c). This was not the principal–agent relationship of the 1990s. Instead, it cast patients as fully-fledged health consumers, able to make choices for themselves about the best location to be referred to. Patient information leaflets were produced by Primary Care Trusts to this end, but a number of problems remain. First, that patient information leaflets contain remarkably little in terms of relevant information for patients and have a tendency instead to focus on non-clinical measures, such as car parking and the availability of public transport (Easington Primary Care Trust, 2006). These are clearly important issues, but patients often lack awareness about where they might find clinical data. The Healthcare Commission's rankings of healthcare organisations gives only a crude rating for the whole organisation, which may not be at all relevant to the service the individual patient will receive. Equally, patients often appear to be given a telephone number to ring in order to make their choices without any paper-based information about the choices on offer, and are then expected to make the decision on the telephone about where and when to be treated. Other patients are making care choice decisions during GP appointments; while GPs are having to negotiate with a complex computer system, patients are having to make decisions quickly, often in the timeframe of a normal consultation (which is usually a little less than 10 minutes). In all, it is hard to see how any of these mechanisms creates the empowered, sophisticated health consumer the government appears to envisage.

General practitioners have found policy going full circle, not only in terms of the re-establishment of a marketplace for healthcare, but also in terms of their role within it. Their practices are becoming practice-based commissioning ones (DH, 2004) in the name of making them more responsive to patient needs, one of the same justifications that led to the creation of GP fundholders in the 1990s (Greener and Mannion, 2006). However, practice-based commissioning practices still seem to face many of the problems that fundholders did earlier in the decade with little power individually to influence hospital behaviour when commissioning care. There are also problems over how individual practice contracting is meant to interact with primary care commissioning more generally, with GPs having to absorb additional time costs as a result of the new contracting arrangements. At the same time as all of this, GPs are being encouraged to be more entrepreneurial in local health economies, offering to take services out of hospital care and to put together new care pathways across public, private and not-for-profit providers to better meet their patients' needs. However, the lack of time and infrastructural capacity available to GPs (Health Policy and Economic Research Unit, 2006) surely limits their capacity to achieve these goals.

There is continued pressure to move care away from hospitals, but they are sites with a great deal of resistance. The appeal of acute medicine remains strong, and new hospital builds financed under the Private Finance Initiative (PFI) means they are likely to remain in use for some time to come. Acute hospital productivity improvements, such as day surgery, have led to greater flexibility, and the use of treatment centres means that NHS capacity as a whole should increase, even if treatment centres do not prove to offer greater value for money.

Hospitals have been encouraged to reform their governance arrangements under Labour to form themselves into Foundation Trusts. Foundations Trusts are promised greater independence from the Department of Health, having their own inspectory body called Monitor, as well as having greater freedoms in the way they can conduct their affairs. They are also a remarkable experiment in trying to achieve greater local democracy in care by advertising to local people to become members. This can be read as a rather cynical attempt to create greater legitimacy for public organisations that appear rather less transparent than their predecessors (Klein, 2003) or as a potential participatory revolution (Birchall, 2003). Health Trusts have been allowed to become Foundation Trusts where they meet criteria laid down by the government with regard to achieving standards of performance, creating what became known as 'earned autonomy' (Mannion et al, 2003). Government has portrayed this as a sensible process by which minimum standards for healthcare delivery are guaranteed (Barber, 2007), whereas for some academics it is instead a process by which health organisations become free to do whatever the government wants (Hoque et al, 2004). The massive resource inheritance hospitals have, however, means that they usually remain the dominant care actors in any health economy. Foundation Trusts are explored in greater depth in Chapter Nine.

In public health there is an odd situation where the state promises increased resources and investment (Secretary of State for Health, 2006), with health providers offering a wider range of services to support the public's lifestyles from the possibility of Reiki healing and gym membership through to counselling and acupuncture to deal with stress and hypertension (Toynbee, 2008), but at the same time requires individuals to take greater responsibility for dealing with these conditions (Peterson and Lupton, 1996). Public health shares with primary care and social care the ambition of moving more treatments out of hospitals and into communities, where most public health interventions necessary take place. At the same time, it has a sense of being preventative, either trying to stop patients from getting ill (and so presenting the illusion of saving the NHS money, because most costs to the NHS occur in the first and last year of life, both of which are unavoidable) or to attempt to prevent pre-existing conditions from becoming any worse. What is less clear is which health organisation is meant to be driving the move to an increased public health focus; is it the role of GPs, Primary Care Trusts or even public health doctors employed in hospitals?

Local authorities were granted the power to 'scrutinise' local health services in 2000, giving them the potential to better represent local people in demanding improvements from the NHS. However, they have often simply been so immersed in their own problems that they have not managed to develop this role seriously (Edwards and Fall, 2005, p 188). Community care became 'social care' in the late 1990s, possibly to try to signal a broader agenda that encompasses social inclusion as well as care services (Taylor, 2006). The main area of reform has been to revisit the mixed economy of care that emerged in the 1980s and 1990s in two particular respects. First, eligibility criteria have been steadily raised so that the number of people able to receive funding from the state has declined (Glendinning et al, 2005). Second, there has been a steady trend towards moving budgets away from care managers and finding mechanisms, such as direct payments and individual budgets, for giving the money direct to social care clients (Glendinning et al, 2000). This can be an empowering experience, as care may be purchased from friends and family who previously gave their services for free, as well as from care agencies (see, for example, Le Grand, 2007). However, take-up of direct payments has been extremely low in most areas of the country, suggesting either that care managers are trying to protect their positions, or that the policy is not as popular with users as its advocates suggest. It is certainly too soon to generalise about the potential for direct payments policies in social care to be tried in healthcare.

Equally, the barriers between health and social care services still prevent users from receiving a seamless service, especially with respect to contentious areas such as hospital discharges. When patients with long-term social care needs leave hospital they need care in their community setting, but hospitals often regard these patients as being 'discharged', ending their responsibility to them (Glasby, 2007, p 79), whereas recent policy has tried to recast the relationship between health and social care as a 'transfer'. With respect to patients with long-term care needs, the boundary between health and social care also emerges, with the NHS tending to focus increasingly on acute care, and social care being expected to pick up the bill. The Royal Commission on Long-Term Care (1999) provoked a rather circumspect response from the government (Secretary of State for Health, 1999), concerned about the expense of paying potentially substantial amounts towards the cost of nursing and personal care. Definitional issues abounded between the difference between long-term care, nursing care and NHS continuing care (Glasby, 2007, p 80). There is a marked disparity between English and Scottish practice. In England, long-term care is means-tested and a part of the social care budget, while nursing care is free to care home residents; NHS continuing care is also free. In Scotland, older people receive free personal care at home (which is means-tested in England), as well as free care in care homes (where in England nursing care only is free). If this sounds confusing, it is because it is. It will be intriguing (and disturbing) to see the implications of it for those who live close to, and regularly cross, the border between England and Scotland.

An additional change that has occurred across the entire tripartite split has come through changes to both the class structure and the gender balance within the medical profession. In the case of the former, the ability of the Royal Colleges and the BMA to represent the medical profession has become increasingly stretched (Klein, 2006). In the 1960s and 1970s, this resulted in the appearance of a raft of new medical representation groups and an increased militancy for the profession as a whole, as the next chapter will demonstrate. In terms of gender, more and more women have been entering the medical profession since the foundation of the NHS, and we have now reached a point where more women are entering general practice than men. This has resulted in a number of changes to the profession. First, it has resulted in tensions in specialties such as gynaecology, where women doctors often feel 'caught between their loyalty to the profession, and partial alliances with feminists, midwives, natural childbirth advocates and women's health activists' (Pringle, 1998, p 66). Additional problems are the result of old-fashioned practices in training and working that result in the pressure to change jobs regularly and move around the country (Allen, 1988). There is a need for medical training to be shortened to accommodate the needs of both men and women, for consultant appointments to be made at an earlier age and for allowing the possibility of part-time work and more flexible hours, otherwise women will continue predominantly to occupy the lower grades of medicine.

Whether consultant medical practice is changing as a result of increasing numbers of women entering the profession is difficult to assess. Studies from overseas indicate that women doctors are often more careful and considerate in examining patients' needs, and that they are more likely to work closely with nurses (Wicks, 1993). It seems that there is a gradual improvement in gender equality in consultant medicine as a result, but things are still moving very slowly.

In general practice, more significant change has occurred, and evermore women are entering the profession (Calnan and Gabe, 1991). There is a greater availability of part-time work, and an environment where women doctors can work closely with other female-dominated professions in community settings, so that women have the potential to avoid male-dominated hospital specialties. Many new entrants regard general practice as a career rather than a vocation, and consider that a balance between work and family life must be achieved (Allen, 1997). However, there is the problem that general practice, as noted above, still occupies a subordinate position in medicine as a whole, and so it may be the case that women, even if their conditions are improved in general practice, will still be occupying a junior role in the medical hierarchy.

Table 3.6 summarises Labour's approach to the tripartite health organisations.

Table 3.6: The tripartite split under Labour

Tripartite actor	Situation
Consultants	Still dominant, but under threat from more organised purchasing (with money following the patient) and from moves to locate more care in primary care settings. Increasingly monitored through clinical governance, and encouraged to adopt entrepreneurial role to offer services as widely as possible
GPs	Budgetholding under practice-based commissioning, but with limited leverage to get consultants to provide better care. Required to be entrepreneurial in setting up new services, but without time or facilities to do this. Increasingly subject to health consumerism where offering alternative and complementary therapies is acceptable, as well as being expected to adopt a health promotion role. Expected to be part of a primary care team
Social care	Still outside of the NHS and non-purchasable using NHS funds. Provides possible future directions for healthcare from individual budgets and direct payments. Confusion over boundaries between health and social care, often mired in definitional problems

Conclusion

The tripartite split in healthcare was the result of negotiations and concessions in the period leading up to the creation of the NHS, but has continued to exist to a remarkable extent today. Hospitals remain the dominant providers of care, where high-technology medicine is practised by specialists, who also often educate other doctors. The attempt to move more treatment to primary care settings is having an effect, but it remains very much at the margins, and the PFI hospital-building programme calls substantially into question the commitment of policy makers to reconfigure health services within the community. If community services are meant to be the way of the future, why are large hospitals with 35-year maintenance contracts being built? This does appear a little contradictory.

General practice has undergone a number of transformations. General practitioners have gone from being lone practitioners and family doctors to primary care team leaders, with Tudor-Hart's model of epidemiologically oriented care appearing to currently be holding sway as the dominant discourse of practice. General practitioners, however, remain firmly at the head of primary care teams, with their clinical expertise providing the legitimacy for the continued importance of their role. Somewhat strangely, there appears to be considerable confusion over the future employment status of GPs. At exactly the time that GPs began to be salaried employees in the 2000s as a result of the GP contract, there was also a push towards recreating an independent practitioner role by allowing GPs to become self-employed, effectively private providers of care. Equally, the rather circular story of whether GPs should be budgetholding care purchasers, and the path from GP fundholding to members of Primary Care Groups, to Primary Care Trusts, and back to practice-based commissioning again, makes it difficult to see whether GPs will embrace their new purchasing roles or simply wait for them to be taken away from them again. This continual change in policy gives politicians little credibility with health professionals, while at the same time making it extraordinarily difficult to plan local services. General practitioners are meant to be not only care providers in the NHS, but also service entrepreneurs, looking for ways of offering new services into the mixed economy of care. However, they appear to lack the infrastructure (Health Policy and Economic Research Unit, 2006) and the time to perform such a role. They are positioned increasingly as being contingently related to their consultant colleagues, but the lessons from the internal market of the 1990s suggest that they will struggle to achieve equal influence in that role because of the relatively small size of their budgets (Greener and Mannion, 2006). Only by acting together or by influencing the purchasing decisions of Primary Care Trusts can GPs hope to influence purchasing decisions.

Local authority health services have also had a difficult time. From being stripped of their hospital assets in the creation of the NHS, MOHs had just about put in place a coherent range of services by the time they were largely removed from local authority control in 1974, with the discourse of community care dominating instead. There was then a dramatic rise in social security payments to fund the largely accidental growth of the mixed economy of residential care in the 1980s, followed by an attempt to get local authorities to cut back on payments in the 1990s through the appointment of care managers and the introduction of more rigorous eligibility criteria. The movement towards individual budgets means that the local authority role can now be potentially undermined (much as it has been for local education authorities), with payments going direct to users to contract for their own care. However, it is still too early to assess the results of direct payments policies because of their low take-up rates. Local authority health services remain remarkably at the margins of care despite the increased emphasis promised for public health (Secretary of State for Health, 2006), largely because of the orientation of the NHS towards GPs leading developments in local communities through the discourse of a 'primary care-driven NHS'.

In all, the tripartite relationship between health services has remained remarkably intact over the history of the NHS. There are pressures for change from the mixed economy of care, and from the current government's obsession with health reform of other kinds. However, the divisions in British medicine have so far proven to be extremely difficult to overcome.

FOUR

The double-bed

Introduction

This chapter explores the relationship between the state and the medical profession characterised by Rudolf Klein (1990) as the 'double-bed'. It is one of the distinctive organisational features of the NHS identified in Chapter Two.

The 'double-bed' relationship between the state and the medical profession is one of mutual dependence (Klein, 1990). The creation of the NHS gave the state an effective monopoly on the employment of the medical profession because of the relatively small size of the private healthcare sector. As such, the medical profession became effectively dependent (as a group) on the state for its employment. On the other hand, the state was also dependent on the medical profession because, in order for a health service to work, it clearly needed doctors. Doctors are highly qualified professionals with a long training and considerable expert knowledge, and so they are scarce within the economy. The state hardly has the option of simply employing new doctors if it does not like those it has inherited. In addition to this, doctors are archetypal professionals, having high status in society because of their high pay, their strong social connections with the great and the good, and their unique ability to literally be able to save lives. If medics and lawyers are the elite professionals, then the medics are perhaps the most prestigious of all.

The state was dependent on the medical profession not just to run the NHS, but also to ration care within it. Because healthcare systems cannot provide every possible treatment for every single person, especially in a cash-limited health system such as the NHS, it is doctors who are implicitly given the role of working out who gets access to its care and resources. General practitioners have had a gatekeeping role in deciding who gets referrals to hospitals and who does not, as well as being responsible for limiting prescriptions. Hospital consultants, on the other hand, have often had to work with out-of-date equipment in crumbling buildings, with access to their services limited by long waiting lists. Rationing for much of the NHS's history has not been explicit, but instead has operated as a function of the system by limiting access to care through the gatekeeper system, then through waiting lists if a referral was made. In addition to this, rationing effectively occurred through the state limiting opportunities for capital investment in new health equipment, so limiting access to new health technologies. Throughout the history of the NHS, rationing has been widespread although implicit.

Klein suggests that the reason why the double-bed relationship has been so enduring is because of its very real symmetry. The state, because of the medical profession's compliance in running and rationing care, receives a 'best buy' healthcare system, remarkably inexpensive in international terms. The price of this has been almost continual arguments over pay since the creation of the NHS in 1948, a healthcare system where cost was to be kept down. However, what the doctors have not done is to challenge the legitimacy or principles of the NHS – they have argued about their pay, but not over whether the NHS should exist in the first place. Indeed, doctors have increasingly tried to position themselves as the guardians of the patient within the healthcare system (Crinson, 1998), challenging reforms that they believe to be threatening care (Greener, 2006). This is a little ironic considering the extent of doctor opposition to the NHS at its creation, but understandable as doctors' representatives were faced with getting their members the best possible deal on entry into the new health service.

Doctors, in return for running the NHS and for rationing care, have received an assurance of employment within it. As the state is effectively the monopoly employer of medics, it has considerable potential scope for interfering in medical politics and training. However, for much of the history of the NHS it has refrained from interfering in these areas, perhaps conscious of what the medical profession is providing in terms of its part of the 'concordat' (Klein, 2006). Table 4.1 summarises the double-bed relationship.

Table 4.1: The double-bed relationship

Party	Dependence	Payoff
Medical profession	Dependent on the state for employment as it became the monopoly employer with the founding of the NHS	Run health services on behalf of the state in return for working in the NHS
The state	Dependent on medics to deliver organisational care and to ration it	Decide overall budget for the NHS

As such, there was an implicit 'deal' at the founding of the NHS: the state would give the doctors considerable autonomy in running health services (Cox, 1991), but in return the state would keep control over the total sum allocated for healthcare (Moran, 1999; Klein, 2006). As well as this, a core policy community was established between the Ministry of Health, the Royal Colleges and the BMA, which was responsible for health policy (Smith, 1993), giving the medical profession a close involvement in national policy as well as local dominance over the running of health services (Gillespie, 1997).

The relationship between the state and the medical profession

The relationship between the state and the medical profession has been an enduring topic of academic investigation throughout the history of the health service. From the theoretical perspective utilised within this book (see Chapter One), the relationship between the state and the medical profession can be characterised as one that is necessary (Archer, 1995), being based on mutual dependence, with the state needing the medical profession to participate in health services and run them, and the doctors needing the state as, with the creation of the NHS, it effectively became the de facto monopoly employer (because of the relatively small private sector) of medical staff (Brazier et al, 1990). However, it is harder to work out whether the relationship between the doctors and the state is a compatible or incompatible one. In some ways it appears to be a compatible one, as neither party has challenged the legitimacy of the NHS for much of the service's history – the state has continually reasserted the principles of the NHS during each reform period, and the medical profession has presented itself as the guardian of both the health service and the patient in opposing reforms it deemed to be against their interests (Greener, 2006). However, in any given time period, there are issues where the two interests also appear to be incompatible. Pay is one – the state generally wishes to keep the cost of the NHS to a minimum, and with pay representing a significant portion of its overall cost, it is clearly in the state's interest to keep pay down (Le Grand, 2007). However, it is in the medical profession's interest to maximise pay. So, from the long-term, high-level perspective, remarkable continuities and compatibilities appear, but looking at the short term, and in more detail, there are clearly areas of dispute (Ham, 1980).

Chapter Two showed how, in the creation of the NHS, GPs wanted to preserve their autonomy while continuing to work in the NHS.

However, it was in the state's interest to attempt to minimise this autonomy and to control the referral and prescribing habits of GPs. In terms of the consultants, issues of control were also significant – if the state was to put in place a 'national' health service, there had to be some consistency in treatment from one area to another (Powell, 1997). However, this might be seen to impinge on the doctrines of clinical autonomy and clinical freedom – the right of a doctor to treat, in confidence, the patient before them according to the best of their knowledge. The more guidance for treatment is centralised, the greater the control the state is able to exert over treatment, but the greater the potential for doctors to regard the state as interfering where it does not belong.

In sum, the relationship between the state and the medical profession is a necessary one and it is in the interests of both to preserve the dependent relationship between them at the heart of the NHS, at the system level, and it is at this level where the relationship is compatible. However, in relation to individual issues, those in the short-term it can be regarded as incompatible. Out of short-term conflicts over issues such as pay and conditions a long-term order appears that has remained remarkably unchallenged for much of the NHS's history. From the state's perspective, the bargain could be undermined if it were able to find another group to run health services, or perhaps if it could increase the supply of doctors to the NHS, which would create the opportunity to reduce medical power by replacing low-performing or non-compliant medics. Equally, if the state were able to find an alternative means of rationing care, it would be less dependent on doctors as their gatekeeper role would become less significant. From the doctor's perspective, the basis of the bargain with the state would be undermined if there were alternative employers available, which would reduce their dependence on the NHS for employment, or if the state found ways of intervening in clinical practice, reducing the professional autonomy enjoyed by doctors.

The situational logic between the state and the medical profession was therefore somewhere between protection and compromise. Both parties had a great deal to lose if the NHS was undermined, so there was a mutual need to preserve the relationship, and to be seen as protecting the health service. Doctors claim to speak for patients, and even the most radical politicians are keen to stress that the NHS is safe 'in their hands'. However, there was also a need for compromise, as both sides recognised that there were day-to-day problems and disagreements that they had to work through in order to make the service function. Table 4.2 summarises this argument.

Table 4.2: The logics of the double-bed relationship

Party	Relationship
Medical profession	Necessary relationship with the state as long as it is dependent on it for employment – if alternative employers appear, danger of undermining. Compatible relationship as long as left alone to run health services and given the resources it demands
The state	Necessary relationship with the doctors as long as medical expertise remains in short supply, and as long as it depends on the doctors to ration care on its behalf. Compatible relationship as long as medical profession works within the resources it makes available and does not criticise policy

At the creation of the NHS, there was a remarkable fit between the ideas of both parties as to how to organise healthcare. On the state side, there was a fit between the economic ideas of Keynesianism, which justified state intervention, and the socialism of the Labour Party elected in 1945, with its commitment to bring key national industries under state control. This created an environment in which Bevan's plans to nationalise the hospitals was seen as justifiable, as well as being compatible with the greater role for the state that Keynesianism suggested. In terms of the medical profession, Bevan's favouring of the consultants' representatives was certainly convenient in terms of them being able quickly to reach binding agreements, whereas the GPs, represented by the BMA, could not. But the emerging ideology of the hospital, representing the epitome of high-technology medicine and the site of exciting medical breakthroughs, was a compatible fit with the tendency of socialists to place their trust in experts to engineer solutions to society's problems. The hospital doctors represented an ideal type of the group the Labour government was most likely to trust.

As such, ideationally, the NHS was a remarkable coincidence of interest. The Labour government was able to have a clear basis for its interventionist tendencies through Keynesianism, and had a professional group it could utilise to run its healthcare organisation. If the state were to have its reasons for intervening in the economy undermined, however, it would significantly threaten one of the key ideas underpinning the NHS, as that would be a threat to the Keynesian orthodoxy that also provided part of the justification for the state's involvement in healthcare. Equally, if there were a loss of faith in medical expertise, that could lead to new ideas threatening the legitimacy of the state's appointed experts in that field. Finally, socialism might be a neat fit with both Keynesianism and modern medicine, but governments of a different persuasion might be rather less committed to running healthcare system based on redistributive principles unless there were other good reasons for supporting it (Klein, 1986).

National accountability with local paternalism

The relationship between the state and the medical profession can also be characterised as being one of national accountability with local paternalism (Greener and Powell, 2008). This reflects the settlement between the doctors and the state at the time of the NHS's founding. The Minister of Health was to be held accountable for the public delivery of healthcare in the UK, but the doctors were to be responsible for delivering health services at the local level. Local doctors were remarkably insulated from central policy makers because of their medical expertise and the autonomy this gave them, but also because of the lack of ability of politicians or central policy makers to be able to measure or examine what the doctors were actually doing. Equally, policies could be made centrally, but had to be implemented locally by doctors in order for the delivery of care to change, and given the lack of formal management control there was in place over doctors, the reality of the situation was that doctors were probably more accountable to their profession than to the organisation that employed them or the NHS as a whole.

The NHS was therefore nationally accountable, with the Minister of Health being expected to deliver health policy and to answer for it in Parliament, but locally paternalistic, because health services were run by local doctors who made the decisions that most affected patients, and who were insulated to large degree from the demands of central policy makers. It is not accurate to characterise the NHS, at the time of its founding, as a 'command and control' healthcare system, as there were no levers with which to exert central command. As Klein (2006, p 38) describes the role of the government, 'it could educate, it could inspire and it could stimulate', but it could not control. This was policy making through exhortation. Equally, the government knew very little about what was going on in the NHS in its early years. Smee (2005) repeatedly stresses the lack of analysis and expertise in the Department of Health, even in the two decades up to 2002, despite the emphasis on managerial reform at that time. As such, the lack of mechanisms for influencing what was going on, coupled with a real lack of information about it, conspired to give central government relatively little influence over the NHS. This argument is summarised in Table 4.3.

Table 4.3: National accountability and local paternalism

National accountability	The state is politically responsible for the NHS – it is electorally vulnerable to claims of failing to provide adequate resources to the NHS or of failing to run it appropriately
Local paternalism	The medical profession effectively runs health services at the local level, insulated from any central demands

The development of the double-bed relationship

Klein (1990) suggested that for the period from the 1950s to the 1970s, state–medico relations in the UK could be characterised as being 'corporatist'. This meant that the leaders of each group effectively met and worked with one another in order to decide on policy, which was carried out (to quote the phrase used at the time) in 'smoke-filled rooms' (Moran, 1995). Corporatism meant that policy was decided by elite groups who were, because of their expert knowledge or privileged position, given special access to the policy process (Alford, 1975). Policy, according to Klein, was therefore a process of 'engineering consensus', of trying to get sufficient agreement between the state and doctors, to make sure that the health service could work sufficiently well. This effectively meant that both parties were given an effective veto over policy.

However, this does not mean that the double-bed relationship developed smoothly and easily over this time period. As Klein makes clear, there was a built-in tendency within the NHS, because of its relatively low cost, for there to be continual conflict over medical pay. In Chapter Three, this was explored in greater depth in terms of the conflict within the medical profession, especially between GPs and consultants, over the relative status of different medical groups. This chapter examines state–medico relations without assuming all doctors to be the same, and treating the dynamic from the outside, from the perspective of the state.

Developments in the 1950s

The 1950s were significant in terms of the story of the double-bed relationship for helping to set the scene for health policy until the 1970s. A number of themes that were to be significant in the NHS's history appeared. Within a relatively short period of time, the NHS was exceeding its expected costs, earning the service an unjustified reputation for being profligate, as well as giving legitimacy in public expenditure rounds for demands for better control of health expenditure, and eventually the introduction of the prescription charge. The prescription charge was legislated for by Labour (and was one of the factors that led to the resignation of Aneurin Bevan as Minister of Health), but was not introduced until the succeeding Conservative government. A fundamental problem at the heart of health service organisation – the gap between central control and local autonomy – was noted by a senior civil servant, Sir Cyril Jones, who was asked by Bevan how expenditure might be better brought under control. Jones challenged the right of doctors to prescribe expensive appliances without the approval of managers and argued that doctors should be excluded from membership of the management authorities of the NHS (Klein, 2006, pp 35-6). This was foresight of a remarkable kind – two years after the creation of the NHS, many of the problems of subsequent decades had been predicted. However, Jones' diagnosis was too much for Bevan, who did not wish to antagonise the doctors.

The first pay disputes in the NHS were with the GPs. The basis for rewarding GPs was a complicated formula based on practice size and smaller, rural practices appeared to be suffering real financial hardship in the early 1950s. The NHS also reduced the scope for GPs to engage in private practice, leading to a reduction in income for many of those working in urban areas. The Danckwerts award for GPs in 1952 began to address these problems, and GPs at the time appear to have believed that they had managed to secure a rather good deal.

On the state side, the election of a Conservative government in 1951 meant that the socialists of the Attlee government were no longer in power. Instead, there was a 'one-nation' approach to Conservatism, whose leaders had famously voted against the creation of the NHS in debates leading up to its legislation, and who might have been expected to take a more sceptical approach to the overspending health service. As well as this, there appeared to be the beginnings of a groundswell of opinion that the public provision of healthcare might not be the best answer. A *British Medical Journal* editorial of 1950 suggested that the NHS was financially bankrupt 'because of the Utopian finances of the Welfare State' (*British Medical Journal*, 1950, p 1262). The Conservatives began a review of expenditure in the NHS, which led to the Guillebaud Report of 1956 (named after the Cambridge economist who chaired the inquiry) and which, to some government consternation, cleared the NHS of the charge that it was inefficient (Ministry of Health, 1956).

Instead, the report showed how, compared to other healthcare systems, the NHS was remarkably inexpensive, and it suggested an increase in capital expenditure for the service.

The clean bill of health given to the NHS did not prevent a serious attempt to move health financing away from the general taxation method towards a greater use of the national insurance contribution and a significant increase in charges (Webster, 1994). There is some irony in all of this change, given that a contemporary understanding of financing suggests that the general taxation method is probably the cheapest way to pay for the service. However, general taxation appears to have run against Conservative principles of the better-off paying contributory charges for their own care, and of a general preference for an insurance-based system because of the increased independence it was meant to bring. By 1960, however, the period of Conservative radicalism in relation to finance appears to have died off amid concerns that the government was attempting to undermine the basis of the service (see, for example, Titmuss, 1961). In 1958, Minister of Health Ian Macleod wrote that 'The National Health Service ... is out of party politics'(Goldman and Macleod, 1958).

Pay disputes rumbled on. In 1957, a Royal Commission into doctors' pay was announced, which reported in 1960 (Royal Commission on Doctors' and Dentists' Remuneration, 1960). The report concluded that doctors' pay had tended to lag behind comparable professional groups, and recommended all-round increases, but also a permanent review body that would inquire into medical pay on a more regular and systematic basis. As such, pay was, on the one hand, moving outside of state control, but, on the other, giving the medical profession a means of potentially securing significant increases through a review process that stood outside of government. However, because the pay body was independent of it, the government was not compelled to honour any recommendations that it made.

By the end of the 1950s, the doctors had not been particularly successful in securing increased pay, but there was a review body that might promise better rewards in the future. Furthermore, doctors, particularly in hospitals, had managed to become significantly involved in decision-making bodies, having about a third of members in regional hospital boards, and around a quarter of members on hospital management committees (Ministry of Health, 1956). Medical representation was therefore institutionalised within the NHS, effectively medicalising management in the process. Medics therefore had not only a corporatist role in health policy at the national level, but also an institutionalised voice in the implementation of that policy.

The 1960s and the first organisational reform of the NHS

In the 1960s, the budget allocated to healthcare increased in real terms by around 25%. However, the demands placed on the budget grew dramatically as well. Medical knowledge was growing and new treatments coming available that significantly increased the costs of the sites of high-technology medicine – the hospitals. But more importantly, the new techniques of medicine created, in turn, new demands for services. Drug therapy for people with mental illness increased in use, and the potential of renal dialysis began to be explored, offering patients with these conditions the opportunity for very different lives, free from institutions in the former case, and with new possibilities of a more normal life in the latter. However, with these new treatments came increased costs. At the same time as this, an ageing population, with around 10% more people over the age of 60 by the end of the decade, put increased demands on health services.

The increased militancy by the medical profession with regard to pay in the 1960s made sense in that, unable to exit from the NHS, the profession exercised the only other possible means of engagement – voice (Hirschman, 1970) – and with an increasingly assertive tone. Industrial action became a significant part of healthcare as the 1960s wore on. As new interest groups emerged (such as the new College of General Practitioners), a kind of competition emerged in which medical representative bodies, in order to attract new members, were keen to demonstrate their bargaining power and negotiating muscle. This clearly had implications for the relationship between the doctors and the state.

However, the 1960s are probably best remembered for an act of remarkable collaboration between the state and the medical profession – the formulation of the Hospital Plan (Minister of Health, 1962). Following the recommendations of the Guillebaud Report with respect to capital expenditure (Ministry of Health, 1956), a group of BMA consultants called for a 10-year capital building plan in 1959, leading to a series of research seminars and workshops where details began to be fleshed out. This led to the Hospital Plan. The Plan was a deliberate attempt to face the legacy of the inheritance of the poor and inequitable capital infrastructure of 1948. It envisaged the building of 90 new hospitals and the substantial remodelling of another 134. The details of the Plan were worked out entirely within the medical consensus, and little apparent concern for consulting patients or patient groups was shown. The Plan appeared to fly somewhat in the face of the

Conservative government that created it – the same government that in the 1950s was increasing patient charges and moving the NHS closer to a contributionary basis for financing. However, the Conservatives justified the capital building programme on the basis of the improved efficiency it would bring to the NHS, alongside a general belief that improved administrative technology made it possible for the state to commit on this scale.

If clinical autonomy was the means by which doctors guaranteed their considerable local discretion, central government was beginning to find ways of at least gathering information about what exactly was going on in the NHS. The government also hoped that, by integrating doctors into planning processes, they might begin to understand the impact that clinical decisions had on the total resources available, and so might become more aware of those constraints in their practice.

Planning health services required information be gathered, and a new information system called Hospital Activity Analysis was born. Built on this was the 'Cogwheel' system, which attempted to demonstrate the link between resources and decision making in order to try to make it clear to individual consultants that, if their colleagues were wasteful in their usage of resources, this had an effect on them. However, little impact seemed to have been made and the new management information systems worked poorly, producing little material that might allow government to challenge clinical practice (McLachlan, 1971).

More disputes over pay

On Labour's election victory in October 1964, Kenneth Robinson became Health Minister. For the first two years of the Labour government, GP numbers actually fell, and unfavourable reports from the pay review body, which was not prepared to increase pay in order to boost recruitment, led to further antagonism between the GPs and the state. The chair of the General Medical Services Committee, James Cameron, wondered aloud whether it was in the profession's best interests to remain within the NHS, and demanded an entirely new contract for GPs, asking for members to send undated resignations to BMA House. Within a fortnight, 14,000 were received (Klein, 2006). Cameron drew up the Charter for the Family Doctor Service, which was subsequently adopted by the BMA (Webster, 1998b). Pressure was growing on the government to do something. even though in retrospect we might wonder about the credibility of the threat of mass resignations from the NHS because of GPs' dependence on the health service for employment (Rivett, 1998, p 171).

Kenneth Robinson found it difficult to negotiate with undated resignations pouring in, but an intensive period of discussions ensued. Robinson wanted to get something from the GPs in return for improved pay and conditions, and initially would not budge from insisting that GPs become salaried employees – a longstanding Labour principle that went back to Bevan's negotiations in the 1940s, but which was dropped because of medical opposition at that time. As in the 1940s, GPs did not give their leaders negotiating power, so all proposals had to be taken to the membership for approval. This created a lengthy negotiating process that did not help the tensions between the profession and the state. Gradually, however, a number of proposals were agreed, and taken back to the pay review body to be priced. Labour then called a General Election (to try to improve on the small majority it had achieved in 1964), which it subsequently won, but which delayed things further. Robinson came back as Health Minister, and found to his dismay that the pay review body suggested a rise in pay for GPs of about a third. At the annual Labour conference, the Socialist Medical Association demanded that private practice should be removed completely from the NHS, and conference carried the decision (Stark Murray, 1971), further provoking an air of confrontation between the government and the doctors. But by now the government was increasingly being overtaken by economic crisis, and it was less than clear what it would agree to do with the review body's recommendations. A tense period then ensued, after which the government agreed (possibly under threat of Robinson's resignation) to fund the pay rise over two years (Glennerster, 1995). Robinson's compromise also managed to introduce incentives for the increased use of health centres, which again showed that, when the doctors and the state found a way of working together, substantial improvements in medical practice and investment could be achieved.

Reorganising the NHS

The difficulties experienced in governing the NHS forced a change in the attitudes of policy makers by the end of the 1960s. In 1968, Robinson put forward proposals for restructuring the NHS in a Green Paper that would have resulted in more managerial control over health services (Ministry of Health, 1968). What is remarkable about the discussions both before and after the publication of Robinson's proposals is the power of the veto the medical profession held. There seemed to be a consensus between the Labour and Conservative Parties that an organisationally unified NHS would be the ideal solution.

This was not surprising; the split between the two had existed since the founding of the NHS and had led to a disjointed administrative boundary between them (see Chapter Three). However, more radically, they also agreed that the best way of achieving this was to transfer health services to local government (Klein, 2006, p 67). But this option ruled itself out of court immediately because of the anticipated reaction it would meet from the medical profession. Even the local government lobby, which stood to gain hugely from the power and influence it would achieve from taking control of the NHS, did not campaign for it in a concerted manner because of the opposition such a proposal would encounter from the doctors.

The 1968 proposals suggested the founding of 40-50 area health authorities, and the complete removal of the regional tier of services. Significantly, the representation of 'special interests' was specifically excluded, with the Managing Director of the Board to be the Chief Administrator. Glennerster (1995) regards the 1968 reforms as a preemptive strike against the likely recommendations of the Seebohm Committee that was investigating the boundaries between health and social care. Klein (2001), however, sees the Green Paper in slightly different terms: as the beginning of the introduction of managerial ideas into the health service. This, understandably, upset the body with most control in the existing system – the doctors. The local government lobby was not pleased either, as it too believed that the implementation of the Green Paper would mean it would experience a loss of power.

In 1970, the new Secretary of State for Health and Social Services, Richard Crossman, put forward a further set of proposals for the future of the service (DHSS, 1970). The efficiency and managerialism proposed by the first Green Paper disappeared, and a new tone of cooperation was established. Labour lost the 1970 General Election, and its plans for reform never came to fruition. The impetus for reform was now strong, however, and the new Minister of Health, Keith Joseph, published a consultative document in 1971 (DHSS, 1971). The tone was similar to that of 1968, with Joseph stating that effective management was the tool necessary to bridge the gap between the underfunded chronic services and the prestigious acute services. There was an absolute belief in the ability of state managers to solve the problems of the health service through rational planning techniques. A chapter title in Klein's (2006) book describes this process well: 'The politics of technocratic change'. However, there was mounting criticism from the right of the Conservative Party that the NHS was now 'incurable' and that Beveridge's approach to the creation of welfare services was 'cloud–cuckoo land' (Powell, 1972). The political Right was becoming increasingly disenchanted with the NHS, and began the process of a radical critique of public services more generally that was to come to fruition a decade later under the Prime Ministership of Margaret Thatcher.

The 1971 Conservative plan encountered opposition because managers appointed by the Secretary of State were to be put in control, not doctors or local authority members, and area board members would be appointed by regions, and so had no guarantee of representation from the 'right type of people' from either interest group. This removed the regional tier from doctors' control, and so took away one of the concessions they had been granted in the original NHS by Bevan. The doctors reacted strongly, and the Conservatives, as Labour did before them, bowed to their objections (Secretary of State for Health and Social Services, 1972). These events give a feeling of déjà vu; doctors were also given representation at the regional level, setting in stone the role of the expert in the new structure. The new design of the NHS was 'the product of committees, it spawned yet more committees in an attempt to ensure that every interest in the NHS would be represented' (Klein, 1990, p 701).

The reforms, finally implemented in 1974, can be seen as protecting and perhaps even enhancing the position of dominant groups within the NHS. Doctors moved from covertly running the NHS to having a role formally institutionalised within it, and Keith Joseph managed to reform the NHS, even if his reform became the subject of one of his many later recantations (Halcrow, 1989). They were an attempt to keep all parties happy, but caused disaffection and frustration because of their complexity and their institutionalisation of the veto role for professionals throughout the service (Klein, 2006). Table 4.4 summarises the effect of the 1974 relationship on the double-bed, with an overall logic where both parties still sought to protect their roles within the NHS, but with an increased capacity for conflict resulting from cumulative mutual frustrations with regard to funding (on the side of the medical profession) and lack of organisational control (on the side of the state).

The 1970s

In the 1970s, there was a marked increase in militancy in the NHS. Medical representation splintered making it more difficult for the government to negotiate settlements to disputes, also increasing rivalry between representative groups in the process. At the same time, economic conditions declined further, with inflation apparently out

Table 4.4: The 1974 reorganisation and the double-bed

Party	Relationship
Medical profession	Institutionalised control as doctors gain rights to representation at all levels of the NHS. Consensus decision-making teams mean that medics have veto power over organisational decisions. Relationship with state still necessary and compatible as able to continue to operate largely independently within health organisations while depending on the state to finance the NHS
The state	Put in place greater capacity for planning, but also greater capacity for any professional group represented on decision-making teams to block change. Relationship with the medical profession still necessary and compatible as medical profession required to implement reforms, but concern over lack of central control of the NHS

of control (Oliver, 1996), and the government's Keynesian approach apparently unable to deal with the economic problems before it (Pierson, 1998). This resulted in taken-for-granted assumptions about the NHS beginning to be openly questioned. If economic growth could no longer be assumed, there was a far greater pressure to reduce health expenditure, and politicians would have to deal with the conflicts generated by the organisational form of the NHS inherited by the politicians of the day.

As economic problems began to hit home in the 1970s, the government attempted to try to find ways of reducing expenditure and getting control over inflation, putting in place a National Board for Prices and Incomes, which attempted to impose limits on pay rises. In the NHS, local productivity deals were allowed to try to make such pay deals self-financing. This went against the principles of national pay bargaining, which were also under stress because of the government's often crude attempt to impose pay increase limits, and undermined preciously guarded differentials between public sector workers.

As inflation rose, so, of course, did the cost of living. Substantial pay settlements were required, especially from 1974 onwards, to avoid workers becoming worse off in real terms. Lower-paid workers tended to fare better under Labour's attempts to regulate incomes, and the doctors' pay review body estimated that living standards of GPs and consultants had fallen by some 20% between 1975 and 1977 (Klein, 2001, p 86). For the first time in the NHS's history, doctors took industrial action. General practitioners had sent in undated resignations to the BMA in the 1960s, but now, allied with their consultant colleagues, they went one step further. In October 1975, junior hospital doctors in Leicester went on strike over pay, and the dispute quickly spread to the rest of the country. The strike action was actively promoted by medical unions – the increase in medical heterogeneity we noted in the 1960s was now beginning to tell as the BMA appeared to be actively competing with the Medical Practitioners' Union for medical membership, and, in the climate of the 1970s, the most radical organisation tended to attract new entrants into the medical profession. Junior doctors got an improved pay settlement, but to the annoyance of their senior colleagues, who saw an erosion of the pay differentials between themselves and this group, and the settlement was criticised in the *Lancet* as representing a movement from being workers in a profession to workers in an industry (Klein, 2001, p 87).

The fragmentation of medical representation of the 1960s continued, and led to a radicalisation of all the groups purporting to work on behalf of the doctors. The Royal Colleges and BMA no longer represented the medical profession (if they ever did) – they were elitist and out-of-date institutions that must have appeared like dinosaurs to new doctors from very different social backgrounds. These new doctors looked for new bodies to represent them, fragmenting the medical profession further, at once making industrial action more likely (as medical representative bodies attempted to reinvent themselves as being more radical), but also possibly less successful (because they could no longer speak with one voice for the whole medical profession).

In 1979, in the middle of what became known as the 'winter of discontent', the NHS appeared to be in turmoil. Nurses stopped short of strike action, but many worked to rule, refusing overtime or additional duties. Ambulance workers went on strike and the military attempted to offer cover in its own outdated vehicles. The government attempted to engage in low-profile, local negotiations to avoid any further industrial action, but this apparently only made things worse. Unions attempted to impose additional work-to-rules, and in some locations emergencies were only treated if hospital admissions were cancelled. Doctors then became angry at the intrusion of unions into what they perceived as their domain and entered into conflict with the unions, even resulting in the blacklisting of operating theatres in Northampton, where surgeons could only continue to work by bringing in their own supplies. Unions attempted to draw up guidelines to ensure that patients did not suffer as a result of industrial action, but almost invariably they did. Waiting lists rose and the government offered a pay rise of 9% at a time when pay rises were meant to be limited to 5%.

Perhaps most significant about this period was the demonstration that NHS workers could effectively bring the service to a standstill. This was remarkable on the side of those working within the service, but frightening to those who were attempting to run it. It appeared as if industrial relations in the NHS (and indeed across the whole of the public sector) had come to a head.

The pay-beds dispute

Dispute over pay was not the only industrial action involving doctors in the 1970s. In 1974, the newly elected Secretary of State, Barbara Castle, effectively engineered a conflict with the consultants over 'pay-beds', the beds located in NHS hospitals that consultants were allowed to use for private practice. Castle clearly felt that pay-beds represented the unacceptable side of the compromises Bevan had made in the 1940s, and now had to go – Labour had promised it in their manifesto, and Castle's hand was forced as members of the National Union of Public Employees (NUPE) went on strike at Charing Cross Hospital to attempt to force closure of the hospital's private wing. A wave of sympathy strikes broke out across the country, attracting media attention, and the ever-present requirement that 'something must be done'.

Castle attempted to head off the industrial action by approaching the Labour movement's traditional ally, the Trades Union Congress (TUC), but was told that the Congress was in favour of getting rid of private practice. The health service trade unions took advantage of the situation by pressing Labour on its manifesto pledge to get rid of private practice in hospital services, putting Castle in a position where she had to be seen to press ahead with Labour's commitment.

The timing of the pay-beds issue could not have been worse. Minister of Health David Owen was attempting to renegotiate a new contract with the consultants, a process that had already been going on for two years. The pay-beds issue meant that Labour attempted to bring a new item to the table – additional financial incentives in return for consultants agreeing to work solely within the NHS. For the consultants, this represented a potential loss of the private practice concession granted to them by Bevan, and they sought reassurances that Castle was attempting only to separate private practice from the NHS, not remove it completely. At the Labour Party annual conference, however, a vote was carried for the outright abolition of all private medicine. Despite Castle attempting to distance herself from this, the BMA and, in this case, the Hospital Consultants' and Specialists'

Association, appeared to be engaged in a race towards militancy, and threatened industrial action.

The government did not want a long dispute with the consultants, but found negotiations impossible to even enter into. Castle's less-than-radical consultative document on private practice (DHSS, 1975) was ignored, and eventually the Prime Minister had to offer arbitration through the appointment of Lord Goodman as mediator, and the promise of a Royal Commission on the NHS. Goodman's proposals were not that different from Castle's, suggesting that there should be a separation between private and public practice, but that doctors should have the right to work in both. In addition, Goodman suggested a limited reduction in private beds, with a complex process for additional reductions without specified time limits or specific numbers. So a deal was struck over pay-beds, but the consultant contract negotiations begun under the Conservative Heath government in 1972 were never completed, and were left to the Thatcher government, demonstrating the remarkable inertia over negotiating with the medical profession. This was not helped by Wilson promising a Royal Commission on the NHS as a part of a strategy of delay in negotiations, which made long-term planning even more difficult in an environment where it was already problematic because of the economic problems and militancy of the 1970s.

In sum, the 1970s represent an era in which those representing doctors sought to flex their industrial muscles, and the bargain between the state and medical profession appeared to be becoming eroded. If the state and the medical profession were still a part of the double-bed, their relationship was becoming noticeably frosty. The medics found themselves willing and able to criticise the state, and the state seemed to have spent most of the 1970s fighting the doctors over pay and conditions. The incompatibilities brought to the fore by inflation and medical pay seemed to be undermining the need for the state and the medics to get on with one another. Even though neither party could imagine a future without the other, both were engaged in a series of bitter disputes, unable to find an alternative to the unsatisfactory status quo.

The 1980s

The 1980s represent an era of both continuity and contrast with the 1970s. It was a decade of further medical protest, but in response to a government no longer prepared to engage in corporatist policy making rather than over the pay and conditions of members in the health service.

The Thatcher government of the 1980s had what it thought was a set of worked-out policy responses to the problems of the 1970s. In Thatcher's eyes, consensus and corporatist policy making was a failure, and a contributor towards the institutionalised mediocrity that was ruining Britain. The state had to be 'rolled back' to allow business the space to invest in the economy (as per the diagnosis of Bacon and Eltis, 1978), and Keynesianism held no legitimacy for a government that felt that public sector intervention was part of the problem, not part of the solution.

An immediate change that had little directly to do with government policy was the dramatic rise in the numbers of subscribers to private medicine in 1980 and 1981. The pay-beds disputes of the 1970s appeared to stimulate the demand for private medicine (Berridge, 1999), with a rise in numbers of private subscribers of 26% in 1980 and 13% in 1981 (Le Grand et al, 1991). Despite subsequent falls in the growth of the number of subscribers during the decade, private medicine continued to expand during the 1980s so that by 1990 the number of subscribers had risen from around 1.3 million (covering 2.75 million people) to 3.3 million (covering 7 million people) (Berridge, 1999).

The Thatcher government was sceptical of the need for nationalised industries, and withdrew financial support from private industry that had become dependent on the government. Rapidly rising unemployment did not deter the government, which deemed that tough love was necessary to solve the economic problems of the nation. Thatcher announced this time that there would be no 'U-turn' on policy. 'You turn if you want to. The lady's not for turning,' she announced at the Conservative Party conference in 1980. The medical profession was no longer a valued partner in the policy process, but rather more closely resembled, in the government's eyes, a vested interest such as a trade union that was blocking the efficient organisation of healthcare.

Restructuring and management review

The Conservatives' instinct was to decentralise the NHS, but this quickly ran into the problem that allowing greater local diversity potentially clashed with parliamentary accountability for the service (Peckham et al, 2005a). The government simplified the 1974 organisational structure, effectively abolishing a tier of management deemed unnecessary (the area health authorities). Next, it sought an external view on how best to manage the service and turned not to an independent review as it had in the 1950s. Instead, perhaps learning from the unfavourable response that independent review had given, Thatcher asked Roy Griffiths, the Chairman of Sainsbury's, to look at the service. His management review (DHSS, 1983) introduced a new element into the relationship between the medical profession and the state.

Griffiths suggested that the problem with the NHS was that no one was in charge. He famously suggested that were Florence Nightingale alive at that time, she would be wandering the corridors of the NHS trying to find out who was responsible for it. The NHS had to devolve responsibility to local managers and to be held accountable for the delivery of services to both local people and the national government. The government, in turn, had to let local managers do the managing, devising clear criteria for measuring their performance, and then being accountable to the centre for that performance. What the centre should not do was to attempt to micro-manage the NHS.

Griffiths' proposals were something of a problem for parliamentary accountability, suggesting a service that was to become significantly devolved. However, the government took up Griffiths' recommendation of putting a manager clearly in charge of hospital services, and general managers, later chief executives, were appointed to be accountable for their part of the NHS. The 'corporate rationalisers' (Alford, 1975) were entering the NHS and with them an explicit challenge to the medical hierarchy. More significantly perhaps, the language of management was entering the NHS, and becoming the reference point through which discussions of resources now had to be negotiated (Bloomfield and Best, 1992).

Limited-list prescribing

The government was particularly concerned with being able to reduce public expenditure, especially in a period when unemployment was rising dramatically. Of special concern in the NHS was the potentially open-ended expenditure commitment that was in place in primary care. General practitioners had no theoretical limits on their writing of prescriptions. Family Practitioner Committees had been made directly accountable to the Department of Health and Social Security as a part of the package of reforms in 1982 that had resulted in the abolition of area health authorities, and so the government now had a far clearer idea of the remarkable differences in prescribing practices that appeared to exist. In 1984, Secretary of State Norman Fowler and Minister for Health Kenneth Clarke decided to instigate a review of family practitioner services, displaying a readiness to challenge the medical profession, which in some ways was a rehearsal for disputes with the profession at the end of the decade.

The result of Fowler and Clarke's review was the 'limited list' of items that GPs were allowed to prescribe. It was announced in November 1984 and provoked a furious reaction from the pharmaceutical industry and the BMA. The government backed down a little, extending the list of allowable items and agreeing to confer with the medical profession about its consultation, but the argument over the limited list was significant in that it was about the content of the reforms rather than the government's right to impose change. The government had effectively imposed a change in NHS policy on the medical profession without consulting it (as Clarke did again at the end of the decade). The medical profession had shown itself to be remarkably fragmented in responding to the government's imposition; some Royal Colleges appeared to rather like the idea even though they had not been consulted and the BMA and pharmaceutical industry were rather 'unimaginative' (Klein, 2001, p 140) in their response to the government's almost overt challenge. Overall, it appeared to the government to demonstrate that it could challenge the medical profession without incurring political unpopularity or being faced down by a coordinated and concerted body of high-profile medics. It had shown that the state could assert itself in health policy without coming away wounded by the medical response.

Performance indicators and the Resource Management Initiative

A second example of the state's increased involvement in health policy came with the widespread introduction of performance indicators into the service. The lack of information about the NHS's activities had been highlighted by the Guillebaud Report in the 1950s (Ministry of Health, 1956), but remarkably little had been done to overcome the problem since. The Conservative government's obsession with securing better value for money from public services meant that it wanted to measure the NHS's activities in order to search for potential savings, as well as to begin to examine whether medics were behaving efficiently. The performance indicators introduced in 1983 were primarily concerned with activities that were easily measured, and although they increased in sophistication through the decade, little progress was really made. The performance indicators did allow, however, simple comparisons of medical practice to be made, and offered the potential for the investigation of significant differences (Pollitt, 1985). The Department of Health was acquiring a reason for getting more involved in the day-to-day operations of the NHS. This meant that the NHS was gradually moving towards being a system where ministers could at least begin to measure the impact of their policies on the NHS, and where it would be possible for political priorities to be systematically introduced into the NHS. This meant there was a greater capacity for the centralisation of decision making.

Alongside the increased use of performance indicators, health economists, particularly those at the University of York (Mooney, 2003), began to examine how tools such as Quality Adjusted Life Years could inform policy making by demonstrating which areas of expenditure were better investments in patient care than others, offering a challenge to the medical profession to make its work more evidence based and to consider how it might make the best possible use of public resources. This approach was important because it challenged the individualism of medical decision making, and suggested instead that a more collective, resource- and evidence-informed view was necessary in order for the NHS to meet its obligations in terms of being fair to everyone it was meant to serve.

The increased use of managerial technologies also allowed other innovations to take place. The Resource Management Initiative (Buxton and Packwood, 1991; Brown, 1992) attempted to get clinicians more involved in decision making and more aware of the costs of their practices. Even though it had a rather difficult inception and eventually changed emphasis and became known as clinical audit, it created space at the local level for managers to begin to ask questions of doctors about their practices. The extent to which local medics were able to co-opt the technologies of resource management and medical audit, however, meant that a dramatic increase in doctor accountability did not occur (Harrison and Pollitt, 1994).

The introduction of general management, performance measurement and the Resource Management Initiative, even though change was slow, both challenged the dominant medical group and threatened the organisational compromise between the state and medicine on which the NHS was founded in 1948. In the first case, general managers were placed in hospitals with an agenda of challenging medical practice in the name of accountability and efficiency. This was a challenge to the medical power at the heart of the NHS for nearly 40 years. In the second case, the organisation compromise or 'concordat' (Klein, 2001) between the state and the medical profession was being eroded by the state intruding in the operational running of the NHS. To be fair, the medical profession could hardly claim to have kept to its side of the bargain by letting the state set the overall budget for the NHS without criticism – the industrial action of the 1970s and the increasing frequency of criticisms of the government by the Royal Colleges and BMA meant that both sides were growing more antagonistic. But it appeared as if a confrontation between the state and the medics was becoming more and more likely.

Despite the numerous changes to policy described above, the Conservative government's impact on the NHS by 1988 was rather less radical than commentators often suggested, and owed as much to political pragmatism on the part of Thatcher, who did not want to mobilise the medical profession in protest against her, as it did to any real enthusiasm for the ideals underpinning the NHS. For all the radicalism in areas such as housing, where council homes were sold to their tenants, Thatcher was extremely concerned about being seen to be dismantling or privatising the NHS for fear of the electoral consequences this might bring. This did not, however, mean that the government was not prepared to challenge and question the 'established rules of the game' (Klein, 2006, p 109).

The move to more radical reform

By the end of the 1980s, a series of less-than-generous budget settlements for healthcare appeared to be beginning to take their toll. As the decade wore on, it became clear that further NHS reform was certainly on the agenda from a government perspective, as health services had become a substantial source of frustration. The NHS was at that time still combined to form a huge department that included social services, and so absorbed a massive amount of government funding, especially at a time of high unemployment. It was also, ideologically, an obvious target for a government placing public sector reform at the heart of its policy agenda. But the NHS remained remarkably popular, despite the long waits it imposed for many treatments and the often ramshackle facilities in which clinicians were required to work. It was still free, and the British public was still grateful to receive its care.

The Conservative election victory of 1987 represented the highpoint of Thatcherism – a third term in power for a Prime Minister who briefly appeared unassailable. But by 1988 and 1989, the economy was sliding into recession, the Chancellor was clearly in dispute with his Prime Minister over the future of Britain in Europe, and health was becoming a battleground deliberately chosen by Labour with which to confront the Conservatives in Parliament. The Conservatives had increased NHS funding year on year in real terms, but the pace of medical technology and the increased demands made of health services meant that it was possible to construct graphs showing a cumulative shortfall in health expenditure during the 1980s of £1.8 billion (King's Fund Institute, 1988). Thatcher herself came to regard the NHS as a 'bottomless financial pit' (Thatcher, 1993), an area where she clearly wanted something done, but feared the public consequences of radical reform. Prime Minister's Question Time became an ordeal of having to refute allegations of ward closures, avoidable deaths and postponed operations, and then the presidents of the Royal Colleges publicly condemned the government's policies. Apparently harried into either admitting to or instigating a review of the NHS on a popular news programme, the discussion leading up to the publication of *Working for Patients* (Secretary of State for Health, 1989) led to many of the legacies of health policy and organisation identified in previous chapters as being faced head on. The government had reached a point where its pragmatism over challenging the medical profession in the previous decade had now become more politically expensive than the possible cost of launching a radical reform.

The review of the NHS made little progress at first. Secretary of State John Moore, regarded at the time as a possible successor to Thatcher, was ill, and facing an onslaught in the Commons at the hands of Labour Shadow Minister Robin Cook. Thatcher split the Department for Health and Social Services into two, giving the social services brief to Moore, and the health brief to Kenneth Clarke, not a man she liked very much but she aware that he had worked as a junior minister in health in the early 1980s. Health was something of a poisoned chalice because of the high risks associated with reforming the NHS – no Secretary of State for Health has gone on to become Prime Minister since the health service's creation. Clarke's behaviour in the run-up to the formulation of the *Working for Patients* document has parallels with Bevan's in the 1940s – he did not consult the medical profession in a concerted way, preferring the counsel of a few sympathetic ears instead (as Bevan did the consultants in London; Rintala, 2003).

The exact source of the idea of an 'internal market' for healthcare remains a contentious one – it had been mooted by visiting academic Alain Enthoven (1985) years earlier, who had famously remarked that the NHS was based on 'perverse incentives' that should be remedied through the introduction of competition for treatment contracts by health service providers. Clarke, however, claimed he came up with the idea himself while on holiday soon after his appointment. Regardless of its origin, the system Clarke proposed, one in which some GPs would be given budgets to purchase care on behalf of their patients (GP fundholders) with the rest of care being purchased by district health authorities on behalf of their populations from hospitals and community health providers, was certainly the most radical health organisation proposal ever to make it into law. Thatcher balked at the idea, and she and Clarke proceeded with the NHS reforms 'by argument' (Timmins, 1995b), but, with the Prime Minister weakened by the debacle of the Poll Tax and seemingly out of touch with her own Party in the Commons, Clarke was able to have his own way in a manner that would have been unimaginable even a year earlier (Timmins, 1995a; Greener, 2002a).

Working for Patients (Secretary of State for Health, 1989) was given a million-pound launch and was front-page news. Clarke had squared up to the medical profession, a politician unafraid of confronting established professional groupings. He had gone directly against the medical profession's expectation of being consulted over major policy changes, a feature of policy making in the NHS in the 1960s and 1970s that appeared to have become institutionalised through governmental reliance on the doctors to deliver health policy. The internal market represented the beginning of a change in the dynamics of health policy from a system based on trust between the state and the medical profession (albeit increasingly frayed trust) to one based on contract, where outputs and standards could be specified in writing between purchasers and providers in the NHS (Klein, 2006, p 155). In this sense, the Conservatives' proposals were challenging to the medical profession, not only in the way the reforms were planned, but also in their potential results.

Clarke's reforms met with a furious reaction from the BMA, which launched a campaign against them with posters showing a bulldozer labelled 'Mr. Clarke's plans for the NHS', and leaflets asking 'What do you call a man who ignores medical advice? Mr Clarke'. But the internal market became law – even in the face of public campaigns by the doctors and the danger of unpopularity this caused, the government stood firm. New contracts were introduced that specified consultants' job descriptions far more fully than ever before in order to be able to measure their performance against them, a change that was also made to GP contracts when their governing body was changed in 1991. Clarke, however, did pay a price for his reforms – he was not permitted to implement them, with the situation between him and the doctors adjudged to have deteriorated to such an extent that he could no longer remain in charge of the Department of Health. The more conciliatory Waldegrave succeeded Clarke with the view that the idea of an internal market perhaps signified a 'muddle between what was metaphor and what was reality' (quoted in Ham, 2000, p 30; Timmins, 1995a). Waldegrave's approach appeared to be less about confronting the medical profession, and more about getting the reforms to work in a less radical way than Clarke's plans – the reforms were going to be more about strengthening the hand of health managers than introducing competition into health services. Waldegrave was told on assuming office that 'Kenneth has made all the changes and stirred them up, and you have to quieten things down' (Edwards and Fall, 2005, p 92).

After a period of radical policy change, the status quo appeared to be reinstating itself. The government found itself wounded by the very public loss of a Prime Minister (albeit an increasingly unpopular one), facing a General Election, and on the receiving end of a concerted campaign by a highly credible professional group against it. The more concessionary outlook of the new Prime Minister may also have been a factor in the gradual climb-down over the internal market. A dilution in language occurred – purchasing became commissioning, competition turned into contestability (Sheldon, 1990). What appeared to be a hugely contentious and radical programme of reform was implemented in a cautious and concerned way.

The result of the internal market reforms was rather ambiguous (Le Grand et al, 1998a; Le Grand, 1999) – GP fundholding appeared to be the most dynamic element, but there is less evidence to suggest that, as a result of the introduction of the internal market, contracting patterns among healthcare purchasers and providers changed significantly from the situation pre-reform (West, 1998). A great deal of change had occurred in the accounting functions of district health authorities and hospitals to deal with the obligation to contract in such a different way, but the government had left itself wide open to accusations of introducing 'red tape' into the NHS with the introduction of an unnecessarily complex bureaucracy. Again, this is ironic considering that the specific agenda of the Conservative governments of the 1980s was to 'roll back the frontiers of the state' in the name of greater public sector efficiency.

What the Conservatives had shown was that is was possible to undertake health reform without consulting the medical profession. The corporatism between the state and the doctors present in the reforms of the 1960s and 1970s had been abandoned, first in the Griffiths management reforms, and second and most decisively in the period leading up to *Working for Patients* (Secretary of State for Health, 1989). The Conservatives had introduced reforms in the face of concerted medical opposition. Despite this opposition, the reforms had gone ahead, the NHS remained popular, and the government got re-elected.

Politicians might have been beginning to reconsider the discretionary space they held in policy making – they appeared to have far more options than they had previously suspected. Even though the retreat after the introduction of *Working for Patients* signalled a calming down of relations between the state and the medical profession once more, things were never going to be the same after the government had so visibly challenged the doctors' right to participate in policy. Table 4.5 summarises the state of the double-bed after the internal market reforms, with a logic of compromise increasingly necessary, as the state still required the medical profession to implement its reforms, but had found it could effectively ignore the doctors in the process of policy formulation.

Table 4.5: The double-bed after the Conservative internal market reforms

Party	Relationship
Medical profession	Necessary relationship with the state, as still dependent on it for employment. Incompatible relationship, as internal market reforms legislated for in the face of concerted medical opposition
The state	Necessary relationship with the medical profession, as still requires its cooperation to make reforms work. Incompatible relationship, as medics feel increasingly free to criticise government and policy

The 1990s

Klein first coined the phrase 'the double-bed' in 1990, so we are now in the position of being able to assess his claims, as well as to take the argument on from 1990 to 2007.

First, Klein stressed the 'real symmetry' of relations between the state and the medical profession. With the benefit of hindsight, this seemed to be overstating the case for the medical profession. The NHS reforms of the 1980s had seen the state challenging vested interest groups, among which it counted the doctors. Secretary of State Kenneth Clarke had been abrasive and swaggering during the process in which his reforms were formulated and legislated for, suggesting that every time he talked to the doctors about his reforms he saw them reaching for their wallets, and that he would not pilot the reforms before trying them out across the country because he felt the medical profession would sabotage them. This was an extension of the approach to reform taken by the government following the Griffiths Management Inquiry, in which consultation with professionals appeared at best optional and at worst entirely missing. The NHS reforms of the late 1980s were carried out by a closed group of senior politicians and advisers with the medical voice almost entirely absent.

If the medical profession had lost its voice in terms of policy making, it still, however, held something of an iron grip over the implementation of any reforms. Any reform would have to work through the NHS's most significant interest group in order to be successful, and would therefore require their cooperation. The symmetry of the relationship between the state and the medics was still in place, but now lay between the state dominating policy making, and the medics dominating implementation. This was an unhappy impasse – unless the state could secure 'hearts and minds', it was unlikely to be successful in its reform, and the medics were unlikely to cooperate with reforms, the content of which they had little or no influence over. The medical veto had moved from one over both policy and implementation in the 1960s to one over implementation only in the 1990s. Treatment decisions remained very much in the hands of doctors rather than state-appointed managers (Harrison and Wistow, 1993). Equally, GPs at least had the consolation that they did rather well out of the reforms financially, with their incomes exceeding the intended level by around £6,000 per doctor. Militancy was doused not only by the government standing firm, but also by money.

Recognising that potentially radical policy had been made, but that it still required medical compliance to work, the government appeared lukewarm in its support for radical change, moving Clarke away from healthcare and putting conciliatory figures in his place. There were therefore low expectations of significant change from the top, and little buy-in from the bottom. The government emphasised the importance of a 'smooth take-off' (Edwards and Fall, 2005) for the internal market, not disrupting established contractual patterns for fear of the radical results that might occur, and aware that a General Election was going to have to occur in the near future. If health services were in disarray, or if doctors were running a visible campaign against the government at the time of the election, this would give Labour a valuable line of attack against the government. Local doctors, having seen their national leaders fail to influence policy in their high-profile campaign against *Working for Patients*, subsequently found themselves facing, despite the structural reform of the NHS into purchasers and providers, very few reasons why they had to change their established practices.

The relationship between the state and the medical profession was still structurally necessary in character, both parties still needing one another for health services to function. But the tensions highlighted by the campaign against the internal market, and the increasingly long history of antagonism between the two parties, meant that the state, no longer in thrall to Keynesianism and instead trying to run an economy stressing supply-side reforms (Minford, 1991), regarded the NHS as difficult to reform, not because of ideological reasons, but because of its popularity and political sensitivity (Witness Seminar, 2006). The government regarded the medical profession not as a partner, but as a labour market inflexibility, a vested interest much as the same as a trade union (Ham, 2000). If the structural relationship between the two interests was still necessary, the medical and state cultural ideas now appeared incompatible, making any kind of resolution extremely difficult.

One of the flashpoints over which relationships were put under strain in the 1990s came through debates over the rationing of care (Hunter, 1997). As health authorities were required to publish plans that made clear their purchasing and made explicit the care that they were prepared to purchase for their populations, lists began to circulate showing differences between what some authorities were prepared to purchase, and others were not. For example, in Cambridgeshire, a child was refused treatment for her leukaemia on the grounds that any further treatment was likely to be ineffective and inappropriate, but the child's parents disagreed, and launched a national media campaign that eventually resulted in her being offered experimental care by a Harley Street doctor. The health authority argued that the child was being denied care on clinical rather than cost grounds, but the case fuelled the debate on the extent to which a 'postcode lottery' of care might develop in which some authorities were prepared to fund treatments such as IVF (in vitro fertilisation), whereas others were not. The government, in response, declared in favour of allowing individual doctors to make diagnosis and treatment decisions rather than intervening at a national level (Secretary of State for Health, 1996).

Between 1992 and 1997, the period of the last Conservative administration, the relationship between the state and the medical profession went through a 'becalming' (Wainwright, 1998) in which disenchantment with reform led to neither party wanting to disrupt the fragile equilibrium that had been established by allowing the least contentious interpretation of the 1990 reforms to prevail. The last White Paper of the Conservative era *A Service with Ambitions* (Secretary of State for Health, 1996), is remarkable for its lack of mention of reform or markets and for its invocation of partnerships instead. The government had either run out of ideas, or wanted a more conciliatory relationship with the medical profession.

One place where a muted challenge to the doctors was made by the Conservatives was in the area of audit. Clinical audit had been largely co-opted as a clinical matter up to 1996, but the rise in the evidence-based medicine movement (Muir Gray, 1996; Sackett et al, 1997) led to a gradual challenge to the way that medicine was practised, which occurred within the profession as often as outside of it, and which could be linked to the debates of the 1980s around the need for medicine to be more cost-effective. The issue of guidance regulations as to the 'best practice' for treating a range of medical conditions followed, with mixed results from the doctors, who appeared to regard them sometimes as a crude managerial tool, and sometimes as a legitimate means of improving practice for their patients. In this sense, they represented a continuation of debates around how medics might use performance management more generally to raise clinical standards (Bloomfield, 1991).

Labour back in power

On its election in 1997, the New Labour government initially appeared to continue with this more conciliatory approach, releasing a White Paper that stressed the importance of professionals of all kinds in the running of the NHS (Secretary of State for Health, 1997). At the same time as this, arguably the most dynamic aspect of the internal market – GP fundholding – was abolished, although the internal market was retained, camouflaged through the use of longer-term contracts and a new language of partnership (Powell, 1998). The Labour government appeared to believe that public reform could be achieved through a process of consensual change, with professionals recognising the need for reform and improvement and relishing the chance to work with the New Labour government. Labour also had a problem, however. In its election campaign in 1997, it had made a series of public service pledges designed to show itself to be accountable to the electorate (Labour Party, 1997). In terms of the NHS, waiting list reductions were promised, meaning that the government would be put under increased pressure as the next election approached to take a more top-down approach in demanding improvements from the service.

Labour's major innovation in terms of state–medico relations was the move towards Primary Care Groups working with what it called a 'single cash-limited envelope', which meant that their budgets were calculated so that they would have to cover the whole of their population's share of NHS resources, including prescribing. The government was effectively asking GPs to police one another, as overspending by one of their number could lead to the service as a whole running at a deficit. This was a new form of accountability for GPs – they were expected to accept collective responsibility for each other's prescribing decisions. Perhaps wary of crossing a new government with a huge electoral mandate, or worn down by the arguments of the 1990s, the BMA accepted, even welcomed, these proposals.

Malpractice and medical regulation

The 1990s ended on something of a sour note, however. High-profile medical malpractice cases dominated the media and resulted in criticisms from the media of the doctors' internal regulatory mechanisms, questioning the ability of medics to regulate themselves (Leys, 2003). On 29 May 1998, the General Medical Council (GMC) ruled that two surgeons from Bristol Royal Infirmary were guilty of continuing to operate on children with heart defects when they knew these operations had unacceptably high death rates (Salter, 2004). A doctor manager was found guilty of allowing the operations to proceed, even though he was aware of the likely high mortality that would ensue. The government announced a formal inquiry, which cost £14 million and took three years, and was linked in the public mind to other medical negligence cases that appeared over the following years, such as those involving the Royal Liverpool Children's Hospital Trust, Alder Hey, and most seriously of all, the serial killer GP Harold Shipman (Smith, 2002). In November 1999, the Labour government published *Supporting Doctors, Protecting Patients* (DH, 1999), which suggested that 'Present NHS procedures for detecting and dealing with poor clinical performance are fragmented and inflexible. There is a strong impression that some doctors who are performing poorly are slipping through the net' (p 39). Labour's favouring of managerial solutions to health service problems appeared to be evaporating, to be replaced by a more overtly interventionist regulatory approach (Salter, 2004). Both the Royal Colleges and the GMC found themselves on the back foot, and accepted the principle of revalidation for their members, meaning that the competence of their members should be regularly tested.

Labour also introduced the policy of clinical governance in response to the problems (Secretary of State for Health, 1998), requiring all Trusts to set up a system for monitoring the performance of clinicians and to identify poor performance, and poor performers. Clinical standards were further developed into National Service Frameworks, and all doctors were required to take part in audit, removing its voluntary aspect. The rhetoric of quality hid what was, in effect, an attempt to increase the accountability of medics for their clinical performance through a bureaucratic means of control (Flynn, 2004).

The 2000s

Within the space of its first term, the Labour government appeared to become increasingly frustrated by the lack of progress towards targets on waiting lists and by organisational change within the NHS. In 1999 new semi-autonomous organisations were created to evaluate present and new treatments to see what worked, and decide which treatments should be paid for within the NHS (the organisation now known as the National Institute for Health and Clinical Excellence, or NICE), and an inspectory organisation was set up to examine healthcare organisations (the organisation now known as the Healthcare Commission).

NICE immediately found itself occupying the position of a rationing body for the NHS, embroiled in controversy regarding its judgements on Viagra, Rulenza and Beta Interferon. The Healthcare Commission (then the Commission for Health Improvement) put in place a rolling programme of clinical governance reviews that were to cover processes for monitoring and improving services, patient and public involvement, risk management, clinical audit, clinical effectiveness, staffing, education and training and the use of information (Commission for Health Improvement, 2001). The Commission could issue reports that allowed the Secretary of State to sack the Board of a Trust if necessary. Both of these organisations firmly emphasised that the NHS was now going to be a national service, where local organisations were expected to tow the line. This meant doctors as well as managers (Davies, 2000).

Funding promises and continuous revolution

By 2000, Labour's frustration with the NHS had grown further. Labour peer Lord Winston proclaimed the NHS to be in crisis in an interview in *New Statesman*, and focused Prime Minister Tony Blair's mind on the difficulties the NHS was experiencing. Shortly after this, Blair made a pledge to David Frost on television to increase healthcare funding to the average European level, to the surprise of both the Department of Health and the Chancellor. The momentum for health reform was growing, and in July 2000 the NHS Plan was published (Secretary of State for Health, 2000), making increased resources available for healthcare, but only if significant reform followed. A new performance measurement system was put in place, based initially on traffic lights and then on star ratings, in which poor performers were to face public censure and their managers a possible sacking. Within a year a consultative document on patient choice had appeared (DH, 2001a), followed by plans to move care away from secondary providers into community settings (DH, 2002c), then a follow-up to the NHS Plan examining its delivery (Secretary of State for Health, 2002), and finally a moving of the NHS back towards a marketplace for care again through a new billing system called 'payment by results' (Department of Health, 2002b).

The private and not-for-profit sector was encouraged to enter the NHS as a co-provider so that, by 2005, around one fifth of all private sector activity was funded by the NHS, a figure that is likely to have doubled by the time this book is published. Labour has reinvented fundholding under the name 'practice-based commissioning' (DH, 2004) and published a White Paper on public health giving a vision of public, private and not-for-profit medicine working across boundaries of western and complementary therapies, and where exercise might be as likely a prescription as valium (DH, 2006b). Increased patient choice has been hailed as being in place across the NHS (DH, 2006c), and healthcare organisations have run up considerable financial deficits, despite the NHS as a whole being given a considerably improved financial settlement. The deficits were brought back under control again in 2006/07 by not replacing posts and by finding considerable savings, and a significant surplus was forecast for 2007/08. The PFI has built an unprecedented number of new hospitals, but has been criticised over concerns about its value for money (Pollock, 2004). High-performing organisations have been encouraged to apply for the new status of Foundation Trusts, with greater autonomy promised than other healthcare organisations, and with a new governance structure that has attempted to extend their local democratic accountability (Birchall, 2003; Klein, 2003; Healthcare Commission, 2005). By 2003, the GMC had been reduced in size and had 40% rather than 25% representation from lay members. This did not stop more radical proposals for medical reform appearing in 2006 (DH, 2006a), which included calls for a significant overhaul of postgraduate medical training (DH, 2006a), on the grounds that medical scandals in both hospitals (DH, 2002a) and general practice (Smith, 2002) meant that significant changes were now necessary.

It has been an exhausting and remarkable seven years. What effect has this hyperactive policy making (Maynard, 2001) had on state–medico relations? A number of themes seem apparent.

First, the entry of private and not-for-profit providers into healthcare has meant that the NHS has increased its capacity, creating the potential to reduce waiting times, but also reducing the state's dependence on doctors working in the public sector at the margins. The structural relationship between the two parties, necessary for so long, is becoming increasingly contingent. The Conservative government's attitude to health policy in the 1980s marked the beginning of this, where Kenneth Clarke effectively ignored the doctors during policy formulation, and showed that it was possible to legislate for reform without consulting them. The reforms proved less radical in their implementation than in their policy making, with the doctors still carrying an effective veto, but Clarke still created an important principle that policy makers almost routinely follow today – that it is not necessary to consult organised doctor groups when planning NHS reform.

Second, the state has become far more assertive in utilising the language of management in its interactions with the medical profession, demanding that doctors are accountable to their institutional employers as well as to their professional bodies. This has resulted in some odd hybrids, with NICE, for example, attempting to make sure that health treatments are 'clinically cost-effective', questioning whether the medical and state discourses automatically need to be incompatible. It would probably be fair to say, however, that most doctors still regard themselves as clinicians first and foremost, and even hybrid postholders such as clinical directors have struggled to embrace managerial roles (Kitchener, 2000). Whether the medical and state discourses of management are incompatible in any local setting depends on their particular context, but at the national level a greater degree of polarisation often appears with doctors demanding that patient care must come before the need to balance budgets.

A third trend is that doctors are being held more locally accountable by their healthcare organisations than ever before. Programmes of clinical governance have required doctors to discuss mistakes and examine problem service areas to attempt to learn from them and improve, and managers have increasingly been deployed to check on whether doctors claiming to be on call for the NHS are on the premises and available to work. The Labour government had attempted a 'direct invasion of medical territory and the profession was ill-prepared' (Salter, 2004, p 140). Medics have found that, whereas as recently as the 1990s they were accountable only to their peers, they are now increasingly expected to be accountable to their employers, and can face disciplinary hearings both locally as well as nationally. Performance management has been a key driver of this at the organisational level. As Trusts are forced to account for their activities in a more precise manner, managers have become more sensitive to differences in clinical practice where they affect treatment time and cost. Statistics now exist that show differences in the length of consultation episodes between providers and between specialisms, offering managers a tool for demanding explanation of outliers (Maynard, 2006). Some commentators claim that the extent of control established over the doctors can been overstated (Salter, 2004), but the direction of policy is clear, and it seems important that doctors are increasingly being co-opted into managerial roles and the disciplines and behaviours associated with them (Greener, 2005c). The discourse of 'evidence-based medicine' (Evidence-Based Medicine Working Group, 1992; Muir Gray, 1996) is instrumental in attempting to create standardised means of treating medical conditions (Harrison, 2002), and the issuing of National Service Frameworks by NICE, while increasing the capacity for evidence gathering and so greater medical knowledge, clearly reduced doctors' local discretion in the treatment of patients with specified conditions. This carries with it advantages in making sure that where medicine can be standardised, it is, but also represents a considerable challenge to doctors practising non-standard medicine and having to exercise their clinical judgement, as they may find themselves having to justify their decisions to human resource departments (Watkins, 2004) when it is 'not obvious we want doctors to be narrowly rule-following creatures' (Harrison, 2004, p 59).

These changes can be characterised as moving the NHS from a state–medico relationship of national accountability with local paternalism, where the government is accountable for the running of the NHS, while the medical profession effectively runs things locally, to one of national paternalism with local accountability, where local doctors and managers are required to take responsibility for any health service failings, while the state increasingly argues that the delivery of health services is a local issue. At the same time, the state has managed to increase its effective control of health organisations to an extent far greater than that in the past through the use of performance management and clinical governance. The state is able to measure outcomes and intervene where it perceives things to be going wrong, but devolves the day-to-day responsibility for the management of healthcare away from itself. The government is thus able to claim that medical behaviour is a local issue on the one hand, with control being in the hands of the GMC and with the managers of health organisations, but on the other make personal interventions by the Secretary of State where a well-publicised incident appears to be politically damaging. In the case of the breast cancer drug Herceptin, Secretary of State Patricia Hewitt overruled a local Primary Care Trust that had refused to fund the treatment, even though she was simultaneously demanding that health organisations balance their budgets and that local health managers take greater responsibility for decision making. This change is summarised in Table 4.6.

Table 4.6: National paternalism and local accountability

National paternalism	The state has increasing control over policy formulation and implementation through performance management, clinical governance and the use of semi-autonomous organisations such as NICE and the Healthcare Commission
Local accountability	Local health organisations, including both managers and doctors, find themselves responsible for delivering national reforms within the budget set and held to blame when this does not occur, despite limitations on their discretion, including the national setting of pay budgets, PFI, and having little say in the target-setting process

The Department of Health finds itself in the position of knowing more about the day-to-day operations of the NHS than ever before, and the government is therefore better able than ever before to try to fine-tune policy and incentive mechanisms to obtain local conformity. It has a greater capacity to interfere in the local running of the NHS, while at the same time reducing its accountability for the final outcome of policy, and having the ability to overrule local managers when it suits politically. The creation of an independent regulator for Foundation Trusts – Monitor – means that unpopular decisions about the governance of health organisations can be passed to a separate organisation (Walshe, 2003a), as was the case at Bradford Foundation Trust. Here, budgetary problems were resolved between the Trust and Monitor without the apparent involvement of the Prime Minister or Secretary of State. Ministers are more able than ever before to 'take credit for generosity, even while seeking to avoid blame for parsimony' (Klein, 2006, p 231). The double-bed relationship under Labour is shown in Table 4.7.

Table 4.7: The double-bed relationship under Labour

Party	Relationship
Medical profession	Necessary relationship with the state giving way to becoming contingent, as medical profession has greater opportunity to practise in private and not-for-profit providers Incompatible relationship with the state but doctors no longer active in protest against health reform, perhaps because of perceived powerlessness, perhaps because of considerable pay settlements
The state	Necessary relationship with doctors giving way to becoming contingent as private and not-for-profit providers enter, and the state gains increasing control over medical regulation and education. Incompatible relationship with doctors and the state increasingly able to get its own way in both policy formulation and implementation through performance management and clinical governance

Conclusion

The politics of the double-bed have undergone a transformation since the establishment of the NHS in 1948. At the creation of the health service, a necessary and compatible relationship appeared to be in place, with policy makers being accountable for the delivery of the service despite their lack of control over it. There was therefore also a dynamic of national accountability and local paternalism.

The subsequent history of the relationship between the state and the medical profession has been one where each party has gone about undermining the implicit bargain within the organisational form put in place at the NHS's creation. The state has attempted to become more involved in clinical practice on the grounds of achieving greater accountability and improving clinical practice by reducing geographical variations in treatment. The doctors, in turn, became evermore vocal in their criticisms of governments, culminating in their campaign against *Working for Patients* on the grounds that it went against the patient's wishes, but also because they were not consulted in its formulation. For the first time in the health service's history, the state went against the wishes of the doctors in reorganising healthcare, demonstrating that policy reform was possible even when it went in the face of medical opposition.

Labour, after an initially conciliatory start, appears to be attempting the most significant programme of reform in the NHS's history. It has reinstated the internal market, this time encouraging private sector involvement in order to create competition for public hospitals, given doctors' significant increases in pay, but instigated significant changes in working practices. In hospitals, consultants have been brought far more under management control through clinical governance reforms that make them more accountable for their decisions than ever before, and in general practice, a points system of incentives has been created in order to shape practice along the grounds required by the state. The language of management, from being vilified by doctors (Lee Potter, 1998), has become evermore widespread, and consultants increasingly find themselves as service managers and clinical directors with responsibilities not only to deliver care, but also to make efficiency savings and generate a surplus from their activities.

The wider private participation in the NHS means that the relationship between the state and the medical profession is more contingent than before, as both now have an alternative to the straightforward government–public doctor relationships of the past. As private contracting using public funds extends, so will the contingency of the relationship, although for the near future it will remain structurally necessary and mutually dependent, as before. The most significant transformation seems to be that, at the same time as the state has been able to measure and interfere with local health organisation activity, it has passed responsibility for delivering high-quality and on-budget care to local managers. The NHS has become an organisation with national paternalism and local accountability – a reverse of the situation in 1948. At present, it is local managers rather than local clinicians who are held to blame where health organisations fail to deliver according to performance measures, but it is surely just a matter of time before the finger of blame begin to point to local clinicians as well.

FIVE

Funding the NHS

Introduction

The third distinctive organisational feature of the NHS comes from the choice policy makers made at the time of its founding in terms of the way it would be financed. The general taxation method of funding health services means that those on higher incomes make a greater financial contribution to the cost of their treatment than those on lower incomes, but with no guarantee of better access or superior treatment. The principle of funding health services from general taxation is therefore redistributionary – the richer in society are helping to subsidise those who might not otherwise be able to afford healthcare (Webster, 1988).

At the same time as this, those in government have become increasingly aware that they gain a great deal from funding health services through general taxation (Klein, 1986). This is because it creates an effective brake on healthcare expenditure that is not available in health systems based on insurance principles. Because funding healthcare through general taxation means that the government effectively decides the overall budget for it (as long as it is able to subsequently control actual expenditure against that budget), funding is effectively supply- rather than demand-led. Insurance systems, in contrast, are demand-led, with expenditure being incurred on the basis of the health services treated in a particular year. In the NHS, care is budget-limited – it has to be provided within a set sum of available funds. When the money has run out, wards have often been closed and operations postponed. This should not happen in an insurance-funded system, which is, theoretically at least, driven by the capacity of health organisations to provide care rather than the budget of the overall system.

This implies that the NHS is not giving care on the basis of need, which seems to directly contradict one of the key principles for setting up the NHS. This apparent contradiction has been overcome through the NHS offering to treat the public, but often making them wait for that treatment. Thus, the NHS does treat people according to need, but only within the resources that are available. This has inevitably meant that services have had to introduce waiting lists.

So central policy makers decide the overall budget available for healthcare, and for much of the NHS's history, this has meant waiting lists. However, there has also always been a way to circumvent the waiting list – by opting instead for private care. Private care can be funded either through the patient having an insurance policy to which they contribute, or through a one-off payment. The irony of this is that private insurance in the NHS has not often given access to an entirely different set of doctors working for a parallel private sector that has nothing to do with the NHS. Instead, it often gives private patients access to the same doctor they would have seen had they waited their turn through the NHS. They may see the doctor in a different healthcare setting (such as a private hospital), or perhaps even in the NHS hospital they would have been referred to had they waited. As time has passed, GPs have become used to giving private referrals not only to doctors, but also to other healthcare professionals such as physiotherapists, for whom long NHS waiting lists have become established, making it possible for such professionals to work entirely privately, or for them to practice both inside and outside the NHS.

In the postwar period, funding problems have been exacerbated by the increased range of treatments and drugs that have become available in healthcare. This means that, even if healthcare settlements were generous year after year (which has often not been the case), the money available for the NHS would struggle to keep pace with improvements in medical care. Equally, there is the problem that around 75% of the costs of the NHS are staff costs (Doyal, 1979), so any increase in NHS budget will have a tendency to lead to increases in pay without necessarily improvements in patient care. Where those working in the NHS are underpaid, there is some justification for increases in NHS budget going to the staff. This seems particularly true in the case of nurses and in professions such as laboratory technicians, who are often highly qualified but poorly paid, both of whom would seem to have legitimate grievances over pay. However, this can lead to frustration on the part of policy makers, who, in response to increases in budget, often expect improvements in NHS care rather than the money going to improve staff pay. Of course, the two may be linked, with improved pay leading to improved morale and better productivity, but this would seem to presume that staff are not yet working at capacity and therefore that there is slack in the system, when it is not entirely clear that this is the case.

In any given year, healthcare demand in the NHS will almost certainly exceed available capacity. Because the NHS is financed from general taxation, citizens receive healthcare effectively at a price of zero (with the exception of prescription charges). Economists tell us that any good with a price of zero will have infinite demand. This does not seem entirely to apply to healthcare – most people, even though healthcare is free, do not find themselves taking recreational trips to doctors' surgeries when nothing is wrong with them. However, it does mean that the state requires the medical profession to make decisions about who gets care, who has to wait and who does not receive care. This typically occurs through GP surgeries, where initial assessments of patients take place and decisions are made about who gets prescriptions and who gets referred on to other health services (Lewis, 1999). Consultants ration care, too, deciding the order of their waiting lists (Pope et al, 1991) as well as their availability within the NHS to provide it. Doctors, then, effectively ration the scarce resource of NHS care. This creates a problem for the state because it has come to depend on them for this role. However, it does mean that the state does not to make difficult and contentious decisions about who should receive care and who should not, effectively concealing the rationing process (Pollock, 1995).

All of this has led to some strange local dynamics in healthcare. A cynical reading of the behaviour of some consultants in their private practice would give us reason to suggest that they have an incentive to create long NHS waiting lists because that simply adds to the potential for their private practice (Richmond, 1996). It is easy to see how some politicians have become suspicious of medical motives and so tried to reform care to prevent this potential conflict of interest from emerging. Where both NHS and private treatment are given by the same doctors within NHS facilities, recurring battles have ensued with Labour governments over the right of consultants to practise using NHS 'pay-beds' (see Chapter Four), and challenges made to consultants' right to practise in both the public and private sectors (Klein, 1983).

The way that healthcare is financed matters because it clearly has a redistributionary effect when general taxation is used, but the price of redistribution comes with the state often limiting the amount of care available, and requiring doctors to ration care on its behalf. Equally, there is the potential for odd incentives to appear in local healthcare settings, especially where particular consultants have significant private practice commitments. Finally, there is a concern on behalf of the state that, because so many healthcare costs are made up of salaries and wages, any increases in funding do not simply better reward staff without an improvement in care. These are the tensions present in the history of the NHS when considering funding. The following account describes their development and the difficulties present in each decade.

The 1940s

The first few years of the NHS led to it being regarded as a service that was unable to keep within its budget and so it acquired a reputation for inefficiency. The original budget and final out-turn figures are shown in Table 5.1.

Table 5.1: The cost of the NHS in England and Wales, 1948-51 (£m)

Year	1948/49 (9 months)	Annual rate	1949/50	1950/51
Original	198.4	268.0	352.3	464.5
Final	275.9	373.0	449.2	465.0

Source: Ross (1952)

The creators of the NHS quickly found themselves having to fight a rearguard action as a backlog of demand for health services emerged, from glasses to false teeth and GP services. During the early days of the NHS, the public went from service to service, enjoying their right to receive care free (Hennessy, 1994). It was a time of great optimism as the remarkably progressive nature of the NHS became apparent. Those who have grown up with the NHS take it somewhat for granted, but in 1948 the relief was palpable from those who previously had to make difficult decisions about whether to seek medical care or not based on cost rather than need.

Inter-war assumptions about the costs of healthcare falling over time were shown to be rather naive. The reasoning behind these assumptions was that a healthcare system would make the public more healthy, and so it might require fewer resources as time passed. However, this failed to take into account rapidly improving medical technology and the increased range of treatments available, as well as the increased demand for healthcare that a free service would generate (Honigsbaum, 1989). As more drugs and treatments appeared, and as patients became increasingly assertive in asking for them, it is hardly surprising that costs appeared to have an irrepressible tendency to rise. The whole point of the NHS was to eliminate financial considerations that might affect individuals seeking healthcare. In this respect, it was remarkably effective.

The result of overspending in the first year of the NHS led to a shift in the way that finance was planned. From a bottom–up system of generating budgets with local hospital authorities issuing demands, a top–down system of dividing up a fixed total was put in place (Klein, 2006, p 37). Individual authorities were given capped budgets, albeit with a considerable amount of discretion attached to them. But the centre rather than the hospitals was driving the budgetary process, and the need for financial control had become a guiding principle of the NHS.

The 1950s

The 1950s began with a change in government to the Conservatives. The Minister of Health, by now, did not have a Cabinet seat, and was in the process of being moved to the peripheries of Whitehall. The popularity of the NHS meant that if the government wanted to introduce reform, it needed a means of achieving this that provided a legitimate need for change. It set up an independent inquiry to try to provide a solution. In 1953, the Chancellor of the Exchequer told the Minister of Health that he intended to reduce the cost of the NHS to the government (Public Records Office, 1953). An independent committee was set up that took three years to compile its report (Ministry of Health, 1956). It would be fair to say that the government did not entirely foresee the result – instead of, as expected, producing a mandate to impose cuts on the service and introduce widespread charging, the committee acquitted the NHS of the charge of being expensive. In fact, it found that the cost of the NHS was actually falling, and that it was relatively inexpensive compared with health services found abroad (Abel-Smith and Titmuss, 1956). The Treasury was less than pleased: 'The report is very unsatisfactory from a Treasury point of view in that it makes no proposals on how a rising charge upon the Exchequer can be avoided' (Public Records Office, 1955). The report gave the government no mandate for change, and politicians discovered that they had created a 'financial treadmill' (Klein, 2006) for themselves with the creation of the NHS, destined never to be able to finance the service at the level demanded by the medical profession, and so to receive continued criticism even when budget settlements were more generous than those of the 1950s.

The change in government from the socialists of Labour to the less egalitarian Conservatives meant that the redistributionary principle of general taxation funding was less important. Labour had legislated for the introduction of prescription charges before it had left office, concerned about the growing cost of the service and faced with increased expenditure commitments in foreign policy (Morgan, 1990), but never implemented them. The Conservatives introduced the prescription charge, but also systematically increased the national insurance element of funding for healthcare, effectively a regressive movement in funding as it required the poorest to contribute the most, proportionally, to pay their NHS 'stamp' (Webster, 1994). The Conservatives wanted to move the NHS away from a redistributionary system towards a contributionary system – one in which the costs of the service were met more from charges, and where an insurance system was preferred to general taxation.

Between 1949-50 and 1958-59, NHS expenditure rose from £345 million to only £395 million, and the proportion of Gross National Product (GNP) devoted to healthcare actually fell from 3.84% to 3.49% (Webster, 1988). This is an obvious first manifestation of a less-than-warm reception to the NHS from the Conservatives – the amount being devoted to healthcare suffered an historically significant fall when, for most of the postwar period, it has at least remained static. The changes the Conservatives made are clear in Table 5.2, which show that charges rose from being 1.6% of total financing when the Conservatives entered office to 4.4% by 1959, and NHS contribution rose from 8.5% to 14% of total financing by 1959. General taxation, although still overwhelmingly making up the largest element of NHS finance, dropped from nearly 90% down to 81.6%. As such, charging and the NHS contribution effectively doubled their proportion of NHS financing in the decade.

The architect of much of this change was Chancellor of the Exchequer Peter Thorneycroft, who proposed that the NHS be steered away from a system funded by general taxation and towards a contributory system in which patients would have to make private payments to insurance companies or pay for healthcare 'out of pocket' instead. This was done on a gradual basis:

- in 1953, the Conservatives increased charges for school meals;
- in 1956, they increased the prescription charge;
- in 1957, they doubled the flat-rate NHS contribution (the NHS 'stamp'), as well as increasing charges for school meal again;
- in 1958, they further increased the NHS contribution; and
- in 1961, they doubled the prescription charge, increased dental and ophthalmic charges and increased the NHS contribution once again.

Table 5.2: Proportional sources of NHS finance, 1948-60 (%)

Financial year	Consolidated fund and local taxation	NHS contribution	Charges	NHS contribution + charges
1948/49	89.1	10.0	0.9	10.9
1949/50	90.5	8.9	0.6	9.5
1950/51	90.6	8.7	0.7	9.4
1951/52	89.9	8.5	1.6	10.1
1952/53	88.4	7.8	3.8	11.6
1953/54	87.7	7.7	4.6	12.3
1954/55	87.9	7.5	4.6	12.1
1955/56	88.6	6.9	4.5	11.4
1956/57	89.2	6.4	4.4	10.8
1957/58	85.9	9.4	4.7	14.1
1958/59	81.5	14.1	4.4	18.5
1959/60	81.6	14.0	4.4	18.4

Source: Based on Webster (1996, p 806)

These last round of increases were seen by Titmuss (1961) as 'the final charge of dynamite under the welfare state'. The NHS contribution's yield, along with other health charges, to the total financing of health was 6% in 1950, but had increased to over 20% in 1961, representing 'a severe erosion of the principles of social justice embodied in the original decision to provide services without charge and dependent upon general taxation' (Webster, 1994, p 71). A Cabinet meeting on 31 January 1957 recorded 'general agreement that the NHS should now be established on a compulsory contributionary basis' (Public Records Office, 1957), and it appeared that this was with the support of the Prime Minister himself (Lowe, 1989).

Once news emerged that there were plans to reconsider the way that the NHS was financed, however, the Conservatives retreated from their plans. 'Thanks to opposition from professionals and public alike, the NHS was shielded from further attack' (Whiteside, 1996, p 99). In addition to the funding changes that were implemented, serious consideration was given to introducing charges for GP consultations and introducing 'hotel charges' for stays in hospital. Further change to the way the NHS has financed was thwarted by

> the strength of public support for the NHS and the vulnerable electoral position of the Conservative government....

> Official papers are rich in instances where proposals for
> more radical curtailment of the NHS were stifled, either
> because of disunity among ministers, or for prudential
> considerations. (Webster, 1994, p 71)

Because of the reduction in the proportion of Gross Domestic Product
(GDP) devoted to healthcare, funding was tight during the 1950s, and
the NHS evolved from being an 'instrument for meeting needs (as
conceived by the founding fathers) to becoming an institutional device
for allocating scare resources' (Klein, 2006, p 29). This allocation was
largely achieved through the strategy of 'delay' (Baker, 1992), in which
an implicit form of rationing took place as doctors took control of
the allocation of available care to patients (Klein et al, 1995). The end
result of this was the effective depoliticising of rationing in the NHS as
politicians delegated decisions about who should receive care and when
to the medical profession. This worked while patients were prepared to
accept the treatment they were offered by the doctors (Moran, 1999,
p 64), and, in an age when patients were still grateful for free care, was
not often challenged.

The 1950s, then, were a period where policy makers appeared to
be challenging the general taxation system of funding the NHS, but
had to back down from introducing an alternative to it because of the
potential political unpopularity of such a change. The most obvious
alternative – moving the NHS towards a contributionary funding
system – would have moved health services away from being based on
a system where risks were pooled across the population and the poor
paid less than the rich for healthcare, and such a move would have
challenged the most popular aspect of the NHS – that it was free at
the point of need without any check on ability to pay.

The 1960s

The 1960s were significant in funding terms through the removal of
the prescription charge by the returned Labour government, only
for it to have to reinstate the charge because of economic difficulties,
and because of the instigation of the Hospital Plan, which involved a
commitment to a long-term expansion of capital expenditure.

The abolition of the prescription charge on Labour's return to office
was a symbolic gesture, suggesting that the NHS was now back in the
hands of its natural guardians and creators (despite the fact that it was
Labour, rather than the Conservatives, that legislated for the prescription
charge in the first place), and in that it demonstrated a very different

approach to NHS financing than had been seen in the 1950s, when charges, as shown above, increased dramatically. It was a popular policy, designed to show that a change in government had occurred (Mitchell and Wienir, 1997). However, within a relatively short period of time, the Labour government, beset by economic difficulties due to both inherited problems and optimistic overestimations of its own of growth, and constrained by a policy of having to keep the value of the pound fixed against the dollar despite these difficulties, quickly found itself having to find cuts in expenditure to avoid devaluing the currency (Pemberton, 2000). Major spending departments, including health, quickly found themselves under considerable pressure to find savings, and a straightforward, but embarrassing, way for the health portfolio to show that it was contributing was to reinstate the prescription charge, albeit with a substantial list of exemptions. By 1968, three years after the abolition of the charge, it was reintroduced. Even so, the growth in health expenditure between 1958 and 1968 was over 26%, twice that of the previous decade (Klein, 2006, p 49).

The Hospital Plan

The Hospital Plan (Minister of Health, 1962) is significant because it was the first attempt to introduce a concerted plan for raising the level of capital expenditure into the NHS. It began under the Conservatives, and was based on the observation that the NHS's stock of buildings was now ageing significantly – much of the health service's infrastructure had been inherited from the voluntary and municipal hospitals in 1948, and was in need of updating. In addition to this, the rationalistic flavour of the times favoured the bespoke building of new district general hospitals that could serve large areas and have the latest ideas in planning and large-scale medicine built into them (Mohan, 2002).

From a financial perspective, the Hospital Plan represented government attempts to impose a legacy of capital commitment on their successors, with mixed results. Capital expenditure in healthcare did increase as a result of the Hospital Plan, but the economic difficulties of the late 1960s made it increasingly difficult for the Labour government to honour capital expansion in an environment where it was struggling to find funds to meet the day-to-day costs of healthcare (Klein, 2006). This highlights the central problem of funding health services from general taxation. General taxation funding means that health expenditure is linked to the amount of taxation revenue available, and therefore puts health service expenditure in direct competition with all the other public services that must be paid for in the given year.

Health expenditure decisions were a function of both the sums available from taxation and the ability of other services to demand increases in funding. Where economic problems were experienced, such as those in the mid- to late 1960s, public services might have been required to make cuts across the board. Where other services were able to show that their claims on expenditure were greater than those the NHS was able to make, cuts had to be made to the NHS budget.

It is always easier to make reductions in capital (long-term) expenditure than revenue (day-to-day) expenditure. Revenue expenditure pays for people who are ill now to get better, or be seen quicker. Capital expenditure builds new hospitals for the future, or buys equipment to help tomorrow's sick get better. Necessarily, there is always a trade-off between the two, but if placed in a difficult decision, most of us would find it difficult to sustain capital expenditure when funds are limited, and the alternative is cutting funds for services needed today. For politicians, the difficulties are even greater, as they may find themselves caught in the dilemma of making long-term decisions from which their successors will benefit (such as building a needed new hospital) or trying to reduce waiting lists by employing more doctors today. This is not to suggest that politicians are any more selfish or shortsighted than the rest of us. But it does suggest that decisions on how much and when to invest in healthcare inevitably carry a bias that makes it difficult to sustain long-term capital expenditure.

Equally, the Hospital Plan created a dilemma for worker representative groups within the NHS. Because the total sum allocated to healthcare was decided centrally, and any increase in revenue expenditure created a reduction in the sum available for capital building, representative groups had to decide between their members' interests and the need for the NHS to rebuild. Should they press for increased pay for their members (as they had always done) and so limit the potential for capital expenditure, or argue for pay restraint to allow the capital programme to thrive? The question was not a difficult one in practice; representative groups survive by being able to give their members better deals. The process of reaching pay settlements appeared to work directly against capital budgeting within a specified NHS budget. Table 5.3 summarises the dilemmas over cutting revenue and capital budgets in the NHS.

NHS reorganisation

The discussions about NHS reorganisation that ran between 1968 and 1974 were noticeable for their lack of challenge to the general taxation mechanism for funding the NHS. What was perhaps more significant

Table 5.3: Revenue and capital expenditure and the difficulties of cutting each

Revenue expenditure cuts	Capital expenditure cuts
Affect politicians today because services are curtailed, and this may lead to unpopularity	Affect politicians in the future, as services today may be preserved, whereas capacity of the future is compromised
Affect unions, which will be campaigning for the best pay deals for their members	May not be noticed by unions, which are more likely to be focused on pay deals for their members
Likely to result in protests from the public and media as services are cut back	May actually be welcomed by the public when the closure of existing hospitals is avoided

than the proposals themselves was the mood with which they were conducted. Crossman (1969, pp 10–11) gave a pessimistic view of the future of health services:

> The pressure of demography, the pressure of technology, the pressure of democratic equalisation, will always together be sufficient to make the standard of social services regarded as essential to a civilised community far more expensive than that community could afford. It is a complete delusion to believe that if we had no further balance of payments difficulties social service Ministers would be able to relax and assume that a kindly Chancellor will let each one of them have all the money he wants to expand his service. The trouble is that there is no foreseeable limit on the social services which the nation can reasonably require except the limit that the Government imposes.

If the means for funding health services was beyond dispute, there seemed to be growing alarm about the potential for the NHS to consume public expenditure. These concerns were to come to a head in the following decade.

The 1970s

Fiscal crisis and crowding out

In the 1970s, the 'long boom' of economic activity came to an end, not only in the UK, but also across the developed nations of the world, and savings were demanded from high-spending departments such as health. The argument that the end of the long postwar economic boom resulted in an escalating 'fiscal crisis' has considerable persuasive power. O'Conner (1973) suggested that welfare expenditure is made up of social capital and social expenses. Social capital is that expenditure which pertains to an improvement of the stock of labour or its infrastructure in an economy – it is expenditure with a definable return. In terms of the NHS, social capital expenditure is, in crude terms, about getting sick people back to work and keeping healthy people from falling ill. Social expenses, on the other hand, are additional expenditures given by the state as concessions to avoid conflict. This is the area of expenditure that was perhaps undergoing the most considerable expansion in the 1960s and 1970s – as medical science advanced, more conditions were subject to treatments, but often, especially in acute hospital settings, at very high cost. Transplantation surgery, for example, is remarkable medicine, but saves relatively few lives and adds little to the productive capacity of the economy. Fiscal crisis occurs when social expenses expand at a rate faster than the economy is able to accommodate, putting the state in a position where it must raise taxes or reduce expenditure. Government is reluctant to pursue the latter option because social expenses are assumed to have a 'ratchet' effect – once concessions have been given, they are hard to remove without a political battle and risk of unpopularity. But equally, raising taxes is not exactly popular government policy either. The state therefore becomes trapped in a bind of escalating welfare expenditure and reduced means of raising money.

There are strong parallels between O'Conner's argument (coming from the Left) and the diagnosis of the political Right, even if the solution advocated by each approach was rather different. Bacon and Eltis (1978) argued that the public sector in Britain had grown too large – so large in fact that it was 'crowding out' private investment, thus undermining the source of wealth within the economy. As public expenditure as a proportion of GDP rose ever higher, they claimed, taxation levels rose and public investment took increasing amounts of capital to service. The only cure was for the public sector to shrink in size. This is a fiscal crisis of a different kind to O'Conner's argument, based on a decline in investment rather than an inability to withdraw from social commitments. However, it does seem that both Left and Right were suggesting that increasing investment in the public sector was becoming an unsustainable solution in an economy such as Britain's.

The limits of Keynesianism and economic crisis

The creation of the NHS was bound up with Keynesian economic philosophy, with a prevailing paternalistic view and an understanding of the state's role as being interventionist. Keynesian economic thought provided a legitimating body of theory for the state to intervene in the economy and in wider society – it could actually be optimal for it to do so. The Labour government of 1964-70 took Keynesian economic planning to a new level, based on ideas of 'Keynesian-plus' policy (Pemberton, 2000) where the Keynesian model was extended to provide the basis for a concerted effort to strengthen the economy in line with prescribed targets based on the most sophisticated economic models of the day. However, its economic plan failed, and the government became more and more distracted by the constraint of attempting to keep the value of the pound sufficiently high to avoid devaluing the currency in the Bretton Woods fixed exchange rate system (unsuccessfully) by managing the UK's balance of payments problem (also unsuccessfully). Government was beginning to learn that there were real limits to what it could achieve – the economy did not work as its economists suggested, but it was only seen as a matter of time before they worked out the flaws in their models and government regained control. The 1970s demonstrated decisively that this was not to be the case.

Dramatic oil and commodity price rises at the beginning of the 1970s sent shockwaves across the world. Inflation, for most of the postwar period a persistent but not significant economic problem, suddenly rose dramatically as a result of the increase in the economy's input prices (Aldcroft, 2001). Prices rose year on year, and the government appeared powerless to respond. Simultaneously with the rise in prices, the economy contracted. According to Keynesian economic thought, this should not happen – 'stagflation' was a contradiction that appeared to undermine the coherence of the Keynesian economic paradigm (Oliver, 1997). At precisely the time as policy makers most needed to get their models to work, they completely failed. The government appeared like it had lost control of the economy, and that it was 'overloaded' in terms of its commitments to run public services (Le Grand, 1991).

As such, the crisis of welfare in the 1970s was as much intellectual as it was financial (Pierson, 1998) – not only were there concerns about the state's ability to meet escalating welfare costs, but also about its ability to find an intellectual legitimacy for doing so. The combination of fiscal crisis and rising inflation occurred at a time when increasingly militant pay demands were being made by doctors, nurses and ancillary staff. A cycle of antagonism occurred where inflation led to increased pay demands, but undermined the state's ability to be able to afford them as economic recession led to reduced tax takes, which resulted in lower pay offers than workers demanded, and which led to further pay demands.

If there was a consensus about the welfare state between the two main UK political parties, it was decisively abandoned by the middle of the decade. In 1975, the moderate Heath was removed as Conservative leader and, largely as a result of a bizarre election process (Clarke, 1999), Thatcher became leader. The Conservative Party began to articulate a very different way of managing the economy that had been in place in the postwar period, suggesting that a monetarist approach that advocated closely managing the money supply in order to reduce inflation was the right way to proceed. The Labour government, experiencing budget deficits and apparently not at all in control of the situation, was forced to apply to the International Monetary Fund (IMF) for a loan to bridge the financing deficit it faced (although Chancellor Healey later claimed this was down to inaccurate Treasury forecasts; Healey, 1993). This was a humiliation for the government, with one of the most powerful economies in the world being forced to ask for a loan in order to be able to meet its commitments. With the IMF loan came conditions – the government had to cut back on expenditure and engage in a form of monetary targeting not wholly dissimilar to the one the Conservatives were advocating. Keynesian economic planning appeared at an end as the economy adjusted to more uncertain times (Lee and Raban, 1988). The belief, founded on a rather inaccurate but pervasive reading of Keynesianism, that it was possible for government to spend its way out of a recession, was abandoned.

Successive Secretaries of State for Health, in the harsher financial environment of the 1970s, did their best to protect the NHS budget, but were forced to make reductions in the capital programme in order to safeguard the current year's budget. There was also something of a perverse problem in that, as the capital building projects of the 1960s were completed, their increased running costs compared with the old, outdated buildings that preceded them put greater pressures than ever on the NHS. Health expenditure continued to rise between 1975 and 1981 in contrast to the fortunes of education and housing, whose budgets fell in the same period (Klein, 2006, p 79). In an era of scarce resources, healthcare appeared to be at the top of spending priorities. This indicated an increased status for the NHS in welfare services, but at a time when the incoming Conservative government was promising to 'roll back the frontiers of the state', it seemed only a matter of time before significant health reform occurred.

The 1980s

The 1980s saw the beginning of concerted debates about the level of NHS financing. The Royal Commission report on the NHS initiated by the Wilson government published its findings in 1979 (Merrison, 1979), and reaffirmed the principle of funding the service from general taxation on the grounds of fairness, concluding that changing the way in which the NHS was funded would not address its problems. The Royal Commission report was received by a Conservative government led by politicians who regarded public monopolies as anachronistic, anti-competitive and unproductive (Lawson, 1991). However, the NHS was largely immune to funding reform for much of the decade because of its popularity, but also because even radical politicians such as Lawson, Thatcher's second Chancellor, realised that the means by which the NHS was funded may not have been ideologically neat for a government that tended to prefer privatisation as a means of dealing with the 'problem' of public services, but did limit health expenditure rather well (Lawson, 1991). Proposals existed early in the decade that would have placed NHS funding on an entirely insurance basis (Howe, 1994, p 258), but which provoked a near riot in Cabinet because of concerns of what the reaction might be should they leak out (which they subsequently did, to *The Economist* magazine, removing any prospect of such a policy being considered further).

Compulsory competitive tendering and clinical budgeting

Despite the difficulties it was experiencing in changing healthcare finance, the government did make changes to the way in which the NHS contracted for ancillary services. The policy of compulsory competitive tendering was designed to make the NHS contract for services such as cleaning or catering in a more business-like way. Services were put up for tender rather than being delivered in-house, with contracts being awarded to the provider able to provide the most cost-effective solution. This provided a bridgehead into the principle of the NHS being an entirely public sector provider, and, even though relatively few contracts went to outside providers in the first years of the operation of the policy, it had the effect of introducing a greater flexibility into the employment of staff employed in ancillary services, particularly reducing union membership.

The reforms of the early 1980s were primarily managerial (see Chapters Four and Six), but the debate about funding the NHS grew in volume as the decade went on. Funding for the NHS was now lagging behind the level of healthcare expenditure of Britain's economic competitors, but the government argued that it was investing significant sums above the rate of inflation into the NHS, and that the problems of the UK health service were organisational and managerial rather than financial in origin. With a view to resolving this, clinical budgeting was introduced to attempt to get doctors to be more aware of the financial implications of their decision making, and then later renamed the Resource Management Initiative (Buxton and Packwood, 1991) when the approach was extended across the whole of hospital activities. Lines appeared on budgets known as 'efficiency savings' where managers of services were required to find savings each year to demonstrate that the productivity of their service was increasing. It was often left to clinicians to find the means by which such savings could be made, which in turn raised the profile of debates on the rationing of care. Doctors had always rationed care within the NHS, but, in an environment where they were being explicitly asked to cut costs and find savings, these debates carried with them a new imperative as well as often angering doctors, who felt that they were being asked to make a success of policy they disagreed with profoundly, while politicians, remote from the implications of their decisions, took the credit for services being more productive (Lee Potter, 1998).

The 1980s bear strong similarities with Conservative policy in the 1950s in that there was a search for alternative funding arrangements for the NHS (Greener, 2001). Prescription charges rose from 20 pence in 1979 to £5.25 in 1996, an extraordinary increase of over 2,500%. There was a sharp decline in the number of NHS dentists as the period wore on, and free eyesight tests and dental checks were abolished, but the charges never approached the proportion of total NHS funding that they did in the 1950s. In terms of the purchasing of care within the NHS, however, the Conservatives of the 1980s broke with the past. Extra capacity was purchased from the private sector, where the government deemed there was an urgent need to reduce waiting lists and patients found themselves sent to BUPA hospitals 'on the NHS'. The rise in charges, the decline in NHS dentistry and optician services, and the use of private sector facilities to treat NHS patients created suspicions that the government was thinking of wholesale privatisation (Taylor-Gooby and Lawson, 1993). The growth of private sector medicine in the early 1980s added to this suspicion, but is perhaps best seen as offering an increasingly affluent middle class a supplement to the NHS rather than an alternative to it. Private patients still went to NHS GPs and to NHS outpatient appointments; they were behaving more as 'commuters' (Klein, 2006, p 125) between public and private medicine rather than leaving the NHS.

Internal market reforms

After Thatcher's third election victory in 1987, the Conservatives found themselves on the receiving end of the criticism that, although health expenditure had been allowed to expand in real terms, it still had not expanded enough. Analysis suggested that it was necessary, because of the higher inflation rate in healthcare, for expenditure to grow at a rate between 1.3 and 2.3 percentage points above inflation just to keep pace with demography, technology and necessary service improvements, and that there had been a cumulative shortfall on this since 1981 of some £1,800 million (King's Fund Institute, 1988). Thatcher was furious, later claiming in her autobiography that she believed the NHS had turned into a 'bottomless financial pit' (Thatcher, 1993). When put under pressure about healthcare funding in a television programme, Thatcher announced, to the surprise of her Department of Health officials (Witness Seminar, 2006), a wide-ranging review of the NHS.

The reforms introduced as a result of Thatcher's review were based on an 'internal market' (Secretary of State for Health, 1989), and are covered from several different perspectives in this book because of their implications for GP–consultant and state–doctor relationships, as well as their implications for the financing of care. The reforms were still based on the assumption that the overall sum allocated to the NHS was about right. Instead of requiring more funding, a means of making the service more efficient needed to be found. Healthcare organisations were split into purchasers and providers of care, with the idea being that purchasers were to hold providers to account for the quality and quantity of the services they provided, as well as seeking the best deal for the budgets devolved to them. Money was to 'follow the patient' so that popular providers increased their funds, and unpopular ones lost out, even faced possible closure.

However, the implementation of the internal market turned out to be far less radical than the original plan. Much of the contracting turned out to be on a 'block' basis, based on large volumes with few measures of quality attached, and there was little attempt by health authorities to make contracts 'contestable', or subject to potential new entry from alternative providers of care (West, 1998). The sheer complexity of the information system necessary to keep track of patients as they moved through the NHS, to make sure that all providers billed for the care given, was immense. Added to this was the requirement for the patient's purchaser of care to monitor these transactions to make sure they were of high quality, increasing the complexity even further. Little wonder that purchasers of care tended to contract with their already-preferred providers, especially in localities where moving contracts might have involved justifying sending patients to hospitals 20 to 30 miles away when there was an NHS hospital available far closer (Salter, 1993). There was even evidence that the Department of Health actively discouraged 'cross-boundary' contracting because of fear it would lead to redundant bed-space in hospitals not as favourably regarded by patients (Witness Seminar, 2006). Very few referrals outside of patients' immediate localities seem to have taken place as a result (Exworthy and Peckham, 2006).

Equally, in London there were particular problems implementing the internal market because of the existence there of a large number of teaching hospitals with high bed capacity and an expensive menu of services. Attempts to gradually reallocate funds from London since the 1970s through the RAWP (resource allocation working party) formula had been diluted because London hospitals received compensation for their treatment of non-London residents But the internal market, because funds would flow to district health authorities to pay for the care of local residents only, threatened to reduce considerably the funds available to London (Butler, 1992, p 115). There was a delay in the use of the new population-based funding formula until 1992-93, and a further delay in allowing London hospitals to apply for the new Trust status that would allow them greater financial independence, until a commission on hospital care in the capital had reported. Hospital care in London had been fudged – had the market been allowed to work as planned, it would have resulted in a capital-wide funding crisis and had major political implications for the government.

After the drama of the early years of the decade, the 1990s seemed to be a period where, after the very public battle between the government and the medical profession at the beginning of the decade, the main concern within the NHS was getting the health reforms to work with the minimum of disruption rather than the maximum of change. This was partially down to the removal of Kenneth Clarke as Secretary of State, but also due to the different style of Thatcher's successor as Prime Minister, John Major, and the need to campaign for a General Election in 1992.

As such, debates around healthcare financing appeared to have largely calmed down during the 1990s. From a situation where there was potential for dramatic change as a result of the introduction of the internal market, remarkably little change occurred, with no hospitals going 'bankrupt' as a result of the purchaser–provider split, and no wholesale privatisation of the NHS.

Labour and health financing

Nonetheless, Labour campaigned in 1997 on a platform of saving the NHS, even if, after its landslide victory, it made few changes to the service's funding system. The internal market was branded wasteful and inefficient because of the growth in contracting administration that had occurred, and contracts were put on to a longer-term basis to attempt to retain the potential contestability of the internal market, while at the same time reduce its transaction costs (Secretary of State for Health, 1997). This was Labour's 'Third Way' in action – attempting to find a way of keeping the advantages of policies while removing their problems. The government was committed to the spending limits of its Conservative predecessors to try to demonstrate its financial probity (Allender, 2001), and so a significant increase in health expenditure was not possible unless cuts to other services were made, or unless savings within the NHS could be found. The government, believing it could resolve the problems of the NHS through organisational means, assured readers of its first White Paper that 'the pressures on the NHS are exaggerated. Indeed they have always been exaggerated' (Secretary of State for Health, 1997, s. 1.19).

Funding promises

Despite the government sounding remarkably confident in its position on health financing, Prime Minister Tony Blair, in an echo of the pressures placed on Thatcher at the end of the 1980s, quickly found himself having to defend the NHS's funding record on a Sunday morning television breakfast show in the face of high-profile health service difficulties. Instead of committing the government to NHS reform, Blair promised, and without consulting his Chancellor, that the government would increase the level of health service expenditure to that of the average level in the European Union (Jenkins, 2006).

An examination of how Blair's promise was to be achieved was commissioned through the Treasury, with the job being given to Derek Wanless, formerly of National Westminster Bank, while policy moved on apace with the launch of the NHS Plan, which confirmed the commitment of policy makers to funding the NHS from general taxation: 'The way that the NHS is financed continues to make sense. It meets the tests of efficiency and equity' (Secretary of State for Health, 2000, p 334). In what appeared to be a little like post-hoc rationalisation, the proposals of the NHS Plan fitted well with the announcement of the increased funds available for the NHS, and with the subsequent Wanless Report (Wanless, 2002). A significant sustained increase in investment in healthcare was made for the first time in its history, but with the government demanding equally significant reform in return.

No investment without reform

A new marketplace for healthcare was then constructed as a means of driving reform, apparently reversing the claims made in 1997 that such an organisational form was inefficient because of the contract-monitoring red tape it created. Labour gradually attempted to move contracting on to as small a scale as possible through a combination of individual patient choices and larger-scale contracts put into place through the new purchasers of care in the NHS, Primary Care Trusts.

At the time of writing, Primary Care Trusts hold well over 80% of the NHS's budget, and are meant to be responsible for driving improvements in care through their budgetary role in much the same way envisaged in the 1980s reforms that aimed to allow money to follow the patient, but now known as 'payment by results' (DH, 2002b). At the same time, Primary Care Trusts are responsible for providing a range of services in non-hospital settings (such as the care offered by GPs and dentists) and for getting health services to work more closely with social care services. They are therefore both purchasers and providers of care, something that has a tendency to cause considerable concern among senior policy makers. General practitioner fundholding has also been revived as 'practice-based commissioning', with practice-based commissioning practices receiving notional budgets on which to spend on care, and to allocate the individual elements of the block contracts for care already made by Primary Care Trusts. Money was now supposed to follow the patient through the system for the first time in the NHS's history, although a wealth of organisational and technical issues still appear to beset this in practice.

PFI

The most significant innovation in terms of funding under Labour, however, as been the increased use of the PFI. The PFI is important because it attempts to address the longstanding problem of financing capital programmes in the NHS. In the 1960s, the Hospital Plan did not achieve all of its goals because the NHS had to compete annually with other public services for available funds in a time of economic difficulties. The problems of the public sector coordinating and running substantial capital programmes were well documented, with substantial delays and budget overruns being the norm (Watkin, 1978, pp 68–70). In such a situation, capital expenditures were always more likely than revenue expenditures to be reduced because of their long-term nature.

The PFI gets around this problem by getting the private sector to build new hospitals, which the NHS then leases over an extended period of 25–35 years, with the private sector providing maintenance of the facilities throughout that period. At the end of the period, the buildings, then fully depreciated, pass into public hands. The NHS is not required to make an upfront capital payment, but is legally committed to make an annual leasing and maintenance payment to the private partner for the use the facilities (Asenova and Beck, 2003). The discretionary element of capital spending effectively disappears, as there is a long-term legal commitment to make the payment to the private sector, and so cannot be the victim of a later expenditure cut. The investments have been approved quickly in comparison with the difficulties experienced in the past in obtaining public finance, and there has been a rapid expansion of hospital building not seen since the 1960s. This has occurred without the government increasing the national debt, as PFI expenditure does not appear as a debt on government balance sheets. The PFI can be interpreted as a pragmatic response to all the problems of securing public capital expenditure of the past.

However, the PFI also carries with it a number of difficult questions (Pollock, 2004). From the perspective of finance, the most important one is whether or not it represents good value to the taxpayer. Private Finance Initiative schemes involve a long-term commitment of public funds; they 'unquestionably redistributed the cost of financing health care into the future' (Mohan, 2002, p 220), offering very good rates of return for private firms in return for taking the risk of building new public facilities. The question of whether the PFI represents a good investment for the public sector remains contentious, with some builds appearing of poor quality and experiencing substantial problems with their private maintenance partners (Pollock, 2004). Equally, where private firms appear to generate returns substantially above those of the rest of the market from PFI, this leads us to ask questions as to whether public value has been achieved (Andalo, 2004). Finally, in an era where care is meant to be moving from secondary to primary settings, there are questions to be answered as to why so much large-scale hospital building has taken place. Perhaps a more strategic approach would have seen more new infrastructure in primary care settings instead (Peckham and Exworthy, 2003). The arguments for and against PFI are summarised in Table 5.4.

Table 5.4: Arguments for and against PFI

Arguments for PFI	Arguments against PFI
Far more capital expenditure has occurred than would have been the case otherwise	Significant capital cost increases have been incurred by Trusts with PFI builds
Private sector expertise brought in and risk shared on capital projects (although not equally)	Long-term contracts with the private sector signed that allow it to make substantial profits
Some rationalising of hospital infrastructure has been possible through strategic building	Hospital builds may not always have been appropriate in an era when care is meant to be relocated to primary care

Deficits

An additional and interrelated area of some debate over the past three years in the NHS has been the deficits generated by local healthcare organisations, as well those of the NHS as a whole. Historically, it has not been that unusual for local healthcare organisations to be in a deficit situation at the end of a financial year. What has changed is that penalties have been established for organisations in this situation that mean that they have been required to both pay off their deficit the following year and receive a budget cut of the amount of the deficit. This has led to some organisations experiencing substantial year-on-year deteriorations in their financial situation. The response of the Secretary of State for Health has been to blame poor local management and planning for the problem with a level of impatience that is understandable at a time when billions of extra pounds have been allocated to healthcare by Labour. However, the causes of deficits are more complex than this, and may also be the result of poor central policy making. Local managers have been left to implement centrally set pay increases coming from revised consultant and GP contracts. Equally, PFI projects have resulted in dramatic increases in the capital costs of local healthcare organisations, where they may have had no alternative except to use the system in order to secure much-needed infrastructure investment. Managers have sometimes been placed in impossible situations where they have to make the best of policy decisions that impose substantial financial problems on them, while at the same time being expected to keep on top of the new reform agenda and to demonstrate service improvements. Deficits may not always be the result of poor management – sometimes they are very much the result of poor policy making (King's Fund, 2006).

Conclusion

The general taxation method of funding the NHS is one of its defining characteristics. The combination of public funding and public provision makes the NHS almost unique, making it difficult to make comparisons with other healthcare systems (Klein, 1997). As in the past, the NHS remains funded primarily from general taxation, but there is a significant move towards utilising private financing for capital expenditure (through PFI), and incorporating private providers to create competition for care contracts. As such, public money is now flowing to private providers within the new mixed economy of care, and private money is flowing into the NHS for capital projects. Although most financing and provision remains public, Labour's approach to both the demand and supply side clearly has long-term implications for the future of health services. The PFI is a long-term policy, as contracts have been signed for periods of up to 35 years. The introduction of the private sector as competitor, equally, may be irreversible under World Trade Organisation rules, which suggest that healthcare cannot be made less competitive through government intervention (Pollock, 2004). The changes introduced by Labour are with us to stay. How exactly they play themselves out in terms of financing remains to be seen.

SIX

Managing in the NHS

Introduction

Managers are now among the most high-profile actors of all those working within the NHS today. They are often cast as its villains. They do not cure people, as doctors do, or care for patients, as nurses do. Instead they are often accused of cutting services, or as taking up money that could be better spent on care. Managers are overheads in health organisations, blamed by politicians when budgets are overspent (BBC News, 2006a) or wards not clean (BBC News, 2001), and reviled by the media as being responsible when things go wrong in health organisations (BBC News, 1999). They appear as shadowy figures in television dramas about hospitals and healthcare, lurking in the background trying to remind clinicians about finances at times when there are lives to be saved, and cutting services when money begins to run short.

At the same time, however, NHS managers now earn considerable salaries, and are held up (at least within the NHS management community) as exemplars of what it means to balance public values with efficiency and service delivery. They are presented as healthcare leaders who somehow manage to balance the often competing interests of resource efficiency and clinical effectiveness and to organise clinicians without alienating them, and they earn respect from the diverse range of professionals working in health organisations in the process.

Managers therefore appear as rather paradoxical beings – both heroes (Learmonth, 2001) and villains (Greener, 2005d), agents of the state and local preservers of public values against the onslaught of health reform, leaders and pragmatists able to work with the competing interests that health organisations hold within them. Attempting to understand the complexities of the role of managers in today's NHS is made easier by understanding a little history, as well as getting to grips with the changing conceptualisation of management within the NHS.

NHS administration

Accounts of the early years of the NHS are remarkable for often missing out managers completely (Eckstein, 1958; Rintala, 2003). This would be unthinkable today, when chief executives are at least visible in local media and in public meetings of their organisations. It is harder to find those responsible for the 'administration' of the NHS before the 1980s.

In the early years of the NHS, those charged with locally organising health services were placed in what would today be regarded as primarily an administrative role. This comprised trying to coordinate the activities of consultants in their organisation (in the case of hospitals), all of whom believed their allegiance and so accountability was primarily to their profession and so they were accountable only to their professional peers. The memorable phrase that summarises this process of coordination is 'herding cats'.[1] Klein (2006, p 33) quotes a medical administrator as saying that the role was one in which administrators helped 'professional opinion to form itself spontaneously' (a term redolent of the way the civil service operated in relations to politicians in the classic television comedy Yes, Minister).

At every level of the NHS, there were three hierarchies of officers: lay administrators, medical administrators and finance officers. Each health authority appeared to have a different dynamic for the relationship between these groups, with sometimes fierce battles breaking out in which they attempted to secure pre-eminence, but with no single administrative organisation going across the three hierarchies. All officers were employed within their individual authorities, with no national policy for recruitment and selection even if staff were all employed on national pay scales. This meant that local health organisations tended to appoint in their own image; so if a particular authority was run primarily by medical administrators, this group would tend to have access to the best new recruits, reinforcing its own position. Promotion was not based on conforming to national standards, but on running local health services well, so central exhortations for compliance with policy changes did not have to be treated particular seriously.

Administrators faced the formidable task of running local health services during the transition to the NHS. This was all the more remarkable because of the lack of experience many of them had of running health services within a nationalised structure (Godber, 1975, p 18). The absence of planning and management in the NHS was raised by an inquiry into the costs of the NHS in 1956 (Ministry of Health, 1956), but little seemed to be done to try to address the problem. The sheer effort of getting health services operational at the local level appeared to be matched by fatigue at the Ministry of Health (Klein, 2006, p 31), which had to negotiate with professional associations or trade unions that represented staff in the NHS.

However, there were examples of almost parodic levels of bureaucracy present that were recognised by writers of the time as being representative of how health services were run. It is easy to find examples of almost mind-boggling ineffectiveness. The Farquharson-Lang Report (Scottish Home and Health Department, 1966) reported on the situation in Scotland but was 'quickly recognised as having wide validity throughout the NHS' (Watkin, 1978, p 106). There was a proliferation of committees and subcommittees, with meetings often going on for hours to discuss decisions of relatively little importance. Watkin gives examples from Farquharson-Lang that include: 'The Committee selected a suitable colour for the cards to be attached to food carriers at …. Hospitals', and 'The Committee were shown a counterpane which had shrunk to half its proper size. It was resolved to investigate the matter' (Watkin, 1978, p 108). The administrative approach to running the NHS predominant before the 1980s is summarised in Box 6.1.

> ## Box 6.1: The administrative approach to running the NHS
> - Administrators coordinate the activities of other health professionals – diplomat role
> - Three levels of officer, but with no hierarchy between them, so potential for conflict
> - Provided organisational infrastructure that helped establish the NHS
> - Committee-based with a reputation for bureaucracy and trivia

What was remarkable about the administration of the NHS until at least the 1970s is that it represented almost the antithesis of the 'command and control' model that has increasingly been used to describe health organisation at that time (see for example, Secretary of State for Health, 2000). This is because the state effectively had no levers for controlling the local running of the NHS (Paton, 1998). It could send memorandums and demands, but local administrators had little power to put them into effect, and local doctors had the discretion to ignore them if they wished (Klein, 2006). The NHS was run in this period in a remarkably decentralised manner, even if organisational charts made it look as if all lines of responsibility ran back to the Department of Health. Textbooks examining hospital management published as late as the 1970s read like lists of the specific details required in each institutional functional area, including chapters on medical records, housekeeping, and laundry and linen (Grant, 1973). The contrast with contemporary health management texts (see, for example, Walshe and Smith, 2006) could not be greater.

The contradiction on organisational diagrams between the apparent lines of control stretching from the centre of the NHS and the reality of strong medical control has been addressed by medical sociologists, who have suggested that hospitals particularly have a dual system of authority: one following administrative accountability and the other medical lines of control (Goss, 1963). This created medical sites of resistance to bureaucratic management, especially where medics played a strong role in policy formulation, as in the NHS. Hospitals therefore became a 'negotiated order' (Strauss et al, 1963), where professionals, administrators, nurses and patients were required to seek constant compromises in order to keep things going. It is little wonder that administrators of that era found it hard to achieve anything more than a reactive, coordinating role in their organisations.

Local health administrators felt profound frustration at attempts by the government to get more involved in the day-to-day running of the NHS, but those in central government became exasperated at their lack of ability to translate their accountability for the NHS into power to change things. Health service administrators regarded themselves as the glue that held the dominant professionals together and allowed the NHS to function, but were regarded as holding largely unimportant roles by the professional groups within the NHS.

Managerialism

Increased pressure to control health expenditure, particularly from the 1970s onwards, led to attempts by the state to have greater control over the operational level of health services. Medics were now openly criticising the sum of money the state was allocating to the NHS, and the state was beginning collect data on how health services were run, and to seek ways of introducing a stronger role for managers within them. The state's greater reliance on management ideas was not a rationalistic, ideologically neutral change; it was one that threatened the operational control of doctors by introducing a challenge to the mode of governance that had existed in the NHS for its first 25 years.

The 1974 NHS reorganisation

NHS reorganisation in 1974 revealed a lack of clarity over the role that managers were meant to play in health services. An emphasis on the potential of better management to improve health services led to management consultants McKinsey's being brought in to examine the potential for improvement and to make suggestions about how the NHS might be better managed. Even though the proposals in retrospect read like a model of conservatism, they were hidden away in an appendix in the 1972 White Paper (Secretary of State for Health and Social Services, 1972) for fear that the medical profession would object to them, and the notion of any kind of challenge to existing health practices through management disappeared in the reforms. The private sector managers that Secretary of State Keith Joseph and his management consultants sought to woo into the service were less than enthusiastic about joining the NHS, which was hardly surprising given the relatively low rewards and status that health service management jobs offered. Instead, the 1974 reforms were dominated by local authority managers and doctors institutionalising their representation on health authorities (Glennerster, 1995), with those previously employed as administrators transferring to the new managerial roles. This continuity created another force for conservatism.

Another continuity in the 1974 reforms can be seen in the consensus decision-making teams that were set up. The reorganisation required professionals, administrators and treasurers to work together as equals on its committees, representing their respective groups' interests. However, each representative also had an effective right of veto (Cox, 1991), an organisational form that appeared to assume that all decisions would be made unanimously (Carrier and Kendall, 1986), but which resulted in few decisions being made.

The 1974 reforms also attempted systematically to introduce planning into the NHS, with health authorities producing strategic plans that showed how they were meeting the Department of Health and Social Security's objectives and national priorities. The Department of Health and Social Security published its priorities in terms of both norms of provision and expenditure allocation, as well as attempting to address inherited inequalities of resource allocation between the regions. These plans were based on the assumption that economic growth would resume, but the economics difficulties of the 1970s quickly undermined them. On top of this, the first projects constructed under the 1960s Hospital Plan came to fruition only for policy makers to find that they were substantially more expensive to run than the buildings they were replacing. This served only to tighten budgets further. By 1976, regional authority chairmen complained to the Department of Health and Social Security about capital building, interference in day-to-day policy that came from the detailed planning process, the contradictory advice often offered by the department, the complexity of its internal structure that made communication difficult, and the inflexibility of national agreements over pay and staff numbers (DHSS, 1976). Reform seemed to have made things worse rather than better, and national priorities impinged only marginally on local decision making because of the inheritance of local commitments (Klein, 2006, p 93) and the lack of mechanisms for central decisions directly to affect hospitals, GP surgeries and community health services.

Management failures

Nearly 10 years after the scandalous conditions found at Ely Hospital (see Chapter Three), the impotence of the reformed health service was illustrated by the problems of Normansfield Hospital (Committee of Inquiry into Normansfield Hospital, 1978). A consultant psychiatrist who appeared somewhat eccentric in his practice had entered into a running battle with nursing and medical colleagues. The situation had received the attention of the Community Health Council, which had protested against conditions there, and visitors from both the government and the health authority agreed that something needed to be done. But nothing was done until nurses threatened a strike that led to an inquiry being set up and the consultant dismissed. The consensus management approach did not appear to be working, and it seemed as if the Department of Health and Social Security was impotent in addressing clinical failure.

Managerial concerns continued to grow over the perceived failure of the NHS to deal organisationally with significant failures in the way it was delivering care, but an additional area of concern was how better to obtain value for money from the NHS. Discussions about the organisational structures of health services that had dominated the 1960s gave way to explorations of organisational dynamics (Klein, 2006, p 105). If policy makers' increased interest in managerialism was a function of their need to try to secure greater operational control of health expenditures, it was also concerned with the increase in militant behaviour from the NHS's various staffing groups that occurred in health organisation in the 1960s.

The Thatcher government

On its election in 1979, the Conservative government's first instincts appeared to be to try to decentralise health services, and to try to decentralise decision making to make it as near to the patient as possible. In 1982, a tier of health organisation set up in the 1974 reforms was removed to try to simplify things, and district health authorities were encouraged to engage in local fundraising activities in a throwback to pre-NHS days when philanthropy was central to the funding of healthcare.

The Thatcher government began to examine closely public expenditure in its early years in office through Raynor 'scrutinies', which resulted in hospitals evaluating their estates and seeking expenditure cuts (Mark and Scott, 1992). But this created an immediate tension: the implicit concordat between the state and the doctors on which the NHS had been founded meant that the doctors were given operational control of the NHS in return for the state setting its overall budget. Health managers were being asked to cut back on services and the state appeared to be delegating financial problems to the local level.

The NHS Management Inquiry

In 1983, the Chairman of Sainsbury's, Sir Roy Griffiths, was asked to examine how the NHS might be better managed. Griffiths set up a team predominantly of investigators with a private management background (Petchey, 1986), in marked contrast to the Royal Commission or public inquiry approach of the past, where academics or judges oversaw a process of gathering and assessing evidence (Greener, 2001). The resulting Griffiths Report, or more accurately 'letter' (DHSS, 1983) bemoaned the lack of control, accountability and customer focus in the NHS, complaining that it could find no one in charge – a direct criticism of the consensus decision-making process (Harrison et al, 1990).

Griffiths was damning about the lack of performance measures of the NHS's activities, beginning the movement towards a focus on improving the outputs of healthcare and away from debates around the level of inputs entering the service. The Griffiths inquiry resulted in the creation of a new post in the NHS – the 'general manager' – who would be individually responsible for running a hospital site. The general manager was meant to make hospitals more business-like, and receive rewards through performance-related pay if successful.

Griffiths suggested that performance measurement systems should be put in place to make sure that the NHS was still accountable to ministers, but also that the state had to learn to delegate. The apologetic approach to attempting to increase the role of managers in the 1970s had disappeared, and they were now seen as a central part of NHS organisation.

Griffiths, as well as presenting the strongest pro-management message that the NHS had seen, also suggested that doctors might be equipped to fulfil the management role, claiming they were the 'natural' managers of health services, and creating an expectation that clinicians would increasingly be involved in management roles (Pollitt et al, 1988).

The role of the new health managers was conceptualised in terms of them being in place to close the gap between policy and its implementation. This conceptualisation of public management as effectively an agent of the state is one present in Alford's (1972, 1975) classic formulations of health politics. Alford suggests that doctors represent the dominant interest in healthcare. Challenging dominant interests are groups such as managers, described as corporate rationalisers, who attempt to get medics to understand their accountabilities to the organisations they occupy, and that decisions cannot always be based solely on clinical need. Finally, in Alford's scheme, there are repressed interests, which must find ways of being heard by combining with other repressed interests to form coalitions, or by combining with either dominant or challenging interests to avoid being excluded from the policy process. It is hard not to see nurses in this light, given their inability to make the significance of the nursing profession felt in health policy and implementation, despite being the largest professional grouping in the NHS.

NHS managers were therefore tasked with implementing centrally made policy, of making things happen on the ground in the same way as private managers are expected to comply with head office-set regulations and targets. Putting in place general managers was meant to give the centre some local control over what was happening, but at the same time allow local managers some discretion in deciding exactly how central targets and policy were to be achieved. However, politicians found it almost impossible to resist trying to interfere to a greater extent in the running of health services – the stakes were too high, as the government was still expected to take most of the responsibility for them. The Griffiths reforms as implemented were rather more centralising of policy and management than decentralising (Peckham et al, 2005a, 2005b).

Performance indicators

In line with Griffiths' recommendations, the 1980s saw the introduction of a new management tool into the NHS – performance indicators. As far back as the 1950s, a lack of information on exactly what was going on in the NHS was a feature of NHS inquiries (Ministry of Health, 1956) and bemoaned by Ministers of Health (Powell, 1966). A combination of the Thatcher government's concern with value for money and the availability of information technology meant that performance measurement was both viable and desirable. It was needed not only to measure the activity of the NHS and to look for savings, but also to defend the government from a charge that, under its stewardship, the NHS was not improving.

The performance indicators introduced in 1983 were extremely crude, containing little that measured quality or patient improvement and focusing instead on numbers that could be more readily measured and calculated, such as numbers of patients treated and total costs (Pollitt, 1985). As time went on, more measures were introduced along with greater attempts at sophistication, but little progress was really made. What the performance indicators represented was not an innovative and clever use of managerial technology, but a means by which crude comparisons could be made and investigations of significant differences mounted (Bloomfield, 1991). The Department of Health now had legitimate reasons for asking difficult questions of health authorities that were statistical outliers on their returns, and so for getting more involved in the day-to-day operations of the NHS. This increased central accountability gave NHS managers a strong incentive to begin to assert their presence in their hospitals and health authorities, along with a centrally derived legitimacy to do so.

The increased use of managerial technologies allowed other innovations to take place. The Resource Management Initiative (Buxton and Packwood, 1991; Brown, 1992) attempted to get clinicians more involved in decision making and more aware of the costs of their decisions. Even though it had a rather difficult inception and eventually changed emphasis into a programme of clinical audit, the initiative created space at the local level for managers to begin to ask questions of doctors about their activities, tacitly involving them in management processes to a greater extent. Doctors' enthusiasm for their new management roles, however, varied tremendously (Pollitt et al, 1988).

However, it is remarkable that, even after Griffiths, the role of managers in the NHS remained largely reactive, introverted and incremental (Gillespie, 1997). Health management was still concerned with meeting the needs of medical professionals rather than having the authority to run services (Harrison, 1988a; Cox, 1991). Harrison and Pollitt (1994) sum up the role required of managers as that of the 'diplomat', mediating conflicts between professionals rather than leading services for themselves. In 1985, a series of cross-regional case studies examining service changes in the NHS showed a raft of problems with securing any kind of local reform of health services because of the huge number of interested parties from which each change required consent, and even because of the fear of breaking the routines of health service workers in order to reduce waiting times for patients (Stocking, 1985). The first Chairman of the NHS Management Board, Victor Paige, resigned from his job in June 1986, frustrated by political interference and the lack of profile afforded managers in the NHS (Edwards and Fall, 2005, p 43). Harrison reported in 1988 that 'as yet there is no systematic evidence that management initiatives are substantially affecting the behaviour of doctors' (Harrison, 1988a, p 145). It seemed as if organisational inertia was set to continue in the NHS for the foreseeable future, even if managers themselves had begun to believe that they could now begin to adopt a more assertive management style towards the NHS workforce (Klein, 2006, p 120).

The New Public Management in the NHS

The introduction of the new managerial class into public services in the 1980s has been widely written about as representing the beginning of the reforms known as the New Public Management (NPM). The evolution and significance of NPM has been assessed and analysed in a number of ways (see, for example, Hood, 1991; Dunleavy and Hood, 1994; Ferlie and Pettigrew, 1996; Ling, 1998). Clarke and Newman (1997, pp 124-5) present a list of differences between the private and public sectors that they claim highlight the influence of the former on the latter in the creation of NPM, as shown in Table 6.1.

Table 6.1: Oppositions highlighted by NPM

Private sector (as NPM)	Public sector
Management	Public administration
Business values	Public service values
Consumers	Citizens
Individuals	Communities

Source: Clarke and Newman (1997, pp 124-5)

In each case, the NPM-favoured approach on the left of Table 6.1 is contrasted with the 'old' public administration approach on the right. The oppositions presented by Clarke and Newman are useful in that they show the difference in emphasis between the private-inspired values of NPM compared with the 'old' public administration approach of the public sector. The NPM categories were preferred by policy makers in the 1980s because of the increases in responsiveness and efficiency they claimed would come from an increased discipline resulting from market orientation.

Management/public administration is the first opposition, with the former being a driving force for improving customer value through entrepreneurial behaviour, and the latter being characterised as a moribund, bureaucratised service based on the convenience of administrators rather than the needs of service users. There is clearly some element of truth in this negative treatment, but it ignores the need for public services often to have clearly defined rules and procedures. None of us wants an unregistered surgeon before us employed on cost rather than expertise grounds. The second opposition is a favouring of business over public service values. Business values are meant to emphasis responsiveness and efficiency, whereas public service values concerned with fairness and rule-following are regarded as being outdated and inefficient. This, in turn, leads to the third set of oppositions, with users positioned as individual 'consumers' of welfare services rather than publicly oriented citizens who wish to engage with services through 'voice' rather than 'choice' mechanisms (Hirschman, 1970). Consumers are encouraged to exit from services they dislike rather than utilising voice or complaint as a means of securing improvements, as citizens might, and with their relationships with providers becoming far more transactional as a result. This is set up in the final opposition, with a favouring of public organisations dealing with individuals rather than elected representatives or collectivised professional groups.

NPM and the NHS

New Public Management was imposed in the NHS through both managerial change and organisational reform. Compulsory competitive tendering was introduced as an early mechanism for introducing private sector disciplines into the provision of ancillary services in the NHS (such as cleaning and catering). By putting such services up for 'tender' each year, and with the contract going to the provider able to provide the most cost-effective solution, the NHS increasingly found itself contracting with private, for-profit organisations to provide services formerly provided entirely within the public sector. Compulsory competitive tendering was justified by fashionable management thinking of the time that suggested that organisations should 'outsource' tasks that were outside of their 'core competencies' in order to 'stick to the knitting' of their main role (Peters and Waterman, 1982). However, compulsory competitive tendering also served another purpose.

In the 1970s, industrial action was a very visible feature of the NHS. In the 1980s, the Thatcher government approached trade union reform with revolutionary zeal, the most visible manifestation of which was in conflict with the miners and the national strike that it provoked. In the NHS, compulsory competitive tendering reduced the number of unionised workers in the NHS, reducing their capacity for industrial action. Many ancillary workers who were members of the Confederation of Health Service Employees (COHSE) now found themselves having to renegotiate their terms and conditions or even out of a job. The effect of compulsory competitive tendering on the most vulnerable and lowly paid workers in the NHS was huge – many of those working in ancillary services were already on low salaries, and were disproportionately made up of women and people from minority ethnic groups. Ancillary services at the time represented a sum in excess of 12% of total NHS expenditures (Klein, 2001, p 136) but only 18% of contracts did not go to incumbent providers in the first round, and even by 1986 annual savings were estimated at around £86 million. This was not an inconsiderable sum, but hardly one turning around the fortunes of the NHS budget. Compulsory competitive tendering therefore saved the NHS relatively little money and created greater job insecurity for the most vulnerable workers within the NHS. It did this in the name of greater efficiency for the service as a whole, as well as having the effect of substantially reducing the influence of trade unions in the NHS. It also increased the role of the private sector within the NHS, gradually taking ancillary services outside of public provision, even if the new contractors often ended up employing the same staff as had been formally employed by the NHS directly, but on substantially worse pay and conditions.

The new managerial focus of the NHS was also reflected in medico–state relations. The Thatcher government held the assumption that interest groups employed in public services were not partners to be worked with, but barriers to reform. As such, the 'managerial state' was born (Clarke and Newman, 1997). In the 1970s, the Conservative government had interfered in medical regulation, and, in 1984, the Department of Health Privy Council refused to 'nod through' proposals relating to changes in rules concerning the fitness of doctors to practise

(Moran, 1999). This led to the opportunity for a wider debate about the governance of doctors, with references to the Office of Fair Trading and the Monopolies and Mergers Commission following behaviour from the GMC, particularly in terms of the way it handled medical negligence claims, that sometimes appeared to those outside of the confidential discussions to be eccentric. In turn, this led to changes in the way that challenges to the clinical competence of its members were dealt with, as disciplinary hearings became far less internal to doctor regulators, and the NHS itself came to investigate claims of professional incompetence within its organisations rather than relying on the doctors to resolve their own problems behind closed doors (Moran, 1999). The doctors, from being an interest group with power and influence, found themselves isolated from the policy process, expected to participate in managerial practices inside their organisations, and far more accountable to managers in those organisations when things went wrong.

Management and the internal market

By the end of the 1980s, after a series of public spending rounds where Secretary of State John Moor appeared to be attempting to demonstrate his ideological purity in Conservative eyes by accepting reduced settlements in the budget round for the NHS, it seemed as if the media was full, week after week, of stories of closing wards and crumbling infrastructure. The Presidents of the Royal Colleges publicly denounced the government's policies, and Thatcher announced on a popular television programme that a major review of the NHS was under way, to the apparent surprise of her cabinet colleagues and officials (Witness Seminar, 2006). The resulting internal market quickly became less about the markets themselves and more about the increased opportunities they offered managers (Hunter, 1993b). The architect of the reforms, Kenneth Clarke, later described the purpose of the reforms primarily in terms of giving managers additional tools to challenge doctors rather than the market being an end in themselves (Ham, 2000). Managers could now claim increased legitimacy in demanding accountability and reform from medics because of the market disciplines the new reforms were bringing (Hunter, 1994b).

For the first time, there was the theoretical possibility that hospitals could lose contracts where patients were required to wait too long for treatment, or where care was not of the quality required by the internal market purchasers, district health authorities and GP fundholders. Managers could therefore place pressure on clinicians to reform their practices because of the threat of contracts moving to other providers if services were not of the standard required. Consultant merit awards were given not only for clinical excellence, but also increasingly for the demonstration of managerial competence (Hunter, 1994a). However, the contrast between the values of doctors, with their concern with individual patients, and management, with its focus on collective outcomes, was one that was difficult to overcome (Moore, 1990).

The 1990s

The 1990s, after all the furore from the doctors in their opposition to the internal market reforms (see Chapter Four), proved to be rather less radical than expected (Klein, 1998). The Conservative government appeared no longer to want to antagonise the medical profession through further reform, and let managers get on with attempting to make the new organisational structures work, with varying results (Le Grand et al, 1998a). The internal market strengthened the hand of managers, but the bastions of medical power still seemed remarkably in place by the time the Conservatives left office in 1997. Managers became aware that relationships with medics could 'quickly sour but were slow to build up' (Pettigrew et al, 1992). The government may have asserted itself and put in place policy change that doctors opposed, but doctors still held considerable discretion in local health organisations because of the confidentiality of their relationships with patients, and their ability to dominate, despite the increased status of managers, the day-to-day running of local health organisations (Baggott, 1994). Both Griffiths (Hunter, 1997) and Enthoven (2000) distanced themselves from the reforms, suggesting in the former case that market mechanisms were actually distracting managers from their main tasks, and in the latter that the reforms bore little resemblance to Enthoven's (1985) prescriptions for how a market should work in the NHS.

Another force for compromise was that the doctors themselves 'went managerial' (Berridge, 1999), with clinical directorates being established in many hospitals, and doctors having to assume greater collective responsibility for individual medical practitioners. Medical bodies also became co-opted into laying down a number of national standards and protocols for good practice (Klein, 2006). Medical audit, initially conceived as a means for managers to intervene in clinical practice, was taken over by clinicians who retained control over the process and prevented it from becoming a tool for management (Hunter, 1992). Managers recognised that it was necessary to get doctors 'on board' in order to change the way that healthcare was organised and delivered

(Paton, 2005), and so gave medics the ability to co-opt many of the policies that were originally designed to try to give managers greater control over them. Equally, many doctors embraced the promotional opportunities that management positions offered them, using them to evade the bottleneck to consultant posts (Kelleher et al, 1994).

Managers' incomes rose significantly as a result of the internal market reforms but their occupational life expectancy fell as they found themselves subject to far greater employment risk. They increasingly worked on short-term, performance-related contracts, and so found their futures dependent to a very significant extent on being able to deliver government policy. In hospitals, managers who had achieved the transition to Trust status were sought after by organisations applying for the new status, and a transfer market for senior staff began to develop as the average period in office of chief executives, in particular, fell. As managers moved between Trusts, the resistance to the market reforms appeared to diminish as the experiences of those who had been through the reform process first-hand began to spread across the NHS. Within a couple of years, both Trusts and fundholding had become firmly established.

An immediate consequence of the reforms was the rise in numbers of staff listed as having management roles in the NHS. The number of administrative and clerical staff rose from about 117,000 in 1989 to 135,000 by 1992, or a rise from 14.5% to 17% of the total workforce (DH and OPCS, 1994). Alongside this, a number of management consultants were employed to help health managers deal with the changes before them. They have not left the NHS since.

Although the health policy area generally went through calmer waters in the 1990s, health managers probably experienced the decade as one of continual change. They were responsible for getting the internal market to work, and, as they were on short-term contracts, there were considerable incentives for working extremely hard to make this the case. Then, as soon as managers had mastered negotiations with their local health authority, they often found that they had to start relationships with new partners because of mergers, and then that they had to report to new bodies at regional level with the abolition of regional health authorities and the establishment of regional offices of the NHS Management Executive in their place. Throughout all of this, accountability flowed more strongly than ever before to the centre of the NHS; it was becoming a national organisation more than ever before, with managers expected to show how they were meeting national policies and national targets.

New Labour's approach to health management

On re-entering government in 1997, Labour claimed to have abolished the internal market in the name of improved efficiency (because of the vast contracting infrastructure required to support it) and equity (on the grounds that GP fundholding appeared to give some advantages to patients enrolled in their surgeries in terms of waiting times) (Secretary of State for Health, 1997). The market, however, was still present, but was instead recast on to a longer-term basis in an attempt to retain some incentives for efficient contracting, but lose the threat and disruption that could come from frequent changes (Powell, 1998).

In terms of management, the language of conciliation with clinicians presented managers as being to blame for the growth in bureaucracy that had appeared in the NHS during the internal market reforms, and for the need now to pass control back to those closest to patients – the doctors and nurses. This was to be relatively short-lived, however, as the managerial themes of the 1980s were to be picked up again by 2000 in the NHS Plan (Secretary of State for Health, 2000). This put in place a commitment to give the NHS additional resources, but only if significant reform was delivered. Stronger management was clearly a central part of this.

Performance management

In the year following the NHS Plan, the Performance Assessment Framework was developed so that clear penalties could be imposed on hospitals trusts deemed to be delivering a low standard of care. The entire management teams of 'zero star' Trusts faced possible 'franchising' of their function to private sector managers, or managers of more successful NHS services elsewhere (DH, 2001b). Managers were held to blame for the failings of their hospitals (Dawson and Dargie, 2002), despite concerns that they may have had control of only around 40% of the variables for which they were being held accountable and that the efficiency measures themselves were subject to considerable error (Street, 2000). Managers had been increasingly accountable for driving reform in the NHS since the 1980s, while at the same feeling that they lacked the authority to achieve the goals asked of them (Dopson and Stewart, 1990).

The difference in the 2000s was that managers were now facing the loss of their jobs if they failed to achieve centrally-set goals. The cooperative, friendly tone of the 1997 White Paper (Secretary of State for Health, 1997), where collaboration between the state and health professionals was to achieve improvements in the NHS, was now a thing of the past. Labour's second term in office saw the establishment of a Delivery Unit in government specifically tasked with improving the performance of public organisations, and which took a strong interest in the reduction of NHS waiting lists (Barber, 2007), not least because of Labour's high-profile election promise to reduce them.

Instead of the 'hands-off' approach of the 1990s where local contracts were the main tool for the local steering of NHS organisation, more 'hands-on' control had been asserted through the Performance Assessment Framework (Newman, 2002). This involved the Department of Health being required to produce performance plans, having to attend stocktakes of how the NHS was performing as a whole, and then account for any problems that had emerged or for a failure to hit promised improvements in service. In some respects, this is plain good sense – requiring the NHS to meet its commitments and demanding an explanation where it does not would seem to form the basis of a simple managerial control system. The problem was that the sheer complexity of the delivery of health services, the lack of care over the setting of initial targets and the distorted incentives they could produce for managers often conspired to break the link between measurable performance and the actual activities of health organisations (Mannion and Goddard, 2002). Health managers were effectively given incentives to focus only on targets for which they would be penalised or rewarded, and so areas outside of the performance management framework had a tendency, even with the most conscientious managers, to receive less attention (Greener, 2004b, 2005c). Managers were required to deliver policy outcomes (Newman, 2002), or be publicly blamed for failing to do so.

Hospital Trusts were supposed to be given additional freedoms as a result of performing well under the doctrine of 'earned autonomy' (Mannion et al, 2003), but managers often seemed to experience this as a case of being 'free to do what they were told' (Hoque et al, 2004) instead. By 2006, the performance system had evolved, with government claiming it was becoming 'lighter touch' than before, but there was little evidence of this. The number of measured indicators had decreased, but instead of relying on Trusts' reports of their own data, increasing central inspection and collection of data was taking place. This resulted, in 2006, in a dramatic decline in the number of health organisations able to present themselves as performing to the highest standards, and a significant increase in those graded lowest (Healthcare Commission, 2006a). As Primary Care Trusts entered the performance management system, the running of which was passed to the Healthcare Commission, they often found themselves receiving its poorest ratings.

Managers found themselves playing for far higher stakes than had ever been the case before. Those in organisations measured as being high-performing NHS Trusts were held up as examples to the rest of the NHS, with publications such as the *Health Service Journal* offering awards to them. Those in charge of low-performing institutions were threatened with having their jobs, and even the jobs of the entire management team, being taken away (Greener, 2008a). 'Turnaround' directors were appointed to attempt to address the failings of institutions deemed to be in the failing categories and to make change happen. The government demanded that health services underwent 'cultural change', becoming more consumer-focused and responsive instead of the producer dominance and 'clan' mentality that was allegedly still dominant (Mannion et al, 2004).

Deficits

A good case study of the changed pressures on managers comes through the NHS budget deficits in 2006/07. As a result of hospitals and Primary Care Trusts declaring increasing deficits in the first months of the year, increased pressure was placed on health managers to find ways of reducing expenditure, with the Secretary of State Patricia Hewitt declaring that she would resign if NHS finances could not be brought into balance by the end of the year (BBC News, 2006b). As a result, decisions had to be made to avoid replacing posts where staff left, and managers were blamed for incompetence in allowing the situation where their Trusts were allowed to run deficits in the first place (Audit Commission, 2006). There is clearly some truth in this – it doesn't seem unreasonable on the face of it to ask health organisations to keep within the budget allocated to them. However, this was in a context where the government had agreed new contracts for both GPs and consultants the previous financial year while significantly underestimating the cost to the NHS of their implementation (NAO, 2007), leaving local managers to sort out the problem.

PFI

A second problem with deficits came through the PFI, which was now the only real means of financing capital expenditure for health organisations (Pollock, 2004). As many hospitals in the NHS were in a state of some disrepair, managers were understandably keen to embrace the possibility of gaining new facilities, and a rapid expansion of PFI projects took place. However, with these new facilities came significantly increased annual capital charges to the new organisations. Managers could have worked out ways of reducing expenditures when the new doctors, contracts were negotiated, and they could have worked out the effect of building new hospitals and reduced expenditures further to cover the new charges they would have to pay as a result of PFI contracts. Whether they could have kept within budget given all of these constraints, however, is another question. Perhaps they chose to run deficits because they did not wish to scale back services, or because they felt they would rather overrun their budget as a statement of their commitment to the values of the NHS in refusing to go along with centrally imposed problems that they were not party to creating. In either case, it was convenient and easy for the government to hail successful health managers as heroes; those in charge of deficit-ridden organisations were accused of incompetence. The government seemed content to make the claim of deficits being the result of bad management, despite its imposition of an accounting system that demanded deficits be paid in full the following financial year in addition to cutting the deficit organisation's budget by the amount of the deficit.

The new mixed economy of care

The pressures on health managers have also been increased by the return of a market for healthcare. In the 1990s version of the market, a lack of competition among providers was blamed on the lack of change that took place in contracting during the reforms (West, 1998). In the 2000s model, the government attempted to address the lack of competition by encouraging private and not-for-profit organisations to contract to provide care for the NHS (Greener, 2008b). Overseas health providers, as well as well-known UK organisations such as BUPA and the Nuffield Trust, would now compete locally for NHS contracts in the name of increasing choice for patients (Greener, 2005b).

Hospital managers face a considerable new challenge from the increased competition within the NHS. There are at least two levels to this. The first comes from public providers of care remaining comprehensive in their provision in that they aim to offer a full range of health services, whereas private and not-for-profit providers may not. The system by which prices are set in the NHS is based on the national average cost of offering that particular treatment (the tariff), but this may not be at all reflected in the local health economy, where a hospital's costs may be lower or higher (perhaps because of increased capital costs, or local economies of scale or scope). However, hospitals must make sure that the services they offer are viable under the tariff system, with managers facing reduced space for manoeuvre in terms of cross-subsidising activities across the hospital (Paton, 2007). This creates an environment where public hospitals (and public providers generally) have to review the services they are offering as a result of finding themselves competing against specialist providers that do not have the same costs of training or capital associated with them. The competitors, such as small treatment centres, might rely on few facilities and economies of scale in order to have costs well below tariff. Managers therefore have difficult decisions to make – should they compete with the new entrants, or concentrate on services where there is little competition? Should they cut back on 'luxuries' like clinical training in an effort to reduce costs, or fulfil their public duty to provide a comprehensive range of services and train the doctors of the future?

The second problem hospital managers face is the potential for an undermining of their position through the new entrants into the health economy. To give an example, if a particular hospital Trust is in financial balance, losing contracts has the potential to cause a deficit because funds that hospital had access to in the past are now going to other providers instead. Hospital managers then have to reduce costs or increase revenues to deal with the deficit, but increasing revenues might be impossible because it would imply attracting new sources of income to replace those lost from other geographical areas of care. As patients do not, in the main, appear to want to travel very far for their care (Fotaki et al, 2005), increasing income by attracting patients from others areas appears unlikely.

The more providers there are in a particular local area, unless there are year-on-year increases in budget to support the extra providers, the greater the danger that public organisations will have to make year-on-year cuts unless managers can find innovative new ways of providing services at lower cost. Managers may try to achieve this by behaving entrepreneurially and moving their services out of hospitals with high capital costs and into the community, as the government is encouraging them to. This, however, carries the threat of the hospital being left with fewer services to cover its overhead costs (which remain the same), which then leads in turn to the need for further cost reductions the following year. The new marketplace, if allowed to follow its own logic fully, could considerably undermine public provision, and in turn lead to the security of local provision being undermined, with no public services remaining if private providers leave the market.

The role of managers in the new economies of care is fascinating – they must compete with new providers and attempt to win contracts to drive out new providers and keep a constant resource base, or face losing out and so have ever-decreasing resources and difficult decisions to make about how to secure further savings. Either way, hospital management has become an increasingly difficult world.

At the same time, the new role demanded of managers in Primary Care Trusts, who are the purchasers of local care in the NHS, has become that of the entrepreneur. Care commissioning has gone from being an activity that involves contracting with the same public organisations year after year to one where new entrants have entered local health economies, and pathways of provision have to be established between public, private and not-for-profit organisations. The gold standard of service provision is that patients should not even notice when they move between providers or sectors; they should experience their care as joined up and integrated, and if managers find ways of contracting across all the sectors, and are able to implement an information system that prevents patients from having to give their details over and over again, this is at least theoretically possible. However, the move to contracting in an 'N'-form-dominated structure (that is, with care organised around networks rather than by services, all within the same organisation) created huge complexities and there is little evidence as yet that the information systems required are capable of supporting services organised in this way. The Primary Care Trust commissioning manager is now cast as an entrepreneur, working across boundaries to attempt seamlessly to stitch together new services that better suit the needs of patients. As long as patients (or GPs on their behalf) choose the new services, the money should flow to them through the contracts made, and successful new services expand.

Finally, there is the intriguing prospect, shared increasingly by the medical profession, that as more women enter positions of seniority in NHS organisations, and very different management styles appear, the potential significantly to change the dynamics of local health organisations exists (Greener, 2004b). There is evidence that women health managers are more focused on getting 'the job done' (Maddock, 2002) than competing with other managers, and that male doctors in particular often give way more to female managers more quickly than to their male counterparts (Greener, 2007). Equally, it may well be that medicine is practised differently by male and female doctors, and as increasing numbers of women enter the medical profession (Pringle, 1998), especially in general practice, patients' experience of doctors may change (Miles, 1991). This research is still disputed and in its early years, but offers a fascinating insight into how changing gender dynamics have the potential to make a considerable difference to the way in which health organisations are run (Brewis, 1999).

Conclusion

A simple summary of the contents of this chapter is that the role of health managers has become increasingly more diverse and complex as the history of the NHS has unfolded. The caricature of administrative practices in the early period of the NHS, based on bureaucracies that dealt with largely unimportant matters, but with doctors actually running health services, does have some credibility. At the same time, however, it involves the same administrators who dealt with the formidable task of getting the NHS up and running, and so it is unfair to claim that no good at all was done by them. Administration was based on principles of fairness, accountability, probity and service. These are fine virtues that form the centre of the public service ethic. It is wrong always to assume that bureaucracies are self-serving and inefficient (Du Gay, 2000) and the role of mediating between professionals can be shown to correspond to a great deal of modern management theory, positioning managers as coaches and enablers of others (Harrison et al, 1992).

By the 1970s, there was a strong suggestion that public managers could learn a great deal from their private counterparts. Public organisations had become far more expensive than previously, and economic difficulties led to demands for them to reduce their costs, while simultaneously, because of the growing consumerist movement (Haug and Sussman, 1969), to improve the services they offered. Public managers, therefore, as well as being facilitators, were required to be corporation-style managers, running services efficiently and according to their customers' needs. This was made most clear in the 1980s with the Griffiths Report (DHSS, 1983), which demanded that managers become individually accountable for their services, and was given an additional impetus by the introduction of the internal market in the 1990s.

In the 1980s, managers were also told that their job was to implement government policy on the ground. They were the corporate rationalisers of Alford's (1972, 1975) model, doing the state's work by making sure the policy implementation gap was filled. Managers who achieved this were to be celebrated, and those who did not comply were labelled as belonging to the past – dinosaurs who did not support reform.

The reforms of the 2000s have dramatically increased the stakes and the difficulties involved in managing health services. Managers have had to become far more financially aware, acquiring an understanding of the complexities of contracting in the new mixed economy of care, of tariff levels, of payment by results and of the PFI. Deficits in the NHS are not tolerated. Managers have therefore had to become competent accountants, able to balance their books (or even generate a surplus), as well as run their service.

In addition to this, managers at both hospital and Primary Care Trust level have found themselves having to acquire entrepreneurial skills. 'Entrepreneur' is a notoriously slippery word, but, in the sense of health managers acting as brokers to link together pathways of care, it is particularly apposite (Granovetter, 1973; Burt, 1993, 2000). Managers are required to be able to take a view across the network of care presently available within a local healthcare economy, and find ways of combining presently separate services into a seamless care pathway that meets patient needs (Dawson and Dargie, 2002). If they are able to achieve this, and to get a new service approved by the Primary Care Trust as one that can be chosen by patients, funds can flow to it and it has some chance of success.

Health managers are also asked to be leaders. They are required to comply with centrally imposed government targets (as corporate rationalisers) but also to come up with new ideas for how health services can be better run at the local level. They must then lead their organisations towards those goals, taking their employees, both clinical and non-clinical, with them. The leadership literature often has competing notions of what the term actually means, from trait-based models (Roberts, 2003) through to approaches that stress the transformational potential of leaders to delegate and empower those who work with them (Conger and Kanungo, 1998). Policy documents are not clear as to exactly what they mean when they demand better leadership from NHS managers, but the demands are certainly there.

Then there is the NHS guardian role (Schofield, 2001). Many public managers do not do their jobs for financial betterment or for career advancement, but instead because they wish to make a difference (Boyne, 2002). NHS managers may closely identify with the goals of their health organisations, and regard attempts to reform them as crude and clumsy attempts by politicians to interfere in something they do not really understand. In many ways, they have a point. Health policy has a tendency towards being somewhat circular. In the past 10 years, managers have seen the abolition of GP fundholding and its eventual reinstatement as practice-based commissioning, the claimed abolition of the internal market followed by its reincarnation as the mixed economy of care, the amalgamation of GP surgeries in Primary Care Groups and the abolition of health authorities, then the transition into Primary Care Trusts, and finally the merger of many Primary Care Trusts into organisations that might look a great deal like health authorities if they relinquish their role as health providers as well as purchasers. With all of this meddling it is a wonder that health services work at all. As such, the role of guardian appears to be an important one, trying to keep the waters within an organisation relatively still compared with the continually changing policies that may surround it.

Perhaps above all, and following from the Griffiths Report to the present day, managers are required to be accountable. This means that they are heroes or villains (Greener, 2005d). When health organisations work well and are high performing by government measures, they are cast as heroes, the ones responsible for delivering high achievement. When things do not work out, when hospitals or Primary Care Trusts have deficits or deliver care of low quality, it is the manager's fault. There are certainly good reasons for blaming managers when things go wrong – it is they who are meant to be responsible for the governance of their organisations. However, it is also politically expedient. It is a lot harder to sack doctors than it is to sack managers. Doctors are also a lot harder to replace than managers, as they have undergone an expensive and lengthy training period, and are a part of a profession that is still highly regarded. Getting rid of a manager, however, is relatively easy, as a replacement can usually be readily found, and there is unlikely to be much public sympathy for the removal of a poor-performing chief executive. Table 6.2 summarises the roles that NHS managers have found themselves asked to play.

Health managers therefore have incredibly demanding and Janus-faced existences. They are almost guaranteed, because of the variety of stakeholders they must deal with on a day-to-day basis, to be failing on some front or another. They also risk, because of the variety of roles they are required to adopt, appearing inconsistent at least some of the time. How is it possible to be both guardian and corporate rationaliser? To be both an administrator of probity and an entrepreneur? This seems to be the challenge health managers are now required to face – squaring the incompatible and extraordinarily difficult roles now demanded of them by the state. NHS managers have become important and powerful figures in the NHS, but are still derided in the media as an expense that detracts from patient care, and by doctors as interfering in their practice.

Table 6.2: NHS manager roles

Role description	Characteristics
Administrator	Probity Fairness Service Enabling
Corporation manager	'Big picture' management Efficient Customer-focused
Corporate rationaliser	Challenger of professional interests
Accountant	Balancer of budgets or creator of surpluses
Entrepreneur	Care pathway creator Adder of value
Leader	Goal setter Inspiration
Hero or villain	Accountability taker
Guardian	Preserver of the good of the past Stabiliser against unnecessary reform

Note

[1] I am grateful to Steve Harrison for introducing me to this phrase.

SEVEN

Nursing

Introduction

The role of nurses has been largely absent from the account of health policy and organisation so far presented in this book. This is no accident. It is hard to see what role nurses, as a professional interest group, had in shaping the discussions leading up to the creation of the NHS. They were positioned into the new health service in a role providing most of the care that patients required, but having very little say in how health services should be organised. Nursing is significant in discussions in the 1950s in terms of the relationship between GP and local authority healthcare, during periods of industrial militancy in the 1970s and the 1980s, and in debates about professionalism in the 1990s and 2000s. However, nurses remain, in Alford's (1972, 1975) terms, a repressed rather than a challenging interest in the NHS, despite being overwhelmingly the largest professional grouping within it. Why is this the case? This chapter tries to explore this question by giving an account of the development of nursing since the creation of the NHS.

The 1940s and 1950s

The effect of the creation of the NHS on the nursing profession was to remove a considerable amount of its autonomy. The rise of hospital medicine, and the dominance of consultants within it, institutionalised the position of doctors as the most significant interest group in the NHS. Nursing, in contrast, was a subsidiary profession expected to fill the holes left by other, male-led professional groupings in healthcare (Davies, 1995). This was perhaps clearest in the midwife role, which was effectively a community-based profession in its own right before the NHS, with midwives practising largely outside of the control of doctors and delivering children for the 50% of women who chose to have their babies at home (Lewis, 1990). The creation of the NHS, however, meant that midwives were now under the control of doctors, organised around medical units of administration based on hospitals, and much of their autonomy was lost (Jones, 1994). Midwives were required to report anything out of the 'normal' process of childbirth to consultants, with only 'natural' childbirth remaining under their remit.

At the same time, the GP was now the first port of call for women seeking midwifery services, making it clear that, in the community, midwives were subservient to GPs (Dingwall et al, 1988). The creation of the NHS continued a longer trend of the medicalisation of motherhood, bringing maternity services under doctor rather than midwife control (Oakley, 1984). Dingwall et al (1988, p 169) suggest that this should not be seen as a deliberate attack on midwives, however. Instead, they suggest it was a pragmatic solution to the problem of low midwife numbers.

As midwives had to defer to doctors, they became assistants to medics rather than independent community nursing professionals, now being called 'maternity nurses' (Dingwall et al, 1988, p 171), losing status and autonomy in the process. Giving birth in hospital became the norm rather than giving birth at home, based as much on the convenience of doctors as on safety grounds. The hospitalisation of childbirth deferred greater prestige on the relatively new Royal College of Obstetricians and Gynaecologists, which was instrumental in reinforcing the view that hospital was a safer place for women to have children, despite the lack of medical evidence to support this view (Lewis, 1990).

The nursing profession now depended on doctors for its legitimacy; doctors were responsible for the care patients received. Consultants, in turn, it could be argued, needed nurses in order to deliver the everyday care that patients required and doctors did not wish to give themselves. However, as consultants represented the elite of the doctors employed in the NHS, the relationship between nurses and consultants was one of deference towards the doctors on the grounds of both gender and class.

Nursing in the 1940s and 1950s was widely regarded as women's work. In this, it represented the continuation of a number of roles women had traditionally occupied; nursing was a 'distinctive secular occupation' for unmarried women (Turner, 1987), nurses were regarded as being 'spiritually equipped to bear the pains of drudgery on behalf of the helpless and the dependent' (Turner, 1987, p 147). Nursing's subservient role to male doctors suggested to sociologists of the 1950s a parallel between mothering and nursing (Schulman, 1958). The low pay, low prestige, unsocial hours, high staff turnover and lack of job autonomy were very much associated with the gender of nurses, and as such, many nurses entering the NHS in its early decades regarded it not as a permanent career, but instead as a precursor to marriage and having a family (Davis and Olesen, 1963). On the one hand, nurses used the female identity of their occupation in order to gain access to professional status in the sphere of employment and occupations at a time when opportunities for women were limited. On the other, however, doctors deployed the rhetoric of femininity to restrict the expansion of nursing and to safeguard their positions of patriarchal dominance (Gamarnikow, 1991).

Nursing was a career that was regarded as bringing out what was then perceived as the finest elements of the distinctive female personality. Nursing training was meant to help women cope with all the human emergencies they might expect to face in their lives as wives and mothers, and to render services selflessly to others (Hallam, 2000). All was not well within the profession, however. The Wood Report of 1947 into the training and role of nurses found some stark statistics; 'wastage' in the training of all nurses ran at some 54%, largely as a result of student discontent and the harsh discipline imposed during training (Rivett, 1998). This discipline, in turn, was something of a function of the simple fact that there weren't enough nurses in post to train students. There was a constant shortage of trained staff to oversee those training to become nurses, and those who did supervise training often had to take it on as an additional responsibility rather than being given any time to do the job properly.

A study by the Nuffield Hospital Trust in 1953 found that senior nurses spent very little time teaching student nurses (Nuffield Trust for Research and Policy Studies in Health Services, 1953). The problems of nurse recruitment and training led to recommendations that they needed to be dramatically overhauled. Nursing colleges were set up, with each region having an organisation independent of the hospitals there. Nursing education was to be given independence – a remarkable achievement at a time when nursing was presumed to be women's work, and women's work was ranked as inferior to that done by men.

The effect of the NHS on nursing was also very apparent in the role of the matron. In the 1950s, the value of the matron went from being 'one of service to the patient to one of service to the NHS' (Hallam, 2000, p 95) in the name of the 'common good'. This meant that the good of the nursing profession as a whole was often lost in debates about the future of nursing (White, 1985) as the notion of service to the NHS through nursing vocationalism became an intrinsic part of the nursing identity. Nurses became positioned as servants to their organisation rather than to their profession, in distinct difference to the way that doctors chose to represent themselves as accountable primarily to their professional bodies rather than to their local health organisations. In contrast, nursing appeared to have a more local and inward-looking focus towards completing the tasks required at their particular organisation rather than an outward-facing role concerned with wider debates about the role of nursing in health services. This was self-reinforcing in that, because nurses' views were not particularly sought in policy debates, they probably had greater potential to influence local health organisations, and so this gave them a strong incentive to participate more at the organisational than national level. However, it did mean that their voice was almost unheard by politicians and during the policy-making process. In direct contrast to the medical profession, nurses also secured very few positions on administrative boards in the new NHS. Doctors held about 30% of total appointments nationally. Nurses held 13 in total in 1947, which fell to seven in 1956 and only one in 1974 (Dingwall et al, 1988).

Two dominant representations of nursing present in the media in the 1950s showed them to be 'human characters rather than ... the embodiments of iconic ideals' (Hallam, 2000, p 45). It was, in these representations, the matriarchal matrons who were in place to run hospitals wards. First, there was the creation of the stereotype of the matron as 'battle-axe' (Hallam, 2000, p 45), being a middle-aged to elderly woman in charge, but with a kind heart, against which was juxtaposed, second, the 'angel' (the youthful and energetic, but occasionally foolish nurse). Hallam (2000) suggests that the battle-axe reflected 'a vocational image of nursing often found in Victorian popular fiction' (p 45), whereas for the younger group at least, nursing was portrayed as the 'ideal preparation for marriage' (p 47) – the 'romantic ideal' (p 62) at the heart of portrayal of nurses at this time. Nursing was therefore publicly represented by a generation of senior nurse spinsters devoting their lives to the service of the NHS, or as a place where young women could attract doctors, or at least prepare them for married life in an appropriate career.

The presentation of nurses in the popular media corresponds uncomfortably with archetypal female identities in the management and organisation literature. Young female nurses were portrayed as attempting to find themselves husbands, as the 'seductresses' (*British Medical Journal*, 1942; Marshall, 1984, p 103) of doctors. The link between care and nursing also suggests a strong link with the mothering archetype (Davies and Thomas, 2002), but with nursing also having strong elements of the 'Hera' (or 'wife') figure (Gherardi, 1995), in which a woman's role is to support and nurture her boss or husband, or in the case of nursing, the male consultant. Nursing carries with it a range of potent images and stereotypes that tend to overwhelm its status as a profession.

Representations of nurses in the cinema, in the 'Carry On' and 'Doctor' series of films for example, further emphasised the stereotypical way that nurses were viewed. As with any caricature, there is a small grain of truth in these images. The vocationalism demanded of senior nurses led to a cadre of older women in charge of local nurse training, and many young nurses still regarded nursing as a career to be pursued until they were married. That nursing was not regarded as a job for married women was partly the force of ideas around male breadwinners, but also because in the 1950s marriage 'bars' still persisted in which women were required to give up their positions on marriage. Nursing recruitment campaigns in the decade did little to try to persuade potential new nurses that these portrayals were anything other than accurate, with nurses pictured as staring admiringly at the side of male doctors while the doctors treated patients. It is remarkable the extent to which these rather vulgar images of nursing remain with us, even today, in popular culture. The characteristics of nursing in the 1940s and 1950s are summarised in Table 7.1.

Table 7.1: The characteristics of nursing in the 1940s and 1950s

Characteristic	Description
Nurses under the supervision of doctors	Nursing loses its autonomy as a profession in its own right (especially midwives)
Characterised as women's work	Nursing positioned as domestic labour for unmarried women, and training for marriage
Difficulties in recruitment and training	Nursing training takes place with few resources until establishment of nursing colleges
Inward-facing, vocational	Nurses work for benefit of their organisations rather than the profession

The 1960s

In the 1960s, many of the stereotypes of the 1950s were preserved, but the challenge of the feminist movement gathered pace, offering a critique of organisations that held women in subservient roles. There is little evidence that this made a great deal of difference to the experience of most nurses in that decade, however. That would have to wait until the 1970s. The 1960s were a decade in which nurses began to challenge their role within health services, particularly with regard to their pay, but their political powerlessness was made forcefully clear.

Problems in nursing recruitment persisted in the 1960s. Nursing had to compete with a number of other professions that young women could enter, with the influence of feminism gradually extending the range of opportunities available to women. However, nursing training still depended to a considerable extent on skilled nurses finding time from their ward duties to look after new recruits. These nurses were women who were pioneers in managing children at home and household responsibilities along with a continuing nursing career after the removal of the marriage bar, or women who had not married and had chosen to work through to retirement. Nursing generally had a very high turnover, and training was still clearly a problem, as even in the late 1950s student failure during training was still over 30%. In 1958, the *Nursing Times* reported that a number of factors made nursing unattractive, including unpredictable duty rosters, long hours, the expectation to attend lectures in off-duty times, strict discipline, exposure to night duty and the often excessive responsibility trainee nurses had to endure, bad conditions – the list went on and on (Rivett, 1998, p 186). Even when trained, and marriage bars removed, nurses often felt ill-equipped to deal with the demands their job made on them, and nurses continued to leave the profession after qualification.

The Salmon Report of 1966 reorganised nursing with the aim of modernising it, in order to achieve a more efficient use of nursing labour (Berridge, 1999). It introduced a managerial nursing structure that put in place a number of grades above the nursing sister and led to the abolition of the matron post. This parallel managerial structure gave nurses, at least on paper, as strong a voice as other vested interest groups in the running of the NHS, and eventually became institutionalised in the 1974 NHS reform through the founding of consensus management teams. Progress was being made in raising the profile of nursing in the NHS, but there were still considerable problems.

Vocationalism

The embedding of the discourse of vocationalism in the nursing profession meant that nursing was presented to its members as being something more than just a job; it was a career choice to which women could devote their lives. This was a double-edged sword. On the one hand, it made clear the considerable dedication that many nursing professionals gave to their jobs: working long hours, the provision of care that doctors refused to perform (such as tasks facilitating patients' basic hygiene), and the provision of a continuity of care for patients that the medical profession, required to see far more patients than nurses, was often unable to provide. Nurses provided the focal point of hospital treatment, the hub around which the rest of care was organised. Nursing could be hugely rewarding, providing a genuine opportunity to make a significant difference to other people's lives.

On the other hand, vocationalism had a downside, because it made it easy to characterise nursing as being women's work, reinforcing the stereotype of it being a natural extension of the mothering role (Kanter, 1977). As such, because nursing could be thought of as offering rewarding work in which women could find their vocation, it was less important to offer good pay and conditions in return. This dedication to the job, combined with the strong identification with local healthcare organisations rather than national professional bodies, meant that nursing had very limited scope for national organisation to challenge the difficulties that many individual nurses faced.

The combination of vocationalism with sexism meant that nursing was not perceived to be as important within health organisations as the medical profession. Given that nurses numerically overwhelm doctors in the NHS, this is remarkable. The lack of prestige afforded nurses was a function of the gendered assumptions about them, but also about their lack of preparedness, despite heavy unionisation, to pursue industrial action for fear of hurting patients. The group with potentially the greatest power to bring the NHS to a standstill was the least prepared to do so, and politicians were well aware of it. Nurses appeared to continue to comply with the 'total obedience' (Turner, 1987) role demanded of them, suggesting that although nurses were encouraged to be engaged in their work, they were also bound by duty to follow doctors' instructions without question, even where it jeopardised a patient's welfare (Gamarnikow, 1991). This unquestioning obedience appeared to be remarkably widespread in the 1960s (Hofling et al, 1966).

Splits within nursing

Nurses were far from being a unified profession. The split between nursing grades led to their separate unionisation, with registered nurses predominantly part of the Royal College of Nursing (RCN) (although the RCN was not officially a trade union until 1977), and enrolled nurses the National Union of Public Employess (NUPE) and the Confederation of Health Service Employees (COHSE). Because nurses belong to collective organisations so extensively, there was a reluctance by the profession as a whole, and specifically the leaders of the profession, to engage in industrial action, even where a single, unifying issue such as improved pay for all nursing groups could be identified. The split between the RCN and COHSE (later UNISON) is very significant in understanding nursing politics.

The RCN was the organisation that nurses with the most training tended to be affiliated with, and can be accused of representing that group only rather than members of the profession as a whole (Hart, 1994). Rule 12 of the RCN constitution meant that its members would not go on strike, and this meant that politicians tended to regard the RCN as a remarkably complicit body in pay negotiations. COHSE, on the other hand, was in many ways the opposite and very much prepared to support industrial action taken by its members. Hart suggests that the 'sherry sipping, middle-class women from the Home Counties complete with twin set and pearls would probably have been most COHSE members' caricature of the leaders of the RCN' (Hart, 1994, p 108), emphasising the difference between the two bodies. These differences are summarised in Table 7.2.

Table 7.2: The differences between the RCN and COHSE

RCN	COHSE
Founded in 1916 (Royal Charter in 1928)	Founded in 1946
Mostly made up of registered nurses, a nursing-specific body	Aimed to have single union representing NHS workers on its creation
Tends to be conservative in leadership, not a trade union until the 1970s, no strike clause for most of its history	Tends to be more radical in leadership, identified clearly as a trade union and prepared to engage in industrial action

As the decade wore on, the RCN opened up its restrictions on membership, especially with regard to male nurses, and this led to wider recruitment in areas such as mental health nursing, where it previously had little influence. Many male nurses, although still representing a small majority of the overall profession, went on to occupy senior roles in nursing unions and hospital administration, suggesting that there is some evidence that the gender split in the profession has divided nurses into separate career paths (Brown and Stones, 1973).

Nursing had also seen a considerable growth in what Abel–Smith (1975) called the 'third portal' – the nursing auxiliary. By 1958, there were 50% more of these 'unqualified' nurses in general hospitals than there were enrolled nurses (Dingwall et al, 1988), but with the registered nurses who often oversaw them denying them training, with the apparent aim of reducing their role to that of hospital domestics. This seems to show a lack of political solidarity on hospital wards, which did not help any of the three nursing groups to improve their respective positions.

This lack of cooperation between the RCN, which tended represent registered nurses, and COHSE, whose membership was made up mostly of enrolled nurses meant that the Whitley Council system set up to decide NHS pay awards did not really work in favour of the profession. By the late 1950s, 26 of the 53 major pay settlements had been to arbitration. The only reason the Whitley Council system survived was that nothing could be thought of as an alternative, and indeed it was working out rather nicely for the government, which had used Whitley Council's 'cumbersome, arm's length machinery … as means of depressing health service workers' salaries' (Sethi and Dimmock, 1982). Governments were able to claim that nursing pay was being decided independently so they were not responsible for it remaining low, even though nursing salary budgets were an obvious target for cost control in the NHS (Berridge, 1999).

Nursing pay

Even though nurses began to try to find ways of drawing attention to their plight in the NHS, it became clear that they held very little influence. In 1961, a 'pay pause' was announced by the Chancellor, effectively meaning no new rise in pay for that year would occur. This was after successive years of deterioration of nursing pay. In 1955-56, nurses earned 13% more than the average wage for women in lower professional groups, but only 2% more by 1960, and nursing pay was 68% of the national average wage in 1955-56, but only 60% in 1960 (Dingwall et al, 1988, p 112). An all-night demonstration was mounted to highlight the issue of nursing pay, with a debate in Parliament occurring soon after. The debate led to very little, and nurses, for perhaps the first time in the NHS's history, began to consider how they might secure more powerful representation without compromising the values on which their profession was based – a difficult conundrum because nursing strike action was likely to lead to patient neglect. It seemed that the state could treat nurses as it wished because it knew they would not respond. As Rivett (1998, p 189) put it, 'The government was teaching the lesson that "power tells" and imposing a pay pause on small people who could not fight back without injuring patients'.

By the end of the 1960s, nurses were beginning to realise how much they lacked influence over NHS policy. The return to power of a Labour government in 1964 had not improved things. Labour itself had pledged to abolish the Whitley Council in opposition, but did not honour this when elected to power, and its own pay policy led to a concerted campaign by the RCN at the end of the 1960s to improve pay through its 'Raise the Roof' campaign.

The 1970s

Chapter Four on the double-bed relationship between the state and the medical profession showed the 1970s as a decade where there were significant industrial disputes over medical representation, junior doctors' pay and pay-beds. Nursing also began to engage with industrial action in a concerted manner in this decade.

Industrial action

The early 1970s saw inflation rising and the government apparently struggling to run the economy (Hall, 1993). By 1972, nurses were losing ground on pay again. Competition for nursing members between the RCN and COHSE was fierce, and COHSE faced further competition from NUPE for the membership of health ancillary workers. Over 100,000 workers followed a call for a one-day strike in 1972, after which industrial action spread to over 750 hospitals. Although they did not win anything of note from the government, ancillary workers showed themselves to be prepared to engage in industrial action, and to interfere with patient care if it was necessary to get a better deal.

Nurses with a more militant voice joined COHSE rather than the RCN, and because of the access COHSE had directly to the government in corporatist politics, especially after 1974 after the re-election of Labour, they could feel that their views were influencing policy in an unprecedented way. Nursing, as a result of this competition over representation, appeared more fragmented than ever. The still-conservative RCN competed with the more militant and diverse COHSE, with the RCN claiming to be the most prestigious body, but COHSE arguably having the loudest negotiating voice. COHSE, however, was also having to compete with NUPE for nursing members, which also was keen to show its credentials in negotiating a better deal for nurses.

The RCN met with Barbara Castle, the Secretary of State for Health and Social Services, in 1974 to present her with its report *The State of Nursing* (RCN, 1974), threatening mass resignations if no improvements in pay and conditions were delivered by the government. While the RCN threatened, however, COHSE implemented a mass programme of industrial action, but again with apparently little effect. By 1978, the Callaghan government attempted to impose a 5% limit on pay, but this would have had a disproportionate effect on the low-paid in the public sector, as a 5% increase on a small wage represented a derisory improvement in pay at a time when inflation was still well above that figure. COHSE instigated a national campaign to attempt a better pay deal.

Nurses demanded an 18% increase in order to re-establish themselves at their 1974 equivalent level of pay, and they heckled politicians at an angry meeting on 18 January 1978. Porters, cleaners and laundry workers in the NHS also demanded a significant pay rise, joining with their co-workers and fellow members of COHSE and NUPE. Over the next two months, in the middle of what became known as the 'winter of discontent', the NHS appeared to be in turmoil. Nurses stopped short of strike action, but many worked to rule, refusing overtime or additional duties.

Industrial action in the 1970s meant that nurses began to challenge the stereotypes that were often used to portray them. Nurses were still described and characterised in the popular imagination as 'female, white, single and dedicated' (Hallam, 2000, p 21) – they were 'angels of mercy'. Salvage (1982) contrasted the militancy among many nurses in the late 1970s with the popular images from Mills and Boon romantic novels of nurses as doctors' handmaidens – an image that continued to appear repeatedly in NHS recruitment material, especially for non-qualified staff.

If the portrayal of nursing was changing only slowly, those who decided to become nurses were going through more significant change. By 1972, it was estimated that 25% of the nursing profession was made up of black and minority ethnic workers, but this group received virtually no coverage and never appeared in recruitment literature – they were 'invisible' (Hallam, 2000, p 118). By 1975, over 21% of all student and pupil nurses were from overseas, usually recruited to be enrolled rather than registered nurses, regardless of their background (Hart, 1994). Nurses from non-UK backgrounds were overrepresented in areas such as mental health and care of the elderly, which were often regarded as the least prestigious nursing areas, and few were to be found in the most prestigious teaching hospitals (Doyal, 1979, pp 205-6). Despite this rise in overseas nurses, they were not represented in the leadership of either COHSE or the RCN.

Perhaps most significant about this period was the demonstration that non-doctor NHS workers could effectively bring the service to a standstill. This was remarkable for those working within the service, but frightening to those who were attempting to run it. It appeared as if industrial relations in the NHS (and indeed across the whole of the public sector) had come to a head – the inclusive Labour government's approach was replaced by a Conservative government with a rather different attitude to trade unions.

Organisationally, the NHS reforms of the early 1970s did achieve a great deal for nurses. Despite the rather cumbersome structures put in place as a result of the rather tortuous process of government proposal and medical complaint that took place between 1968 and 1972, the final 1974 reforms gave nurses an unprecedented role in 'consensus' teams, where each member could potentially veto decisions they did not like. Nursing, theoretically at least, had acquired a voice as strong as that of the doctors in terms of day-to-day decision making within the NHS. Even if the 1974 reforms can be portrayed in retrospect as creating sclerotic structures that almost institutionalised inertia (Glennerster, 2000), nurses were given a much stronger role within health services.

The 1980s and further confrontations with the nurses

At the end of the 1970s, nursing was just beginning to explore the potential for challenging the second-class status it had held in the NHS by taking industrial action. Nurses were attempting to find ways of confronting the stereotypical images of themselves at this time, and come up with means of challenging the basis of their own professionalism – that of the 'carer' – and to find a new source of identity.

More pay disputes

In 1979, the RCN, although a trade union by that time, voted against TUC membership – COHSE, in contrast, was a longstanding member. The RCN held the balance of power on the nurses' and midwives' pay council (the Whitley Council – holding 12 seats out of 41 at its beginning, with COHSE holding just four) and with organisations sympathetic to the RCN also making up a significant part of its representation, effectively leading to the pay body being remarkably conservative.

This conservatism of nursing representation was to change as the 1980s wore on. 1982 saw an eight-month pay battle for the nurses. It marked another period of stark contrast between the RCN, which again refused to sanction strike action and was often openly disparaging of nurses who took part in the dispute, and COHSE and NUPE members, that appeared to want to use the dispute as a means of showing solidarity with the trade union movement (especially the miners) more broadly. With COHSE demanding a 12% pay rise, the Whitley Council found itself with a hung constituency, but with the RCN holding the casting vote (Hart, 1994). The representatives of the RCN voted in line with the government's proposals, even though its own members had rejected them twice. The government offer was eventually revised upwards, but not to the 12% demanded by COHSE. The reasons for the RCN continuing to cooperate with the government are complex. Hart (1994, p 86) suggests that:

> The more flexible approach of the RCN, their willingness to be seen to negotiate and pave the way for a settlement that many nurses wanted, made it easier for them to portray themselves as being in control of events, the architects of victory, particularly claiming the pay review body as their achievement, a claim supported by the Tories and Margaret Thatcher herself.

The divisions between the RCN and COHSE highlighted again the differences between nurses in the pay dispute. The RCN was attempting to position itself as the authentic voice of nurses, especially senior, highly skilled staff, and found its members rewarded for their loyalty in the pay review body's recommendations. COHSE, however, represented a more militant approach, wishing to stand with the trade union movement more generally in its opposition to Thatcherite policies, and prepared to be more radical in pay demands from it. The RCN, however, because of its status and position of power on the Whitley Council, appeared less radical; its role was more about representing the most highly trained nurses rather than the profession as a whole, than in trying to organise a challenge to the government.

Griffiths

The rest of the decade was a story of the voice of nurses, often raised in anger at NHS reform, being ignored. The Griffiths management reforms of 1983 (DHSS, 1983) dismantled the institutions of the 1974 NHS, removing nurses from the consensus decision-making teams. Nurses were allowed to apply for general management posts under the new rules, but then had to become managers rather than nurses (Petchey, 1986), showing the reduction in status resulting from the reforms, which seemed to ask nurses to give up their professional identities in return for seniority. Nurses reported that they felt 'mugged' by the reforms (Strong and Robinson, 1988). Even the RCN balked at this, investing some £250,000 on a campaign of opposition against the reforms, but it appeared to achieve little directly, even if it perhaps raised the profile of nurses in the wider community. The irony that Griffiths had used the imagery of Florence Nightingale wandering the corridors of the contemporary NHS in his report, while at the same time reducing the influence of nurses in management, must have been especially biting. At the same time as nursing appeared to be losing influence, however, ethnographic studies demonstrated the importance of nurses in medical training, where they were often required to give advice and support to junior doctors and locums (Hughes, 1988).

Professionalism

Nursing became increasingly professionalised during the 1980s, with increased professional control of entry coming from the UK Central Council, and the plans for Project 2000, which shifted nursing training towards an academic framework. New nursing roles appeared that created clinical nurse consultants, and in areas such as transplant surgery nurses could appear to have as significant a role as doctors because of the seniority of their roles. Enrolled nurse training, however, came to an end, only to be largely replaced by the new healthcare assistant grade. Nursing therefore remained a two-tier profession, split between its professional nurse and 'handy women' (Berridge, 1999) roles. A further split occurred in the 1980s when, as a part of the policy of compulsory competitive tendering, domestic work such as drink serving and cleaning was contracted out to the private sector, leading to a renegotiation of the boundary between healthcare assistants and privately employed domestics. In this situation, formal boundaries appeared between roles where previously there had been a great deal of flexibility and cooperation. Although costs may have been cut as a result of the policy, efficiency was probably reduced (Hart, 1991).

Strike action

In early January 1988, 37 NUPE nurses went on a one-day strike in Manchester after rumours that the government was recommending to the pay review body that nurses' special duty payments be removed. The official voice of the RCN, the *Nursing Times*, described the striking nurses as 'misguided' and RCN general secretary Trevor Clay condemned the action (Hart, 1994). Industrial action, however, spread rapidly across the country, especially in London where activists were more militant. There was an attempt to form an extraordinary meeting to discuss Rule 12, the rule in the RCN's constitution that the College would not strike. Another 24-hour strike was called on 2 February, and RCN members found themselves in the bizarre situation of being prepared in some locations to work double shifts to allow their COHSE colleagues to strike. Nursing, because of the strong sense of vocationalism among its RCN members, effectively blunted the industrial action and so removed the prospect of a serious challenge to the poor pay and conditions nurses as a whole continued to receive.

When the RCN lobbied against the internal market reforms in the late 1980s and 1990s they were once again largely ignored, but then again, so was the BMA, so this was more a reflection of Kenneth Clarke's wish to face down the NHS professional groupings than the lack of voice for nurses specifically. The nurses had shown increased militancy, even if it had not had the impact that many of its number might have hoped for.

The 1990s and 2000s

Boundaries between nursing groups

In the past two decades, nurses have found their jobs changing considerably. Registered nurses are increasingly moving away from everyday patient care, and finding themselves, through the creation of roles such as the 'nurse practitioner', embracing roles previously reserved for the medical profession – performing increasingly more specialist roles and even prescribing medication within limits. This has meant that the 'unskilled' nursing auxiliary is increasingly taking on the role formerly reserved only for 'skilled' nursing labour – the role is much less about making beds, and much more about providing basic patient care. This is intuitively empowering, but has occurred at a time when nursing is facing another of its recruitment crises. The numbers of nurses are still gradually increasing but this conceals widespread shortages, with temporary nurse recruitment increasing over 30% in the four years to 2004 (Carvel, 2004). The shortages are particularly significant in midwifery, where the 10 years to 2003 saw a marked reduction in the number of trained staff in the NHS (Boseley, 2003). There are also significant recruitment problems that exist in particular areas of the country. In London, it is still often more financially rewarding for nurses not to take on full-time roles in the NHS, but instead to enrol with a private nursing agency, and to work whatever hours suit them. NHS agency nurse bills remain startlingly high (BBC News, 2004).

Gender and nursing

An underresearched, but increasingly important area for research has come through the consideration of doctor–nurse relations where both professionals are women. As more women have entered the medical profession, nurses have increasingly found themselves working with women colleagues. This has introduced a new dynamic into nursing practice. Early studies suggested that nurses found that female doctors had taken on the same ethos as their male counterparts, and that they were treated in much the same way by them as a result (Savage, 1986). It also seems that nurses scrutinise the qualifications and practice of women doctors more closely than they do for their male counterparts, and that this causes those doctors greater stress as a result (Firth-Cozens, 1990).

An additional area where new research has highlighted differences within the nursing profession has come in examining relationships between male and female nurses. Some female nurses have suggested that male entrants tend to be ambitious and middle class, and that it is male nurses rather than doctors who dominate them (Salvage, 1985).

Consumerism

Nursing has also changed considerably through the consumerist movement in healthcare. As patients come to demand better service, it is nurses who face the brunt of their claims. Nurses now not only have to provide a high standard of care, they must also be perceived to be providing it. Complaints against nurses have risen on the basis of them providing inadequate service (Beardwood et al, 1999), and nurses report that the need continually to smile and engage in patient-friendly activities may actually detract from the quality of care that they offer (Bolton, 2001). Considering patients as customers puts nurses squarely in the position of having to provide frontline customer service; nursing professionals are already pressed for time because of the expansion of their roles in the past 20 years. The customer service role that is demanded of them adds to this pressure, by demanding a range of skills other than clinical expertise.

Matrons

Labour has recreated the role of the matron, attempting to place responsibilities for the cleanliness of wards and the efficient running of hospitals under their control, but the language associated with these reforms often frustrates and annoys those working within the profession. Many nurses regard themselves as modern professionals, not as the 'battle-axe spinster'[1] stereotype of this role. Patients (and certainly politicians), however, appear to like the idea of senior nurses occupying matron-type roles, and so they seem with us to stay, perhaps again highlighting the different priorities of the profession and of policy makers. It also seems unfortunate that the matron role has become predominantly associated in policy makers' minds with enforcing hospital cleanliness rather than governance leadership, a role that again seems to link more with gendered stereotypes than having a clear conception of nursing in the modern NHS (Witz, 1994). This is not to say that enforcing the cleanliness of hospitals is not an important role; the rise in hospital infections has shown that it is. But the association between stereotypical roles for women and cleaning suggests that policy makers need to work harder and more imaginatively in considering the future of the nursing profession.

The nursing role

Nursing has become a graduate profession for those entering the 'trained' grades and nurses are increasingly studying for postgraduate qualifications when taking on roles in nurse training and ward management as well. In addition to this, the creation of chief nurse roles has given an increased status and authority to those who occupy these posts, and nursing practice has become increasingly informed by work from the US that seeks to define the nursing professional as an independent clinical practitioner (Kelleher et al, 1994). The philosophy of the 'nursing process' attempts to translate this need for independence into an approach to everyday care (Witz, 1994), and is legitimated by claims to move nursing from a task-based approach to one that more closely meets patients' needs (Baggott, 2004, p 43). But the long hours and dedication that the role demands, often for poor financial rewards relative to those that can be achieved in other jobs that nurses can fairly easily move to, mean that it is hard to see how the profile of nursing can be easily raised and recruitment problems overcome. This shortfall affects both trained and auxiliary nurses, with the NHS having to rely increasingly on immigrant labour to plug the shortfall in trained staff. This is wonderful in encouraging the diversity and plurality of modern Britain, but imperialistic in its deliberate strategy of bringing in staff from abroad more prepared to work for the pay and conditions on offer in the NHS rather than addressing those pay and conditions directly.

Pay and conditions

The reasons why policy makers are not addressing nurses' pay and conditions are perhaps twofold. First, it is difficult not to attach a residual sexist notion to policy with regard to pay and conditions – nurses are overwhelmingly women, and their role has often been cast as that of doctors' assistants rather than autonomous practitioners in their own right. As such, their pay and conditions have always been somewhat down the waiting list of demands, certainly coming after the doctors in terms of priority. The pay awards granted to the GPs and consultants in the 2000s gave them access to significantly better rewards (NAO, 2007), and even though nursing pay has risen by around a quarter since 1997, this was from a low base. Nurses have periodically threatened industrial action and given Labour representatives a hard time when presenting to their various conferences, but industrial action on any kind of widespread basis has not occurred, and nursing, despite a brief period when it appeared to be explicitly mentioned in policy documents (Secretary of State for Health, 1997), still appears to hold very little influence in policy making.

Second, given that there are so many nurses in the NHS, any significant pay rise would have significant fiscal implications for the healthcare budget. In an era when financial probity has become a significant part of NHS decision making (Audit Commission, 2006), brokering a significant rise in pay for nurses would represent a significant challenge. However, the more pressing question should really be whether nurses deserve a significant pay award rather than its potential to cause financial difficulties for a period in which pay might be allowed to get to a reasonable level. But there are strong reasons for nurses having to retain the same poor pay and conditions – the differential pay between nurses and other NHS professional groups cannot be seen to be undermined, and nursing leaders, especially those in the RCN, are often far less radical than their membership. Both nurses and politicians know that nurses withdrawing their labour is unlikely, taking away a key negotiating tool for the profession.

Conclusion

This chapter began with the question of why nurses struggle, given that they are overwhelmingly the largest professional grouping within the NHS, to make themselves heard in the policy-making process. A number of answers have suggested themselves. First, the vocational nature of nursing means that nurses tend to be focused on the very real local difficulties of getting care organised rather than bigger national issues about access to policy makers. While nursing continues to regard itself as a vocation rather than a profession, this will continue to be a struggle. However, nurses in the 1990s and 2000s have become more professionally focused, and the number of nurses taking up managerial roles in health organisations means that barriers and stereotypes about the role of nurses are beginning to be challenged. This will hopefully lead to an increased number of nurses being confident enough to raise their horizons from their own organisations and to demand better national representation.

Second, there is a strong element of sexism in the status afforded to nurses. Nurses are by no means entirely all women, but it remains the case that most of them are. It is easy to cast nursing as women's work, a natural extension of feminine stereotypes, and so not really a proper job in some way. Women are 'exploited as nurses because they are socialised into a doctrine which equates nursing with mothering and sees the hospital ward as merely an extension of the domestic sphere of labour' (Turner, 1987, p 149). Nursing can be presented as a calling, a vocation, a version of the care role historically associated with women. In this line of thought, it would almost be insulting to offer women better pay as nurses, as it might lead to women who are not 'called' to the profession joining purely for financial gain. It is also rather insulting because nursing is hard, demanding work, and those who practise it are often financially rewarded pitifully. Nursing is also becoming a profession that takes on roles that are more associated with one of the most elite professional groups, the doctors, and treating nurses as if they are unskilled, easily replaceable labour is entirely inappropriate. Paying nurses more would involve a considerable financial commitment for the NHS, but one that is surely worth meeting.

Third, there is the conservatism of those who often represent nurses with whom most of the most highly qualified staff affiliate, the RCN. Hart's (1994) claims that the leaders of the RCN are often far less radical than its members has a great deal of explanatory power in considering why nurses have failed to punch their weight in discussions concerning NHS policy. While nursing leaders appear to be delighted simply to be asked to give their views, irrespective of whether or not they are taken into account in policy decisions, it is not likely to lead to a significant improvement for nurses in the NHS. Equally, the threat of industrial action begins to ring hollow from nursing leaders who always appear to back down when a firm decision is needed about whether industrial action is required to improve nurses' lot. In contrast, doctors often appear far more prepared to be radical in withdrawing their labour.

What has undermined doctors' attempts to confront the government has been the increased fragmentation of representation within the medical profession. A similar situation exists in nursing, with the RCN unable to speak for the whole nursing profession, and competition in trade union membership appearing to make some branches of nurses (those belonging to unions other than the RCN) more likely to take industrial action. At the same time, because nurses are unable to speak with a unified voice, this reduces the impact they are potentially able to make. That the RCN has been prepared publicly to condone the actions of nurses taking industrial action really has not helped to unify the profession or secure change.

Nurses must learn to exploit the fact that, in theoretical terms, they are the group most necessary for the NHS to function. They have the ability to stop the NHS in its tracks tomorrow with an organised and concerted programme of industrial action. But without significant change in the way in which nurses are represented, and without a considerable change in the attitudes that policy makers hold towards the profession, it is hard to see how nurses can improve their pay and conditions to the level they deserve. Nursing continues to develop as a profession, taking on roles formerly reserved for doctors, and with increasing managerial responsibilities. But this expansion of roles asked of nurses rarely brings with it corresponding rewards and status for the largest professional grouping in the NHS.

Note
[1] I am grateful to the (nurse) students of my MSc Population Health group at York for the creation of this phrase.

EIGHT

The role of the public in health policy

Introduction

In the past 10 years, there has been a significant increase in interest in the way that policy has positioned the users of public services in relation to professionals and managers (Deacon and Mann, 1999; Le Grand, 1999; Greener, 2002b). From being overlooked in much analysis in the 1970s, which often focused on the relationships between the state, managers and doctors, an interest in the experience of the user of health services has come along with a new emphasis on both consumerism and citizenship in healthcare. The central question this chapter examines is how the NHS, and how NHS policy, has positioned the users of health services. Have they been thought of largely passively, receiving services from professionals, or having their interests looked after by managers? Or are they instead assumed to be active co-producers of their own healthcare, or even healthcare consumers, taking responsibility for making medical decisions for themselves and demanding improved care from doctors?

Position of the public in the early years of the NHS

At the creation of the NHS in 1948, lists of GPs were published to allow the public to choose the GP with whom they wished, in the terminology of the time, to form an 'association' (Ministry of Health, 1944). This means that the public were establishing a long-term relationship with their GPs, and were not expected to change their doctor frequently, or even at all (Greener and Powell, 2009: forthcoming). Doctors initially appeared to be concerned that, as patients were now receiving care free of charge, they would march into practices declare that as doctors were now public employees they had better start improving their service (Webster, 1998b). These fears appeared largely unfounded, however, with patients usually relieved just to be receiving free care for themselves and their families, and so largely happy to accept doctors in their professional roles. General practitioners were regarded as family doctors, trusted local people often held in high regard, in whose presence patients were largely deferential and grateful. Considering that around half of GP practices comprised doctors acting alone, there was the potential for a close and long-term relationship between the GP, who might know families across several generations, and the patient.

The association relationship between GPs and patients was a long-term one not simply because of patients' loyalty. It could, in practice, be rather difficult for patients to change GP once they had made their selection of doctor. This was exacerbated by GPs' lobbying in the early years of the NHS to prevent patients from changing their registered doctor on the grounds that it was 'abusing' the system (Titmuss, 1958) and resulted in a rule change in 1950 that put in place a waiting period before a change could occur, and the written consent of the existing doctor (Ministry of Health, 1950). This created a barrier that patients often found embarrassing and time-consuming, and so limited the scope for patients to change their GPs easily.

The problem with the associational model in place in the NHS between 1948 and the early 1970s was that it effectively ignored the asymmetrical power relationships between GPs and patients. General practitioners, in their gatekeeper role, effectively controlled whether or not prescriptions would be written, and whether patients were referred to hospitals for specialist care. In addition, doctors were usually socially elevated and well educated, and held expert knowledge, that patients would have found difficult to challenge. General practitioners had expertise in physiology and diagnosis that patients were not privy to, and widespread access to medical knowledge was simply not available.

Accounts of doctors dating from the early years of the NHS portray GPs as being dedicated and working long hours, but having few opportunities to display their medical knowledge as their role involved referring complex cases to hospitals and dealing for the most part with relatively common and mundane illnesses. Patients recognised that GPs had long lists of people waiting to see them, and put up with waiting and often poor surroundings for their consultations.

Consultants were portrayed as heads of clinical fiefdoms in hospitals, clever but arrogant, curt and rushed, treating patients more as collections of symptoms, as problems to be solved, than as human beings (Fox, 1993). In film and television portrayals of the period, hospital doctors often spoke about patients as if they were not really there, discussing symptoms with other doctors on 'rounds' and referring to patients in the third person even where they were standing in front of them. Patients appeared rather passive, waiting to be briefly seen by the swarm of consultants and junior doctors, while receiving the majority of their care from nurses. Of course, things were not always like this; some consultants were caring and considerate, and some GPs were prompt in seeing patients and had considerable expertise in their own right, but these caricatures still resonate with anyone who has experienced NHS care.

Knights, knaves, pawns and queens

Le Grand (2003, 2007) suggests that for much of the welfare service's history, users have been treated as pawns, effectively powerless individuals who rely on professionals behaving in a 'knightish' or virtuous and self-disinterested way with them. He suggests that this mode of operating has significant problems. First, if professionals are not knightish, but instead behave in a 'knavish' manner, they may have remarkable scope for pursing these less-than-beneficial ends. Le Grand suggests that it is necessary to devise incentive structures in welfare organisations so that professionals have an opportunity cost for behaving knavishly (Le Grand, 1997). Extending this work, he has come to the conclusion that the best way of organising public services to achieve this goal is to increase user choice, treating users as 'queens' (powerful, autonomous figures), and organising welfare services much more around their wishes (Le Grand, 2007). The use of markets, according to Le Grand, empowers welfare users to the most significant extent; therefore, there should be a greater use of the choice mechanisms that market systems promote. These claims will be discussed later on in this chapter, as market-based solutions were not introduced into UK healthcare until the 1990s.

Considering the theoretical relationship between GPs and patients, it seems that patients remained, unless they moved to a new area, with the GP they initially registered with. Patients were not quite the passive 'pawns' characterised by Le Grand, as GPs worked extremely long hours, often making house calls well into the evening, and offering a remarkably personalised service. Le Grand is right in suggesting, however, that expectations of the role that patients were expected to play in their healthcare were rather low – they were meant to do what the doctor told them. Patients were positioned rather passively, but GPs often worked extremely hard to provide them with care. This seems a like a professional–client relationship in which the client was considered passive, but where the professional was prepared to work hard to meet the client's needs, even if there was little threat of them going elsewhere. Appeals to the professional to provide better service were not based on the threat of the patient going to another doctor, but instead to the sense of professionalism or even vocationalism of the doctor. General practitioners had an incentive to have as many patients on their lists as possible, as they were paid on a capitation basis (see Chapter Three), but as patients could not easily move to a different doctor, they had little incentive to provide good service other than conforming to their own professional standards. However, in most cases, this was probably enough to get doctors to behave as 'knights' (Klein, 2005), despite there being real asymmetries between the needs of patients and the rewards made available to GPs.

The relationship between the patient and the consultant, on the other hand, was likely to be of a different character. Most patients experienced hospital care (outside of long-term care) episodically, in relation to a particular illness or injury that a course of treatment in hospital was meant to remedy. Consultants might have seen patients only once, and treated them only for the time they were resident in the hospital or attending a clinic. It may even be the case that the named consultant never saw the patient themselves, putting patients in the direct care of more junior doctors in their specialism. As consultants worked with teams of doctors whom they oversaw, patients may never have seen the same doctor twice, and when they did see doctors, might have experienced very different bedside manners and so have had very different experiences.

The majority of care in non-outpatient settings in hospitals was (and still is) delivered by nurses, who provided continuity between the occasional episodes when the consultant or their colleagues called. Consultants appeared to patients, as their name implies, as professionals to be consulted rather than to provide care themselves. Patients saw consultants at the doctors' convenience rather than their own, and then the experience may have been a remarkably passive one. Le Grand's notion of the passive 'pawn' fits the bill remarkably in explaining the hospital experience of many patients, who were often uninformed of what was going on, talked past rather than to, and who were expected to organise their time to suit the consultant rather than vice versa.

Before we go too far in deploring this model, however, it is worth reflecting on the sheer busyness of many hospital doctors, who have expert knowledge that might be in short supply, and who may have regretted the transactional way in which they were often forced to behave with patients because of a sheer lack of time to see patients and a pressing schedule (Tallis, 2005). In such circumstances, it is perhaps understandable that patients were expected to fit around the consultant's schedule. There is potentially a clash between efficiency, where doctors, as the scarce resource in the relationship, see as many patients as possible and at their convenience, and good service, where patients would be seen according to their convenience, and in a less rushed and more friendly manner. This clash illustrates the difficulty that public services often have in accommodating consumerism into their practices.

Citizenship at the creation of the NHS

At the creation of the NHS, the public were not only potential clients of health professionals. They were also citizens of the new UK welfare state. Access to the NHS's services free at the point of care represented a new right granted to the public, and can be seen as part of the extension of rights generally, as outlined by Marshall (1950) in his hugely influential work on citizenship. Marshall suggested that civil rights were predominantly given in the 18th century, and were mostly associated with the protections given to the public through law. Political rights were given predominantly in the 19th century, and gave the right to political participation and representation, with the extension of the voting franchise probably being the most significant achievement. Social rights, in Marshall's view, came along in the 20th century, and were based on the state accepting responsibility for guaranteeing a minimum standard of living for its public.

So as well as being clients of health professionals, the public were also citizens with a newly established social right, that of access to healthcare free at the point of need. Citizenship was therefore expressed primarily in terms of the rights that citizens held, rather than any responsibilities they had to fulfil (other than being a member of the nation state in question). This is directly in line with the conventional wisdom about the role of users in welfare organisations (Stewart and Walsh, 1992), where politicians were responsible for the running of services in a way that made them accountable to the public. This discourse was present in Bevan's famous aphorism that responsibility for the running of the NHS was based straightforwardly in Whitehall, where, he suggested, the corridors rang to the sound of bedpans being dropped, but this doesn't really bare much scrutiny in practice. At the creation of the NHS, there were few mechanisms by which user voice could be involved in policy making or local implementation, and it is hard to see how General Elections every five years could achieve any degree of accountability or allow the participation of users in any other significant way. The role of the public at the time of the creation of the NHS is summarised in Table 8.1.

Table 8.1: The role of the public at the creation of the NHS

Role	Description
Associational relationship with GP	Able to choose GP, but supposition of entering a long-term relationship from which it was difficult to move
Asymmetric relationship with GP	Patients need GPs for care, but GPs only need patients on their 'list' to be paid. Patients as clients of GPs
Passive relationship with consultant	Care is episodic and organised at consultants' convenience – patients as pawns
Citizen role	Public has right to receive care, but with few responsibilities in return – effectively passive role

The 1960s and 1970s

Criticisms of care

During the 1960s, feminist critiques of healthcare suggested that it was often organised around what was more convenient for the doctor than for the patient (Nettleton, 2006). Concerns expressed by feminists were particularly focused on maternity services where practices such as episiotomy were especially criticised, with some doctors found to be almost routinely performing the painful operation not in order to make birth safer for the woman, but because it was easier for the consultant. Campaigning and informing women of their rights, the feminist movement helped demonstrate the possibilities for mounting an intellectual as well as political challenge to the medical profession (Stacey, 1998). Alongside feminist groups, disability rights campaigners from the 1960s onwards have been instrumental in challenging medical models of care, attempting to normalise members of the public with missing limbs and learning difficulties, and establishing appropriate and supportive means of care geared to individuals rather than societal norms (Clarke, 2004). Their interest groups demanded that patients be treated as individuals with specific needs – not as representing some kind of generically disabled group who needed to be somehow made whole again through the use of prosthetics or to be hidden away from the rest of society (Welshman, 2006a).

These social movements were important because they created space within which legitimate criticisms of medical practice could be offered, which were combined in the 1970s with mounting evidence that inappropriate and over-medicalisation could actually be damaging to health (Illich, 1977). This period also marks the founding of many health users groups, which were to campaign to improve patient care, typically in relation to a particular condition (Allsop et al, 2002). Initially, the mental health groups appeared to have the most impact, particularly around scandals in the conditions of health institutions at the end of the 1960s (Klein, 2006).

There was also, by the 1960s, concern that hospitals were treating patients more generally in an impersonal and often careless way. Titmuss (1958, p 125) wrote:

> How often one comes across people who have been discharged from hospital, bewildered, still anxious and afraid; disillusioned because the medical magic has not apparently or yet yielded results, ignorant of what the investigations have shown, what the doctors think, what the treatment has been or will be, and what the outlook is in terms of life and health.

Titmuss suggested that the hospital had become isolated from the community it was meant to be serving, and although medics were not conspiring to serve patients badly, this was often the end result. The solution, in his eyes, required administrators to intervene to make sure that their organisations cared far more about patients in order to deal with what he called the 'catalogue of hospital inertia' (Titmuss, 1958, p 131). Many of the same sentiments were expressed from the opposite end of the political spectrum by Enoch Powell during his time as Health Minister, who criticised the 'conveyer-belt' approach of maternity hospitals and of the inflexible practices he found in relation to patient care and patient visiting more generally (Watkin, 1978, p 119).

Community Health Councils

The first concerted attempt organisationally to improve services to patients came in the reforms of 1974 with the establishment of Community Health Councils (CHCs) (Secretary of State for Health and Social Services, 1972). Community Health Councils were often at their most effective in lobbying local hospitals through the media to make changes. Complaints could be escalated outside of the often poor procedures in NHS organisations, but not every case was felt to be deserving and useful to the media, leaving the issues CHCs could campaign about fairly unbalanced because of their inability to participate as equals in the running of hospitals.

Equally, CHCs were not representative of their local communities (if such a thing is even possible) and were bodies at least as much appointed as elected, meaning that they were not bastions of democracy either. Klein and Lewis (1976) label CHCs as 'consumer' organisations, but this is not quite right, as they often had most success in campaigns over systemic rather than individual failings in health organisations, and so in contemporary parlance were rather closer to being issue-based campaigning organisations that attempted to bring about policy changes. They sometimes campaigned on behalf of individuals in their local areas, but then usually to try to get policies changed for everyone rather than to deal with individual failings in health organisations. Community Health Councils held power only in the sense that they could 'throw grit into the normal machinery of NHS decision-making: to impose delays' (Klein, 2006, p 84). They were both an ally of the medical profession, in that they could support it in demands for improved resources and services, and enemy, in that they could be mobilised in complaints against doctors.

Community Health Councils were not attempts to create representative organisations, being based on member appointments, and were extremely variable in their ability to help patients deal with the problems they experienced. Levitt (1976, p 193) described the CHC role soon after their creation:

> The meetings of CHCs are open for members of the public to attend ... who may be given the opportunity to speak. People can also call at the CHC office for help and advice. If they have complaints about the NHS the CHC can explain how to make best use of the official channels and procedures. Although it is not the responsibility of CHCs to judge or investigate individual complaints, by playing an active part they can support people through what may be complex and bewildering encounters with the NHS administration and they can comment constructively on areas of complaint to the health authorities.

As such, health service users were subject to a kind of compulsory loyalty as the NHS was the only potential provider of care, and it was not, from Levitt's quote, organised to be responsive to user complaint or query. Users appeared, for the most part, to be rather passively positioned, and depended on the professionalism of their doctors to receive good care. The client-based model still dominated.

The increasing numbers of consumer groupings in healthcare that appeared in the 1960s and 1970s shared something in common with CHCs in that they appeared to be as much citizen organisations (albeit, again, usually organised around a single issue or illness) as consumer organisations because they made collective representation to healthcare organisations, or to the Department of Health itself, in order to try to make change happen. Health consumer groupings were important in that they provided a means for enabling hard-to-reach or excluded voices to be heard within the healthcare policy context when they might otherwise have been excluded. They also provided a means for those with particular conditions to learn from one another's experiences, to gain access to the most recent research on their conditions, to support one another and to lobby for greater funds or importance to be attached to their conditions (Baggott et al, 2004). They were more citizen-type organisations than consumer organisations in that they might use individual case studies as a kind of exemplar of present policy failing, but their campaigning was predominantly on behalf of collectives to make policy changes that affect whole groups, rather than representing individuals.

A different meaning to participation appeared in the language of health policy in the 1960s and seems set for a comeback under the Prime Ministership of Gordon Brown in the present day. In the 1960s, a call for greater participation through volunteering was a part of policy in the latter half of the decade in which the Secretary of State called on the public to become involved in health services to make a personal contribution to their running. The logic of this was that 'The greater the participation of the local community in its local health services, the greater the response of the service to the community's needs and of the community to the service's needs' (DHSS, 1970). This cast the NHS and the local community in a virtuous circle of improvement. However, writers including Titmuss (1958) regarded the move towards greater participation through volunteering as a 'fashion' that was unlikely to come to anything.

Choice and healthcare

In 1972, healthcare users were presented as having an additional choice available to them in the policy document *The National Health Service Reorganisation* (Secretary of State for Health and Social Services, 1972) that had not appeared in policy documents prior to then, but had always potentially existed. The document specified that it was 'right for people to have an opportunity to exercise a personal choice to seek treatment privately' (s.166). Health users were being conceptualised as something different from the client of a devoted professional – as a proactive chooser of care. Of course, this concealed a great deal. Private care was only available to those who could afford it, or those whose employers paid for private health insurance. However, this seems to be the beginning of presenting health users in a more consumerist way, with health choices being equivalent to those found in other aspects of life. Within the public sector as well, this more consumerist notion was present, with the care available to patients designed to offer 'services best suited to his needs, his convenience and, as far as practicable, his choice' (section 48).

The 1980s and 1990s

Principals and agents

Alongside the growth in managerial thought in the 1970s, a new discourse of criticism appeared that allied well with the feminist and disability rights concerns of the earlier decade. Questions began to be asked about why public organisations couldn't treat their 'customers' as well as private sector institutions did. In the NHS, the clearest articulation of this appeared in the *NHS Management Inquiry* of 1983 (DHSS, 1983). Griffiths suggested that managers had to be put in charge of health organisations to take responsibility for them and to drive up standards of care. In the 1980s, the producer-dominated relationship between doctors and patients began to be reformulated as one that should instead be that of principal and agent. Doctors were *agents*, holding expert knowledge and with access to health service resources. Patients were *principals*, lacking the knowledge to make clinical decisions for themselves, but worthy of consultation from doctors, who were meant to be acting on their behalf to secure the best possible care. This recasting of relationships should have led to an improvement in the care offered to patients, who suddenly found themselves being asked to fill in questionnaires about their experiences in health organisations, but it is difficult to untangle the evidence to work out if this occurred or not. The public in general continued to be remarkably satisfied with the NHS – it was among the most popular institutions in the UK (vying for first place with the Royal Family) – but this may not have been entirely reflective of those who were receiving its care.

More criticisms of care

The feminist critique of organised medicine continued in the 1980s. Although the improved access to health facilities had led to women receiving care far more easily than they did before the creation of the NHS, a reaction against high-technology medicine appeared to grow in momentum (Berridge, 1999). In the US, the publication of *Our Bodies, Ourselves* by the Boston Women's Health Collective in 1971 led to a UK version of the text in 1978, and women having greater access to material about their bodies, allowing them to play a greater role in determining their own health (Jones, 1994). By the mid-1980s, gender politics appeared to coalesce around arguments about maternity care in particular, highlighted by the case of consultant obstetrician Wendy Savage in London, who was suspended from her duties largely, in some commentators' eyes, because her women-centred practices met with disapproval and a campaign of smear tactics by male colleagues.

As the government became increasingly enthusiastic about advertising the benefits of healthier lifestyles on television, the public increasingly chose to visit complementary and alternative therapists (Saks, 1994). There are a number of reasons why this might have occurred: a growing disaffection with western medicine (Le Fanu, 1999), the relatively short times patients spend with doctors in the UK (Payer, 1996) or the increased interest in spirituality coming from affluence (Offer, 2006). This tendency to visit alternative therapists was allied with the growth of self-help groups, and their joint ability to 'address the expressive needs of people' (Kelleher, 1994, p 116). By the 2000s, a Chinese herbalist seemed to be on every high street, demonstrating the remarkable growth of the industry. The number of public visits to complementary therapists is hard to pinpoint, but seems to have risen from around 12 million in 1993, to 15 million in 1997 to, astonishingly, over 30 million by 2003 (Peckham, 2006, p 525).

The internal market

The Conservatives' internal market has already been examined in earlier chapters in terms of the way it changed relationships between the state and the medical profession, between doctors, and between doctors and managers. It also had significant implications for doctor–patient relationships. The reforms extended the principal–agent relationship between GPs and patients further. Patients were meant to choose their GPs (although it continued to prove, in practice, to be difficult to change doctor), and GPs were meant to serve the wishes of their patients in referrals. Patients were meant to exercise a 'real choice between GPs' (Secretary of State for Health, 1989, s. 7.4) – an emphasis not on making a choice of GP for the long term as in 1944, but instead on changing doctor 'without any hindrance at all' (s. 7.7), a more short-term transactional notion of GP selection. General practitioners were now there to serve their patients' needs, and 'fundholding' GPs were given budgets so that those choices carried with them resources. General practitioner fundholders were meant to be dynamic purchasers of care on behalf of their patients, and for whom the evidence suggests reduced waiting times were achieved (Propper et al, 2002). However, this could potentially have created a problem of equity, as if fundholder patients were receiving care more quickly, it might have been at the expense of those non-fundholder patients (Petchey, 1995). However, patients did not appear to be aware that they might be able to get quicker referrals from fundholding practices – there is no evidence of them reregistering and changing GPs in order to receive a quicker service.

The internal market reforms also meant that most health research at that time was busy looking for changes in referral patterns or for new providers appearing; in other words, trying to assess the changes in producer behaviour rather than examining whether patients were more satisfied as a result. Patients seemed, if anything, to have become more dissatisfied as a result of being members of fundholding practices, despite the evidence that they may have been treated more quickly (Dusheiko et al, 2004b). A supply-side explanation for this might be that fundholders had incentives for reducing referrals and prescriptions because they were able to invest any 'surpluses' on their budgets in practice development. As such, patients might have experienced a reduction in referrals and prescriptions as a reduction in service, even if those who actually received referrals were seen more quickly. A demand-side explanation would be that patients registered with fundholders had rising expectations of the service they would receive, and so were likely to be dissatisfied even if standards were raised. Equally, despite the rhetoric about doctors now having an incentive to follow patients' wishes more closely, patients were not granted additional choices by the reforms, and there were no real additional mechanisms for getting doctors to provide better service to them (Maynard, 1993). Table 8.2 examines the patient–GP relationship after the internal market reforms.

Within the internal market increased use of the private sector was again encouraged, and patients were described in an even more dynamic way: 'People who choose to buy health care outside the Health Service benefit the community by taking pressure off the Service and add to

Table 8.2: The patient–GP relationship after the internal market reforms

Actor	Relationship
Patient	Dependent on GP for referrals and prescriptions. Positioned by policy as principals in principal–agent relationship, but with few mechanisms for asserting role. Reduction in satisfaction with fundholding GPs after reforms
GP	Fundholding GPs in receipt of budget, so incentive to prescribe and refer effectively. Positioned by policy as agents, but with few incentives to be more responsive to patient need because of lack of patient assertiveness or threat of changing GP

the diversity of provision and choice' (Secretary of State for Health, 1989, s. 1.18). Those who could afford private care were portrayed as altruists, taking pressure off public resources and allowing greater choice for those receiving care within the public sector. This was meant to work because 'introducing more choice into the provision of services will greatly increase the opportunities for managers to buy in services from the private sector where this will improve the services to patients' (Secretary of State for Health, 1989, s. 9.12).

The evidence from the first internal market reforms appears rather contradictory in terms of the role of the patient. On the one hand, patients did not change GPs to receive the care of fundholders, who might have been able to access quicker referrals on their behalf, suggesting that they did not understand the new way in which healthcare was organised. On the other hand, patients receiving care from fundholders appeared less satisfied, even though they were likely to be referred more quickly than before. The principal–agent model was constrained by doctors not having much of a choice of alternative providers, even if they wanted to contract for the best possible care on behalf of their patients.

The idea of driving health reform through the internal market seemed doubly hamstrung by the lack of a real care market and a lack of awareness and information for patients to make informed choices of GPs. There was less of a change to the role of the patient than the principal–agent model might have suggested. Patients, in Le Grand's (1997, 2003) terms, still appeared to exhibit strong 'pawnish' tendencies, not being sufficiently informed or motivated to choose GPs that might have given them shorter waiting times, but perversely, reporting themselves less satisfied where they had access to this benefit, as stated above. This suggests that the consumerist discourse present in healthcare was beginning to be incorporated into patients' vocabularies in a negative sense in which it acted as a source of dissatisfaction rather than motivating patients to drive reform. Patients were increasingly inclined to challenge doctors where they felt they were receiving poor service (although this might have been predominantly the middle classes), but appeared either unwilling or unable to exercise choice where they were dissatisfied. In turn, 'voice' mechanisms such as complaint remained underdeveloped in the NHS (Allsop and Jones, 2008), despite having been noted as a problem in policy documents since the 1970s (see, for example, Secretary of State for Health and Social Services, 1972). Improvements in care appeared to depend on the assertiveness of the individual patient and the extent to which the doctor before them was prepared to accommodate them, a different form of voice that was far more individualised and reliant on the patient's skill in negotiation, than on any mechanism intrinsic to health service reorganisation. Patients were principals according to NHS reform, but with very few mechanisms for delivering improved service from their agents, and so still locked into a relationship that was more client- than consumer-based.

The Patient's Charter

The 1990s were also significant for the instigation by the Major government of charters (Prime Minister, 1991), with the *Patient's Charter* (DH, 1991) giving patients a confusing list of customer service standards that they were meant to expect, but with little sanction in practice should they not be met (Allsop, 1995). Individual outpatient appointments were given to patients for the first time, rather than them being expected to turn up at the same time as several other people and be seen at the convenience of the consultant. After this, in 1994, the Department of Health published performance guides for the first time, giving star ratings (with the highest scoring five stars, as a hotel might) based on many of the charter requirements (NHS Executive, 1994). Despite the attempt to position patients in a more consumerist role coming from the rhetoric of the *Patient's Charter*, little seemed directly to change as a result of the charter's introduction; the public were generally unaware of the performance of their local health organisations, and they were given few enforceable rights as a result of the introduction of the charter. Although this was a form of top-down consumerism, it came with few teeth and did not appear to be welcomed (or even noticed) by the public.

The 2000s

In 2000, the NHS Plan (Secretary of State for Health, 2000) reminded patients that they had 'the right to choose a GP' (s. 10.5) and that 'to make an informed choice of GP, a wider range of information about GP practices will be published' (s. 10.5). As in 1989, this was a principal–agent approach, in which patients chose GPs and GPs chose care on behalf of their patients. As well as this, however, there was a recognition that professionals had to take their individual users' voices more seriously: 'today successful services thrive on their ability to respond to the individual needs of their customers' (s. 2.12). In recognition of the problems users had in getting their complaints heard, there was a drive to improve procedures, whereby 'the government will act to reform the complaints procedure to make it more independent and responsive to patients' (s. 10.21), specifying that patients should be listened to in their interactions with health professionals, and making it clear that they should complain if they are not.

By 2006 (DH, 2006b), it was no longer GPs who made decisions about where they should be treated, but patients: 'In the NHS, patients now have more choice of the hospital that they go to, with resources following their preferences ... driving down maximum waiting times' (s. 3). General practices were to 'redesign care pathways to match patients' needs and wishes' (s. 6.8), with the relationship between GPs presented as a competitive one: 'To ensure that there are real choices for people, we will introduce incentives to GP practices to offer opening times and convenient appointments which respond to the needs of patients in their area' (s. 1.9). In order to make hospital choices, patients would need support: 'Individuals, their families and other carers need to understand the services that are available in order to make good choices, and they need to receive maximum support in obtaining their chosen service – wherever it is provided' (s. 8.42).

Health consumers

In the 2000s, therefore, a new model of how patients were meant to interact with health services emerged (6, 2003). Since 2001 (DH, 2001a), patients have been increasingly cast not in the principal–agent relationship with doctors, but as fully-fledged health 'choosers', with organisational systems being put in place for them to make choices about who they will be referred to in secondary care, and when. Patients in need of secondary care, or a referral to a practitioner such as a physiotherapist, were meant to make the choice for themselves. A plurality of new providers had entered the health marketplace from the private and not-for-profit markets, meaning that competition between those providers could now happen. Patients were meant to be both willing and able to drive health reform for themselves as active consumers of care. At the very least, they were meant to approach the NHS with raised expectations of the care they might receive (Sang, 2004).

However, it is unclear exactly how patients are meant to make the new choices available to them within the NHS institutions presently in place. Patient choices can take place in surgeries, in which case GPs must either rush through the process of the 'Choose and Book' computer system with the patient, to avoid falling too far behind on the appointment list, offering little time for discussion or information provision, or expect the patient to wait. Alternatively, on leaving the GP, patients could wait for another appointment with a patient choice adviser provided at the expense of the surgery in an era where practices again are required to manage their own budgets. An alternative, popular model is for GPs to provide patients with a telephone number to call to book their secondary referral, again offering little potential for information or discussion of which provider might be best for them. It seems that only if GP practices are prepared to fund patient choice advisers from their own budgets can patients even approach the potential of making informed choices. All of this also assumes that patients want to choose their providers of care, which may not be the case at all (Fotaki et al, 2005). If patients are to be asked to decide 'on the spot', non-clinical factors such as the availability of parking or public transport links are likely to dominate discussions about treatment locations. These factors certainly appear prominent in the first patient choice leaflets (see Easington Primary Care Trust, 2006), and this poses difficult questions of whether this really is the best way for patients to have their secondary care selected.

Equally, the increasing disaffection patients express about the NHS might well be the result of a tendency in consumerism noted by Bauman (2007) to create cycles of raised expectation and reduced satisfaction with services. These, in turn, lead to user disaffection and expectation levels of services that can never be delivered. From having very low expectations, patients may have such high expectations that they will be disappointed no matter how good their care is if they start to view the NHS's services not through the eyes of patients but consumers of care. Patients may now demand access to drugs that are still unproven in terms of their efficacy, expect harried nurses to spend time with them in the name of better customer service, and demand private rooms even though there are none free. Hospitals may be expected to have the same levels of service as hotels, a symptom of consumerism directed not towards improved patient care, but towards non-clinical aspects of service. This is unsurprising; if users are told they must behave like consumers, but are unable to judge the quality of the medical care offered (as they lack the expertise to do so), they will instead focus on those aspects of care they do understand.

The Internet

The relationship between doctors and patients also has considerable potential to be recast through the use of the Internet. Two particular elements appear to be significant in this. The first of these, the use of online support groups, is in many respects an extension of the role of condition-specific support groups and charities of the past. These support groups and charities are often characterised as consumer groups (Allsop et al, 2002; Baggott, 2004; Baggott et al, 2004), but their lobbying role makes them more political than this. The Internet allows patients the ability to look to others who may be experiencing the same symptoms for support, gaining a better understanding of what may be wrong with them, or the opportunity to learn what appears to work for others in terms of treatment. This first role does not specifically apply to NHS care, with patients supporting one another from across the world, and is primarily about conditions rather than about the healthcare system specifically. Equally, users can provide more system-focused support by offering advice on the best way of getting specific health organisations to work for patients with particular conditions, how patients might get referred more quickly, how to complain, what their rights are in terms of waiting times, and how to enforce them. In other words, as well as providing support, online groups can empower patients through giving them a better political understanding of how health systems work and how to make them work better to their advantage.

A second means by which the doctor–patient relationship can be changed is through the provision of what was formerly specialised medical knowledge. In this sense, the medical profession was similar to the priesthood in premodern times, speaking in a language that patients did not understand, and holding expert information that patients found difficult to challenge. The Internet, however, makes medical knowledge available to anyone able to type their symptoms into a search engine. A positive interpretation of this is that medical knowledge has 'e-scaped' (Nettleton and Burrows, 2003), becoming potentially available to all and allowing patients to challenge doctors making sloppy diagnoses and health systems not offering the latest drugs and treatment. This interpretation has a history going back to self-help groups established to deal with HIV/AIDS in the 1980s, where networks of lay advice were established to try and fill the gaps in organised medical provision and provide guidance on alternative therapies (Berridge, 1996).

It is no accident that the agencies now responsible for purchasing care in the NHS – Primary Care Trusts – find themselves being repeatedly challenged by patients who are unable to be prescribed the latest drug treatments because of budgetary limitations. These patients (or increasingly their doctors, who also use the Internet to keep up to date) have found out about these treatments from support groups or medical pages on the Internet. By the mid-1990s, there were over 800 self-help groups related to health in the UK alone (Berridge, 1999; Allsop et al, 2004). As such, it is possible to view the increased availability of medical knowledge as being emancipatory, allowing empowered health consumers to challenge outmoded medical practices and health systems offering sub-optimal care.

Another interpretation, however, is that the mass of information often makes doctor–patient relationships far more difficult because diagnosing illness is not as simple as typing symptoms into a search engine (although GPs do seem to be increasingly using this facility in their surgeries). If this were the case, there would be little need for the extensive medical training doctors undertake. If this training has value, and it seems sensible to assume that it does, it is in giving doctors a far more extensive knowledge not only of particular diseases, but also of their underlying physiology, than patients are ever likely to have. Patients may be able, through an evening's reading, to gain a detailed knowledge of what they think is wrong with them, when someone with greater knowledge and experience will be able to determine quickly that the symptoms actually lead to a very different condition. As such, the Internet risks creating misinformed patients and putting them into a conflictual relationship with doctors where the latter have to explain misconceptions before going on to diagnose correctly.

Equally, it is important to point out that while the greater availability of health information can be welcomed, there is also considerable potential for the availability of misinformation. Websites exist that attempt to explain childhood eczema in relation to how quickly a child was held by their mother after birth, clearly giving the potential for considerable guilt to mothers of children who suffer from that condition, when little clinical evidence is available to support such claims. Equally unproven treatments abound on the Internet, and patients may find themselves on websites for complementary therapies that have never been properly tested, or in the hands of charlatans who may believe they have the power to heal with their hands or exorcise demons that are the root cause of all illness, but could be damaging to both vulnerable patients' health and their finances.

As such, policies such as the 'Expert Patient' (DH, 2001c), which aims to help those with long-term conditions self-manage their care, have the potential to be emancipatory by giving patients the tools they need to look after themselves. However, they can also be seen as a means of trying to persuade patients that they need to see doctors less in order to save NHS resources for other uses (Wilson, 2001), and will not work unless there is a considerable initial investment in patient education, which does not seem to have occurred (Multiple Sclerosis Society, 2003).

Problems with health consumerism

Finally, where patients find new treatments available for their conditions that doctors cannot prescribe for them 'on the NHS', the tensions between consumerism and implicit healthcare rationing are held up to scrutiny. If patients are to be cast as health consumers, they clearly have the right to demand to be treated using the most effective and up-to-date medicine, but this is an individualised model of care with little regard for the resources available to everyone else. Consumerist notions of healthcare are, by definition, only concerned with the treatment available to the individual consumer (Bolton, 2002). However, the NHS has a budget that has to be stretched to everyone needing its care, and decisions to prescribe new treatments or to invest in new technologies have a knock-on effect on others. There is therefore a need for mature and careful debate about what will be funded and what will not, and this is still largely absent from the NHS.

At present, the National Institute for Health and Clinical Excellence (NICE) presents guidelines on how particular conditions should be treated, and makes rulings on which new drugs can be prescribed within the NHS. Drugs that are shown to be clinically cost-effective according to strict criteria are allowed within the NHS, but even then, local Primary Care Trusts have to balance budgets and so have somehow to make NICE guidelines work in practice without being seen to take the blame for creating what the media like to call 'postcode lotteries', where different treatments are available in different places. Turning patients into healthcare consumers brings demands for new drugs and treatments into the public domain where Primary Care Trusts are forced to justify their clinical priority decisions, and this is to be welcomed.

What is less welcome is that, where this debate takes place entirely on consumerist terms, the idea that Primary Care Trusts are effectively a body for the allocation of scarce resources gets lost, and no debate takes place asking difficult questions about the allocation of funds for new treatments and medicines. Equally, there is no discussion of the impact of funding new treatments on those presently receiving health service monies who may stand to lose their care as a result.

There is a gap emerging between the role of the patient positioned as the sovereign queen in Le Grand's (1997, 2003) terms, and the reality of health consumerism in the NHS in practice. The entry of private and not-for-profit providers into the mixed economy of care has meant that, in many areas of treatment, patients may have a genuine choice of treatments or providers. However, the presence of competition does not automatically lead to the possibility of informed choice. If patients are to be drivers of health reform by choosing the best providers, a great deal more information and support needs to be given to them if they are to occupy consumer-type roles. This is assuming (and this is a big assumption) that they actually want this role in the first place.

Equally, there are many possible conflicts between the rhetoric of consumption, the need to ration treatment through limiting the range of treatments available through the NHS and the demand that doctors practise evidence-based medicine. It seems as if the government is attempting to delegate these difficult decisions to the local level, and along with it, the blame when patients raise media storms about not receiving treatments. When this has happened, there has been a worrying tendency for health ministers to step in and demand that local health organisations provide treatment. This means that central policy makers delegate the blame for local decision making, thus divorcing themselves from the consequences of their policy, but then try to take the credit for sorting out the problems caused by the policy in the first place. Patients in the position of being denied care must be wondering exactly who it is that is responsible, and who they need to appeal to in order to try to get care decisions overturned.

In all, patients are expected to choose their GPs and their secondary care, even though it is not clear what criteria they are meant to apply or what information they might be able to gather in making these choices. Where patients have a clear idea of what treatment they want, they may not be able to receive it where NICE or their local Primary Care Trust has decided not to fund it. Equally, when patients demand a treatment that is not evidence based, such as homeopathy, they may have to enter into a complex discussion with their GP, who may feel that such a referral would be a waste of public money, or would run against national guidelines for the care of a particular condition. Thus, patients are apparently expected to be consumers because a marketplace of providers is now present, despite there still being considerable barriers preventing them from occupying this role. It is also worth noting that giving patients a greater choice of treatment in the UK is likely to be hindered by the remarkable lack of knowledge most patients have about their physiology compared with patients in other countries (Payer, 1996, p 112). As such, where there is a choice of treatments available, the principal–agent model of the 1990s may now be far more appropriate than the consumer role, with GPs making decisions in active collaboration with patients, and with GPs having an incentive to get this right from their new practice-based commissioner status. This is necessary, as there is evidence, even today, that GPs discriminate between patients on the basis of their class (O'Reilly et al, 2006).

Health citizenship

In terms of patient representation, CHCs remained in place until proposals in the NHS Plan created new forms of participation through the Patient Advice Liaison Services (PALS), which interestingly was originally going to be about advocacy rather than advice (Baggott, 2005), but this seemed to be too confrontational for policymakers. As well as this, Patient and Public Forums were set up, which were meant to be supported by the Commission for Patient and Public Involvement in Healthcare until it was abolished some two years after its creation, leading in turn to Patient Forums, in turn being replaced by Local Involvement Networks (or LINks), which are larger organisations designed to take over their role. If all this reorganisation sounds confusing, it is because it is – it is hard to see how sustained, consistent and credible patient support can be developed when organisations are changed every couple of years. This confusion seems symptomatic of the problem that throughout the history of the health service there has been a failure to promote public involvement (Mohan, 2002, p 220).

Foundation Trusts have schemes in which local people become members of the organisation in an attempt to extend democracy, and which will either become a remarkable experiment in democracy (Birchall, 2003), or make very little difference (Klein, 2003), depending on which commentator the reader believes. The overall difference these changes will make remains to be seen, but the sheer volume of reform since 2000 means that very little can yet be seen in terms of evidence, and there is a danger of user-representation mechanisms becoming incoherent.

Labour's focus on greater public participation in the NHS can be linked directly to the consumerist ethos of policy running from the 1980s onwards, but is also linked to Labour's promise to rebuild trust between citizens and government in the political process, enhancing the legitimacy of government in the process (Newman, 2002). Participation is viewed as providing greater flexibility than the blunt instrument of party political voting, and a link to a network form of governance that has the potential to build social capital and strengthen civil society (Deakin, 2001). The language of voluntarism in public services is making something of a comeback in the language of Gordon Brown. Unless calls for voluntarism are backed by more than government rhetoric, however, voluntarism may disappear as quickly as it appeared to in the 1970s.

More significantly, perhaps, the public have also increasingly become involved in the decision making of local healthcare organisations through the use of opinion surveys, which have become important because they have performance indicators and star ratings attached to them. But the extent to which these surveys actually involve local people is open to question, and is perhaps most important in Primary Care Trusts because of their care commissioning role. If commissioning is to be locally responsive – one of the reasons for the establishment of Primary Care Trusts in the first place – local people clearly need to feed into the processes through which priorities for healthcare are decided. However, it is remarkably difficult to achieve this in practice.

Labour appears to require hyperactive health consumers: individuals who research the best hospitals, make choices about where to go, what food they require, how often they will access the telephone, and so on; but also hyperactive citizenship, with the public joining the local Foundation Trust as a member and participating in its LINk. This asks a great deal. If the mechanism for making public organisations more responsive is to come from consumer-type mechanisms, they need to work. Equally, if public organisations need to be made more democratic, or at least more accountable to local people, participatory systems need to make this happen. However, whether the public want to make choices about healthcare provision, or are prepared to give up their time to this extent, surely remains questionable. The danger is that local health representation will be predominantly made up of those with the time and resources to be able to attend meetings for free, which will not achieve any goals of local representativeness, and will not achieve the goals of either greater democracy or more accountability when so many people are excluded.

Conclusion

A very brief summary of the above chapter would be to suggest that the public have moved from being clients of health professionals, and rights-oriented citizens at the creation of the NHS, to being consumers of healthcare and having both rights and responsibilities (especially to participate in the running of services), in the present day. This is too neat. The process by which users have been given choices is far more complex than this, and the extent to which most people participate as members of local hospitals or Primary Care Trusts, or as members of LINks, is minimal compared with those who do not. Perhaps more significant in terms of responsibilities has been the new public health (Peterson and Lupton, 1996) movement that demands that the public take a greater responsibility for pursuing a healthier lifestyle, and for making healthier choices in their lives (Secretary of State for Health, 1996, 2006). This has the potential to mean that those with healthier lifestyles are treated more quickly or receive additional services compared with those who do not, and anecdotal examples already exist of this happening in the treatment of repeated alcohol offenders, drug abusers and those suffering from obesity. If healthcare is going to be about taking responsibilities as seriously as rights, it will mean a dramatic change in the way in which patients are treated in the NHS. Patients in the UK, internationally speaking, have been afforded few rights because of the paternalistic way that medicine has been organised (Payer, 1996). Expecting a quick change in doctor–patient relationships appears to be extremely idealistic. Patients still need doctors more than doctors need patients.

Equally, however, the attempt to turn patients into consumers of health appears to be problematic. Patients do not necessarily want to make choices about their care (Fotaki et al, 2005), with there being a considerable difference between patients being asked whether they want care choices before they fall ill, and again when they actually become ill (Schwartz, 2004). It is not clear how patients are meant to choose between potential secondary care providers in the new mixed economy of care, even less how they will make choices that will actually allow health reform to work by driving out poor providers. If patients cannot tell the difference between good and bad providers, and persist in choosing hospitals and other providers based on their closeness to home rather than the excellence of provision, little will change in terms of the financial flows following patients, and the whole basis of the current reforms will be undermined.

Instead, it might be more sensible to treat patients not as consumers, who almost by definition are proactive and informed individuals capable of making the choices before them, but through a more co-productive model in which they might be customers instead (Greener, 2003a, 2005b). What this means in practice is a relationship closer to the principal–agent model in place in the 1980s and 1990s, where patients expect to receive advice from doctors on their care options, and to be able to reach a decision in consultation with them as a result. Patients are able to judge the politeness and respect with which they have been treated, and so it makes sense for them to be asked for their opinion in judging the quality of the service they have received. Such judgements must be treated with caution – most of us would rather a brusque but brilliant doctor than a fawning but incompetent one – but there is little or no excuse for doctors treating patients as something less than human beings while they are in their care. Although there has been a transformational improvement in the manner of most medical professionals, there are still many who appear to regard themselves as providing a favour to patients by seeing them. Table 8.3 summarises the difference between the patient roles of client, consumer and customer.

Table 8.3: The patient in client, consumer and customer roles in the NHS

Client	Consumer	Customer
Professional-dominated relationship	Patient-dominated relationship	Co-production model
Patient effectively passive	Patient drives service improvement	Patient assesses quality of service
Professional makes choices and determines level of service	Patient makes choices (perhaps with professional advice) and assesses level of service	Professional makes choices (in collaboration with patient), patient assesses level of service

In all, the role of the public in the NHS has changed dramatically since the creation of the NHS in 1948. The process by which doctors have come to treat patients as co-producers of care rather than as passive recipients of it has taken longer to come about, but there are signs of considerable improvement. However, the unrealistic expectations of the state in terms of the role, and range of roles, it presently expects the public to occupy in relation to the NHS create considerable problems for the current wave of health reforms. Considering patients as customers of health services offers the chance for them to become co-producers of their care without the extremes of consumerism, but still leaves open the question of the appropriate means of citizen-type, collectivist participation for the public in the NHS – a topic to which this book will return in Chapters Nine and Ten.

NINE

Health policy under Labour

Introduction

This chapter brings together the analysis from other chapters of this book to consider health policy since 1997, when Tony Blair's Labour government was elected. It takes the account of health policy and organisation through to the end of 2007, shortly after Blair retired as Prime Minister and Gordon Brown took over.

The context of health policy in 1997

During the 1997 election, Labour campaigned to 'save the NHS', but its approach to welfare policy during its first term in office faced a significant problem in that, in order to gain credibility with the financial markets, Chancellor Gordon Brown made it clear that he was going to honour Labour's commitment to keep within the public expenditure limits set by the previous Conservative government. This did not remove all possibility of change, but did mean that radical reform, which is not cheap, was unlikely.

The period from 1992 to 1997 marked a period where, after the confrontations between the doctors and the government over the policies in *Working for Patients* (Secretary of State for Health, 1989), health policy went through something of a 'becalming' (Wainwright, 1998). The internal market, radical in policy, turned out to be rather 'bland' in implementation (Klein, 1998) because the government retreated from its more radical promises, recasting the reforms as managerial rather than market-based (Ham, 2000) and so being more about contestability (the potential for competition) than competition (Sheldon, 1990).

Equally, it possibly became clearer to policy makers how little control they had in practice over the implementation of the internal market. With messages about attempting to assure a 'smooth take-off' for the new market coming from the Department of Health (Edwards and Fall, 2005, p 84), and with requests to minimise contract changes for the first year in order to minimise disruption, there was little incentive for district health authorities, the major purchasers of care, to try to contract with the best possible providers. After the first couple of years, contracting patterns seemed to change little in most areas, constrained by the combination of patients not wishing to travel too far for care and the lack of available local competition. Some commentators suggested that a market never existed in any recognisable form at all (West, 1998). It was therefore left to the other purchasers of care in the internal market, the GP fundholders, to try to make a significant difference. Fundholding did appear to bring one-time savings through reduced prescribing and referrals (Baines et al, 1997), but concerns about the reduced waiting times for fundholding patients (Propper et al, 2002; Dusheiko et al, 2004a) led to allegations that the health service was becoming 'two-tier' (Petchey, 1995). There also appeared to be evidence that, because of the increased time and costs of contracting, fundholding actually reduced patient satisfaction (Dusheiko et al, 2004b). This was a serious problem for a reform created in the name of achieving greater patient responsiveness. It is hard to establish whether fundholding was a success or not, but it was certainly an intriguing experiment.

The New NHS: Modern, Dependable

On coming to office in 1997, one of Labour's first acts was to abolish fundholding on the grounds that it was inefficient, that it created a massive bureaucracy to administer the contracts between hospitals and fundholders, and that it was inequitable because of the potential advantages it gave to patients of fundholders. District health authority purchasing was portrayed as bureaucratic and wasteful, with longer-term contracting introduced to cut through 'red tape' and save money. A conciliatory White Paper appeared entitled *The New NHS: Modern, Dependable* (Secretary of State for Health, 1997), which suggested that the problems of the NHS were nothing that a little organisational reform and putting a little more trust in health professionals couldn't resolve.

The Labour government appeared to believe that, as the 'natural' guardians of the NHS had been restored to power, taking a more sympathetic approach to health policy was all that was needed to achieve improvement. The government suggested that problems of the NHS were not to do with its funding, but instead were caused by the way wasteful way in which the Conservatives had organised health services. A three–part rhetorical strategy was presented in which NHS organisation was not to be based on 'command and control' as Labour claimed policy had been the case prior to 1989, nor on the wasteful market, as it had been since then. Instead, it would find another way that took the best aspects of each approach and removed the difficulties. This was to be a pragmatic, evidence-based approach to policy that put decision making back in the hands of those who knew the patients best – the doctors and other health professionals. In what appears almost touchingly naive from the perspective of the present day, Labour's ministers believed that the problems of the NHS were relatively easily solvable (Timmins, 2002); as Alan Milburn later said, there 'was a sense of expectation about us being able to put the NHS right' (Edwards and Fall, 2005, p 157). As a result, and despite the organisational changes mentioned above, it seemed as if Labour's policies in the period up to 1999 at least offered considerably more continuity than change when compared with those of its Conservative predecessors (Clarke et al, 2000).

To fill the gap left by the abolition of GP fundholding, Primary Care Groups were set up, replacing district health authorities as the main purchasers in the NHS. Primary Care Groups, however, were also providers of care. This was an attempt by Labour to begin to cross the boundaries between health and community care, with the plan that Primary Care Groups would take over much of the purchasing and provision of community-based care through the establishment of Primary Care Trusts (Berridge, 1999). The emphasis appeared to be on the integration of services, but the long historical traditions of GP practice, hospital medicine and local authority healthcare meant that simply putting services back together was not straightforward. Labour's emphasis on partnerships to overcome the barriers between services appeared to be confused over the nature of the partnerships required to bridge the gaps between services (Poole, 2000).

New healthcare organisations

Within a couple of years, however, Labour's approach to the NHS had changed. In 1999, new quasi-autonomous government organisations were set up that appeared to be centralising in their tendencies, moving power away from the health professionals so trusted in 1997 (Paton, 2005). An organisation now known as the Healthcare Commission (then the Commission for Health Improvement) was set up with a brief to inspect healthcare organisations and make sure that they were up to the required standard, in a similar way to the functioning of Ofsted in education policy. Another organisation, now known as the National Institute for Health and Clinical Excellence (NICE) (then the National Institute for Clinical Excellence), was set up to standardise treatment and get health services working to the highest standards of evidence-based practice. More controversially, NICE was also responsible for making the decision as to whether expensive new drugs should be licensed for use in the NHS according to the criteria of whether they were 'clinically cost-effective', requiring a strange hybrid of demonstrable clinical efficacy and cost-effectiveness according to measures such as the Quality Adjusted Life Year. Health economics, after a period when it had appeared to lose influence in the 1990s, was undergoing something of a comeback as it provided an established series of tools for assessing whether or not medicines and technologies should be paid for publicly.

Lack of progress?

Concerns were also mounting that Labour had not made much progress in reforming the NHS, and that this should now become a higher priority (Giddens, 2002). The changes put in place in 1997 had not abolished the internal market as Labour had claimed, but removed the internal market's most dynamic purchasers (fundholders), and moved contracting on to a longer-term basis (Powell, 1998). This recasting of the marketplace meant that consultants were no longer dependent on GPs or GP practices for referrals, as resources could not easily be moved away from them. The relationship between the two groups was becoming contingent, as consultants no longer feared losing funds for their services if they did not meet required waiting times or quality standards. The link between the doctor professional groupings was broken again.

By 1999, Labour's belief that a more responsive health service could be achieved without significant reform was coming to an end. When Secretary of State Frank Dobson left his portfolio in an unsuccessful attempt to become London Mayor, despite being the Labour Party's official candidate, he was replaced by the more Blairite Alan Milburn. Milburn is an interesting figure, appearing on Labour's election to office to be hostile to private sector involvement in the NHS (Timmins, 2002), but while in office putting in place policies that went down a very different path for the NHS from those of his 'Old Labour' predecessor. Equally, Labour's 'iron' Chancellor appeared to be beyond reproach for his financial stringency (Keegan, 2003), and the purse strings of the Treasury were beginning to become a little looser. Baggott (2004) suggests that pressures that built up between 1998 and 1999, especially from the media pressure over failures in clinical governance and high-profile cases of care, were a direct consequence of Labour's expenditure parsimony in its early years of government. In 2000, the NHS Plan appeared (Secretary of State for Health, 2000), signalling the beginning of a new phase in health policy.

The NHS Plan

The NHS Plan was remarkable in that it presented a 10-year plan for increased investment, but made it clear that this came with a clear commitment to significant reform (Milburn, 2002). A performance management system was to be put in place to examine every hospital (and later every Primary Care Trust) and give it a rating. Initially, the rating system was to be based on traffic lights, with hospitals being graded as being green-, amber- or red-light institutions. After someone pointed out the potential connotations of branding hospitals 'red-light' institutions, the system was changed to one where instead 'star-ratings' were given out on a scale between three star (the best hospitals) through to zero star (the worst) (DH, 2001b). Organisations coming bottom of the rankings were threatened with the potential of management teams being removed wholesale and those from more successful organisations brought in to replace them, perhaps even in the form of an organisational take-over. Hospitals coming at the top of the performance scale were to be given access to additional performance-related funds, as well as potential freedoms from future inspections through what was called 'earned autonomy' by meeting centrally-set performance standards (Mannion et al, 2003). The policy can be read as giving NHS Trusts the freedom to do whatever the government wanted (Hoque et al, 2004), or as a sensible and overdue imposition of minimum standards of care on NHS organisations. In either case, from the day of the announcement of the new performance management system, local healthcare organisations have had to be far more centrally accountable for their decision making than ever before.

Foundation Trusts

Three-star hospital Trusts were to be given the right to apply to become Foundation Trusts. The introduction of Foundation Trusts represented one of the most controversial aspects of New Labour's package of reforms for the NHS because of concerns that it led to healthcare Trusts moving closer than ever to being run on a not-for-profit basis, and so further way from the initial NHS ideal of a publicly funded and provided health system. Foundation Trusts are a central part of the approach to decentralising health policy (Peckham et al, 2005b) and were designed to give greater earned autonomy to their managers. They were also the result of a significant government row between Chancellor Brown and Secretary of State Milburn, with the latter wanting to grant far greater autonomy to Foundation Trusts, particularly with respect to their financial governance, and the former alarmed that public money would be put at risk if used to fund what were looking to him like semi-private institutions (Jenkins, 2006). Brown won out, and limitations were imposed on the financial autonomy of Foundation Trusts, but this did not mean that they became any less contentious.

The incentive system under which Foundation Trusts operate is not the only area of innovation – from their conception they have also been required to find new ways of organising their governance arrangements to include directly more local participation in the decision making and activities of healthcare organisations than has been the case with hospital Trusts in the past (Healthcare Commission, 2005). Foundation Trusts have responded to this challenge through the creation a range of mechanisms designed to include public consultation and participation (Healthcare Commission, 2005). The abolition of Community Health Councils and their replacement with Patient Forums is one part of this (Allsop et al, 2004).

Foundation Trusts are an experiment in mutual governance, devolving power to patients and employees as members. They follow other mutual models in social rented housing (community-based housing associations, housing cooperatives) and leisure services (leisure trusts). Compared with the rather conservative ways in which Primary Care Trusts have often engaged in public participation (despite commissioning on behalf of them), they are radical indeed. Foundation Trusts have a membership drawn from local people and patients. 'Lay' governors are directly elected by Foundation Trust members and form a majority. It is intended that transparency, trust and 'opinion responsiveness' are more prominent under this 'new model of social ownership', and that 'direct elections of governors ... will get local hospitals better focused on meeting the needs of the communities they serve' (Hutton, 2003).

There has not been such a large-scale move to recruit patients as members of a health delivery agency since the Friendly Societies that existed prior to the creation of the NHS. In historical terms, Foundation Trusts can be seen as a handing back of control to patients, which they lost in 1940 when the state first began to organise a comprehensive healthcare system. However, the circumstances are very different. Only some of the bodies involved in the governance of the provision of care have been mutualised, not the funding of the health system, and the power of patients as Friendly Society members came from their ability to hire and fire doctors on their 'panels'.

The ideas underpinning the governance arrangements for Foundation Trusts are controversial; some commentators claim that public participation in Foundation Trusts is likely to be confronted by the usual problems of participation self-selection and an accountability structure that is so complex as to be unworkable (Klein, 2003). Wilmot (2004) echoes many of these concerns, suggesting that the participation arrangements for Foundation Trusts are incoherent and mutually conflictual, and Hoque et al (2004) state that hospital managers do not believe that the Foundation Trusts reforms will deliver them greater autonomy because of the presence of central targets. Greener (2003b) reinforces this view and points to the tensions that result from attempting greater democratic localism on the one hand while introducing central performance targets on the other. Morrell (2006) suggests that the reforms represent an attempt at creating a narrative of reform only tenuously linked to reality, implying that detailed empirical research is a definite priority in this area.

Other commentators, however, suggest that Foundation Trusts deserve a 'qualified welcome', as they represent an attempt to decentralise and make NHS organisations more accountable to the communities that they serve, even if political pressures, a lack of guidance as to governance arrangements, overselling of the reforms and their rather rushed inception might yet work against them (Walshe, 2003a). Simmons et al (2007) suggest the reforms offer the possibility of democratising the NHS, and point to their remarkable achievement in recruiting nearly 300,000 members in a short space of time. The Healthcare Commission's review of Foundation Trusts in 2005 found that although some concerns remained in that not all Trusts were working to the high standards set by many of their members, 'many of the concerns and fears that had been initially expressed about NHS foundation trusts were not evident' (Healthcare Commission, 2005, p 5; Monitor, 2006). However, the same report also suggested that 'The costs and benefits of the new structures of governance are not clear. Unless these are demonstrated ... there is a danger that governors and members may not be taken seriously' (Healthcare Commission, 2005, p 55).

Care Trusts

As well as Foundation Trusts and Primary Care Trusts, Care Trusts were proposed in the NHS as the latest attempt to bring together health and social care. The idea was that Care Trusts would integrate health and social care in a single organisation, commissioning primary care, community health services and social care if organised around a Primary Care Trust, or having a provider role only (Glasby and Peck, 2003). However, only five were established by 2002, and a further three in 2003 (Baggott, 2004, pp 288-9), with problems over the differing boundaries between Primary Care Trusts and local authorities cited as a difficult problem, and with local authorities themselves opposing the formation of Care Trusts because of concerns that they would lead to a take-over of their social care function. Despite continued enthusiasm from the government for the better integration of services, Care Trusts seem to have largely stalled as an idea, and an emphasis on the new mixed economy of care to cross the health and social care divide has developed.

The Private Finance Initiative

An area of health policy that has proved to be contentious for Labour has been the PFI. The PFI attempts to address a longstanding problem in the NHS: that of capital funding, particularly for infrastructure projects. In the 1960s, the Hospital Plan (Minister of Health, 1962) acknowledged the shortfall in building expenditure in the NHS in its first 20 years, and put together ambitious plans for building new facilities. However, three particular problems seemed to frustrate the Plan.

First, because the NHS was funded out of general taxation, it still had to receive the funds necessary to finance any long-term building plans from the total available from the Treasury each year for public expenditure. Running a sustained public deficit was not an option, as, during the 1960s, the UK pound was a member of the Bretton Woods fixed exchange rate system, and the government was obliged to keep the value of the pound pegged at or around a particular value of the dollar. Any significant increase in public expenditure would act to reduce the value of the pound against the dollar, putting pressure on the currency, so it was not possible to finance increased public expenditure through debt. Concerns about the international financial implications of running budget deficits acted as a strong constraint in the funding of health services – a feature the policy environment shared in the 2000s, albeit for different reasons.

The second reason for the Hospital Plan not taking off was a political one related to the problem of the NHS being financed by general taxation. When the economy does not grow as anticipated by the Treasury, it is usual for government spending departments to be asked to find savings, as the amount of tax revenue will fall short of that which is budgeted. Faced with cutting back on either revenue expenditure (day-to-day expenditure) or capital expenditure (long-term expenditure for buildings and infrastructure), it will always be easier to cut back on capital expenditure because it does not carry with it immediate political consequences. Capital expenditure will come to fruition in several years' time, and it takes a brave politician to cut back on day-to-day spending in the present to allow the building of a hospital for which they may not even be around to take credit on its completion.

Finally, the Hospital Plan struggled because of the sheer scale of the programme, and the lack of expertise and project management skills in place to oversee and organise building on such a scale. Hospitals are significant items of expenditure and are complex and difficult building projects. They require projections about future health needs, a long-term commitment of expenditure that requires detailed costing, incredible amounts of coordination to get the building up in the right order to plan and to budget, and so, considerable building, project management and financial skills, which the public sector often found itself lacking. Hospital-building success stories were apparent, but so were problems of prolonged planning processes, budget overruns and difficulties with building coordination. Little wonder that capital projects in the NHS achieved something of a bad reputation as being difficult to fund, or to manage even if funds were granted.

The PFI was designed to try to address these problems. The roots of the PFI can be traced back to the Labour government of 1974-79,[1] but the policy in its modern form was formulated by the Major government of 1992-97. In its early years, however, relatively little happened because of the difficulty of getting private sector partners to take an interest in working, effectively, for the government. Labour's election saw a change in attitude because of its willingness to expedite the contracting process for the PFI.

Why was Labour so keen to embrace a policy that had achieved only very limited success with its Conservative predecessors? There seems to be two particular reasons. First, the PFI was well placed to overcome past difficulties in getting capital projects off the ground, in that extra capacity could be brought in from the private sector rather than trying to coordinate a complex working arrangement between public and private contractors for new projects. However, the PFI also allowed Gordon Brown to make capital expenditure commitments without losing his reputation for being tough on finance. The PFI works by the private sector taking on the building of a new capital project, and providing maintenance for the facilities for a period of typically 25–35 years in return for an annual fee from the public sector. The public sector gets a new facility without having to pay for it upfront, the private sector gets an annual income stream for taking on board the initial costs and risk associated with a complex building project (Asenova and Beck, 2003), and the Chancellor, because the PFI does not appear in government accounts as creating a debt for the public sector, gets new investment in public facilities without the problems of acquiring government debt. It seems that everyone wins.

The state effectively underwrites private sector risk in PFI. In February 1998, the government announced 11 PFI schemes to a total value of £750 million. The long-term leases given to the private sector led to the first NHS projects being assigned 'AAA' ratings by credit-rating agencies, despite the alleged risks being taken on in the building of the capital projects (Leys, 2003). The PFI has introduced a new type of corporation-like organisation into the NHS that is wholly dependent on government contracts, but still holding the freedoms of the private sector (Gaffney et al, 1999). These new corporations have the ability to have a significant voice in future negotiations over the NHS because of the significant role they now play within it.

Problems with the PFI

There are a number of difficulties with the PFI, both in the present day and in the future. First, the use of the private sector should mean that buildings go up quicker and more cost-effectively than they would do if subject to the problems in the past of public building programmes. New hospital and Primary Care Trust facilities have certainly gone up more quickly than at any other time in the NHS's history, with the Treasury's list of confirmed PFI deals in October 2007 totalling a book value of over £11 billion in both England and Scotland, but that could end up costing the public sector an overall sum of around five times that by the time the contracts are completed (BBC News, 2006c). The size of these figures has led to significant concerns from the Public Accounts Committee that insufficient competition for contracts means that good value for contracts may not be achieved for the public sector (BBC News, 2007).

Jean Shaoul and her colleagues have calculated the average return of hospital PFIs at 58% for the first three years, with the additional costs to the public purse of private finance (as opposed to contracting within the public sector for the builds) at £60 million a year, twice the cost of public provision (Public Finance, 2007). The very long-term nature of the maintenance contracts under the PFI has seen private partners offloading contracts to other providers in a chain of subcontracts that can serve to obscure the exact partner with whom the NHS is now contracting with, as well as creating the potential for services to be less responsive and for changes in building use to be expensive and difficult to achieve (NAO, 2008). Finally, questions have been asked as to whether the PFI is moral, with suggestions that it creates debts for generations to come while it is the present generation that gets to enjoy the facilities it funds.

Performance management

A third significant area of NHS reform has come from the introduction of the performance management system described above. The new emphasis on performance across the NHS has had a number of effects. First, the grading of health providers and the widespread publication of the results has led to it becoming straightforward to construct local league tables of providers. This, in turn, creates the possibility of patients choosing between organisations for their care, in a similar way that parents have done for their children's schools since the 1980s. However, the health data remain rather crude, as the overall organisational performance may not be at all reflective of the particular service a patient is to receive. Equally, it is remarkable how few members of the public are aware of what the rating of their local healthcare organisations are, suggesting that the information, although it is high-profile in the media at the time of its announcement each year, does not really register as being of particular importance for very long.

Within health organisations, performance management has led to a number of problems. First, there are serious ongoing concerns about the accuracy of the data collected to compile the ratings (Audit Commission, 2003; King's Fund and *The Sunday Times*, 2005). If the data collected are inaccurate, it is clear that the ratings will be as well. Second, there is considerable evidence of health managers prioritising services that are measured within the performance measurement system (the so-called 'P45' targets, as managers can be sacked for not attaining them) above other services that are not (Greener, 2004b, 2005c; Mannion et al, 2005). Third, there is also evidence of 'gaming', where health managers attempt to exploit the exact wording of targets to claim they are met, when they have not really been attained at all. As such, there is an occasional tendency for patients to be offered appointments on public holidays, which are likely to be refused, allowing managers to claim that the appointment was offered within the necessary period of time and thus they have met the target. Another managerial ruse has been to admit patients into hospital before they can actually receive treatment, in order to allow managers to tick the box that the patient is now receiving care, even if they are not receiving the particular treatment that they require. These tendencies are clearly perverse, but if an emphasis is placed on the mindless meeting of targets regardless of clinical need, this kind of behaviour can be expected, and is extremely difficult to legislate against (Smith, 2002). A clear priority of New Labour's second term of office was achieving 'delivery' (Barber, 2007), which was shorthand for focusing on hitting precise targets for the improvement of public services, even if sometimes it seemed as if the targets could have been more carefully chosen.

Towards the end of its second term, Labour appeared to begin to accept the limits of the performance management system it had put in place in the NHS. From 2005, attempts have been made to make the system more 'light touch', but it is hard to see evidence of this in practice. The star-rating system has been abandoned and replaced by a new 'annual health check', which rates the quality of services and use of resources for healthcare providers across 24 core standards of care. There is still a four-point grading scale, but it now goes not from zero star to three star, but instead from weak to fair to good to excellent. The Healthcare Commission, which now oversees the performance management system, has made it explicit that the new ratings are not comparable to the star-rating system, but it is troubling that the two systems produced such different results in their first year of operation. In 2005, the last year of the star-rating system, 426 Trusts were labelled as three- or two-star organisations, with only 24 positioned in the bottom category of zero stars. In 2006, the first year of the new system, more than 200 Trusts were graded as weak in one category or another, with one third of all trusts scoring in this category for their use of resources (Healthcare Commission, 2006b), and only two Trusts scoring excellent in both categories of measurement. This would seem to indicate that either the old star system was substantially misrepresenting performance, or that the new one is excessively harsh, as it is unlikely that the performance of so many organisations could have declined so quickly in one year.

The new mixed economy of care and payment by results

The biggest turnaround in Labour policy since 1997 has been the revival of the marketplace for care in the NHS. In 1997, the market was dismissed as inefficient and inequitable (Secretary of State for Health,

1997). By 2001, however, Labour appeared to have come to the view that the NHS should make greater use of private and not-for-profit providers in order to increase the capacity of health services and so reduce waiting times (a key indicator and target in the NHS Plan). There was nothing new in this – the private sector was used in the 1980s as a part of 'waiting list initiatives' to drive down waiting times. What was new was that the private and not-for-profit sector was invited to compete with public providers in the NHS to create a new marketplace called the 'mixed economy of care'. So whereas the internal market of the 1990s theoretically involved public providers competing with one another (although there was not much competition in practice), the market of the 2000s has been about trying to achieve competition between public, private and not-for-profit competitors in mixed economies of care (Clarke et al, 2007).

Healthcare appeared to be taking a leaf out of social care policy since the 1980s, where in both care for the elderly and home care a private marketplace had appeared, initially funded by the social security budget (in the 1980s) and then by local authorities from the 1990s. In the 2000s, Labour has attempted to pass the budgets for those eligible for state-funded social care to the users themselves through 'direct payments' (Glendinning et al, 2000; Secretary of State for Health, 2006). These are meant to empower individuals to be able to contract with whomever they wish for their care, to be able to reward friends and family for care they have previously provided out of friendship or loyalty or to be able to employ local care providers for a wider range of services than in the past. However, the take-up of direct payments remains very low, even if some commentators seem to be getting a little ahead in claiming success for them, and that giving individuals a budget for care should be the future of the NHS (Le Grand, 2007).

In healthcare, the mechanism through which the choice of provider is meant to be made is rather ambiguous. On the one hand, the government appears to have reinvented GP fundholding through its creation of 'practice-based commissioning' (DH, 2004). Practice-based commissioning is meant to try and secure greater responsiveness from healthcare providers and achieve more localised commissioning – much the same goals as were specified for GP fundholding in the 1990s (Greener and Mannion, 2006). Practice-based commissioning, as fundholding did before it, allocates GPs a budget to purchase care for their patients, encouraging them to take greater responsibility for their use of resources as well as giving them a means of driving up standards in local health economies through the careful commissioning of care. Labour appeared to have learned lessons from the market of the 1990s in that, in many local care economies, there is now competition for at least some services because of the entry of new providers and the appearance of innovations such as treatment centres, which specialise in providing a very limited range of services to the NHS in contrast to the general provision of most NHS hospitals. Equally, as every GP practice is a practice-based commissioning one, the problems of equity between fundholders and non-fundholders in the 1990s may be avoided.

However, the problems with getting an information system infrastructure to underpin the complexities of contracting in an environment as complex as the NHS are difficult to resolve, and the 'Choose and Book' computer system meant to underpin the reforms is still far less reliable than the government had hoped. As such, if GPs are to avoid the 'transaction costs' involved in organising and monitoring separate contracts for their patients, as well as to manage their budgetary implications, a significant improvement in Choose and Book will have to occur, and the problems of 'Connecting For Health', the information system meant to be linking GP surgeries with hospitals to provide electronic patient records, overcome.

The other ambiguity around practice-based commissioning is its fit with its policy for extending patient choice (DH, 2001a). If GPs are meant to be responsible for budgets and for increasing the dynamism of local health economies, this would seem to be premised on them making care decisions on behalf of their patients. However, extending patient choice means that it is patients who are meant to decide which of four providers they go to for their secondary care (DH, 2006c). Giving individual patients a choice of their secondary care providers (as well as emphasising the importance of their choice of GPs in the first place) is a significant change from the principal–agent model of doctor–patient relationships in the 1990s. Patients are now meant to choose their secondary provider with less support from their GPs, and more from their knowledge of the local health economy. A significant amount of information is available to assist them in this choice, but it is not always easy to find or to understand this information, and the first patient choice leaflets appear to focus more on car parking and star ratings than on clinical measures (Easington Primary Care Trust, 2006). Even if patients were to receive information comparing the potential hospital providers in their local areas, the bases through which they would make their choices are not immediately apparent. Would the quickest provider be chosen (in terms of waiting time) or the closest? Would patients choose the provider with the cleanest wards or the best clinical outcomes? How patients are supposed to make a 'frame' within which to process this information into a decision is difficult to see. Perhaps there is a good reason why GPs made decisions on behalf of their patients up to now – the decision may be complex, and will often be taken at a time where patients are feeling unwell and vulnerable (Schwartz, 2004).

The new mixed economy of care positions patients as consumers, but also makes it extremely difficult for them to be able to fulfil that role (Greener, 2003a, 2003c, 2005c). The relationship between GPs and consultants is also subject to some ambiguity. If patients are meant to be making referral decisions, even if those decisions bring with them resources under the payment by results funding mechanism (DH, 2002b), consultants and GPs are still contingently related. This is because mutual dependence has not been established – it is patients who are making the decisions rather than GPs. If GPs make decisions, however, and there is an emphasis on the practice-based commissioning system, the relationship is once again one where both parties stand to gain from GP referrals, with GPs able to select the best care for their patients and their choices carrying with them resources, and consultants keen to attract those resources. Referrals will matter again. On both consultant and GP sides, a discourse of entrepreneurship is emerging (Leys, 2003). Consultants are encouraged to find new ways of marketing and delivering their services, perhaps moving clinics into primary care settings in order to be more patient-focused, as well as perhaps reducing the overheads attached to them by moving them out of the expensive hospital setting. General pracitioners, in turn, are encouraged to offer new services to the mixed economy of care marketplace, putting them, as with Primary Care Trusts, in the position of potentially both providing services and referring patients to them.

The new market for care has the potential to be the most radical reform in the NHS's history. The Labour government appears to have made a conscious decision that, having exhausted the possibilities for extracting greater efficiency from the existing system, it would drive forward systemic public service reform in its third term in office (Barber, 2007). However, the evidence for how committed the government remains to radical reform has come under question since Blair stepped down as Prime Minister, with the new Secretary of State, Alan Johnson, appearing more conciliatory than his predecessors, and the new Prime Minister less committed to the imposition of market disciplines than Blair was.

However, the introduction of the market dynamic into the NHS means that the future has become tremendously unpredictable. There is the potential for public provision to disappear for key services in local health economies, making the NHS entirely dependent on private or not-for-profit provision in some areas, or even not providing particular services at all in direct contradiction of the NHS principle of comprehensiveness (Talbot-Smith and Pollock, 2006, pp 179-80). Indeed, in some areas, this may already be the case. At the other extreme, though, private providers could find their margins within the NHS too small and retreat from the new marketplace, leaving the system much as it was before. A middle path where some health economies are fiercely contested (especially urban areas with a large number potential patients, and involving widely needed treatments with low complications) and others predominantly publicly provided (rural areas involving complex or chronic conditions) seems the most likely.

Revisiting the double-bed

The reforms listed above have recast the relationship between the government and NHS professionals in new ways. At the creation of the NHS, parliamentary accountability was placed at a premium, with the Minister of Health acknowledging that every bedpan dropped on the corridors of the new service would echo through the corridors of Whitehall. Health services were centrally accountable, but locally paternalistic, as they were administered primarily through the doctors who ran the NHS's organisations. In the 2000s, however, Labour appears to have turned this logic on its head. Health services appear to be locally accountable, but centrally paternalistic. What this means in practice is that the government sets the context within which policy must work through innovations such as the mixed economy of care and the PFI, as well as retaining control of contracts for GPs and consultants, but when things go wrong, it is quick to blame local managers and doctors (Dawson and Dargie, 2002). On top of this, it is able to present itself as coming to the rescue in overruling local health organisations where they put in place decisions, based on national priorities set by the government, that have become politically unpopular. Two case studies (of the many possible) will illustrate this.

Budget deficits

In the 2000s, despite the additional funding granted by the government, NHS organisations often ran at a budget deficit. This was often sorted out through a series of local fixes, where Primary Care Trusts with surpluses effectively 'netted' them off against hospitals with deficits (or vice versa), so that overall, the budget came in about right. However, as Labour was driving forward market-style reforms in which the flow of patients carried with it resources, organisations were no longer willing (or able) to cross-subsidise one another. Alongside the market-based reforms, the government settled both GP and consultant contracts on what look, with hindsight, to have been extremely generous terms (O'Dowd, 2005; NAO, 2007), and many hospitals or Primary Care Trusts went from having very low capital costs because of the poor infrastructure they had inherited, to very high costs because they had participated in a PFI project. The cost-base of many healthcare providers, because of the doctor contracts, and the use of PFI, increased significantly.

In 2006, the NHS deficit reached £512 million, double the level of the previous year. In the same year, strategic health authorities (the replacements for regional health authorities) generated a surplus of around £500 million, apparently demonstrating the unequal inheritances between hospital providers and administrative organisations within the system. The BMA declared that deficits were due to government 'meddling' (BBC News, 2006d), especially through excessive use of management consultants, PFI and reforms involving the private sector, which meant that public money flowed outside of public provision. The government blamed local hospital managers for budgetary incompetence (BBC News, 2006b). The government has a point – if healthcare organisations are running over-budget by 25% (as did Surrey and Sussex NHS Trust in 2006), that would seem to indicate poor management. However, this poor management occurs in a context where infrastructure and resource inheritances significantly affect the ability of managers to do their jobs, and with the government responsible for pay settlements and for a policy context in which the PFI and a new market for healthcare existed, so they cannot claim to be blameless. The NHS has become a site in which the local attachment of blame has become far more common than it used to be.

Prescribing decisions

An additional tension has appeared in the decision to delegate national guidelines for prescribing to NICE, while at the same time founding Primary Care Trusts on the grounds that they should create more responsive commissioning. However, where NICE has put in place guidelines that have been politically sensitive, or where Primary Care Trusts have refused to fund particular treatments, both organisations have faced a barrage of local press criticism suggesting that the NHS is 'denying' treatment for particular patients, or that a 'postcode lottery' of treatment exists where decisions taken by Primary Care Trusts differ from one geographic space to another. The government has intervened when politically difficult decisions have been reached by NICE or Primary Care Trusts, implying that the NHS organisations had got things wrong, when it was often government policy that created the problems in the first place. This is not to trivialise the desperate claims of patients wanting to receive new treatments where they believe they may be able to make the difference sometimes between life and death. However, government blaming Primary Care Trusts for not being able to afford new drugs conceals the national process through which budgets are allocated, and takes away central government accountability for the way in which services are run within the NHS. Either there should be a standard list of treatments that the NHS is prepared to fund, and which are paid for regardless of the local Primary Care Trust budget, or local health services should have to work within their budgets but be allowed to make difficult decisions about what is paid for without central interference.

As NHS managers of all kinds have found themselves being blamed for the problems of the health service, and doctors told that they must take more extensive managerial responsibilities, the relationship between the state and the medical profession has become more contingent. The incompatibility present since at least the 1960s is becoming more apparent at the policy level, with the BMA and Royal Colleges happy to condemn reforms with increasingly regularity. However, this does not appear to be matched by doctors working within the NHS. Individual doctors appear less inclined to protest against health reforms than they have been for some considerable time (Greener, 2006). Doctors have found themselves increasingly subject to National Service Frameworks, NICE decisions and regimes of evidence-based medicine; radical proposals concerning medical regulation (DH, 2006a) are routinely required to manage the risk of their profession in a more explicit way than ever before (McDonald et al, 2005); and even medical recruits found themselves unable to find places to train in the NHS in 2007. Despite this, there are no national medical protests. Perhaps, after the bruising experience of having the government implement reform in the face of sustained medical opposition in the 1990s, the rank-and-file doctors no longer have any appetite for conflict. Perhaps the rather favourable pay settlements given to both GPs and consultants are ample compromise for the increase in accountability demanded from the state. Whatever the reason, the relationship between the state and the doctors has never been more contingent since before the NHS.

Conclusion

On returning to power in 1997, Labour's approach to the NHS appeared conciliatory and cautious. It abolished GP fundholding, retaining the internal market but recasting contracts on to a longer-term basis in the name of cutting bureaucracy. It appeared to believe that the problems of the NHS were overstated and could be resolved relatively straightforwardly through better cooperation between the government and health professionals. The word 'reform' did not even appear in Labour's first White Paper on healthcare (Secretary of State for Health, 1997). However, by 2000, under pressure to reduce waiting lists because of election manifesto promises, and believing that health services were not improving, a change in Secretary of State for Health from the 'Old Labour' Frank Dobson to the 'New Labour' Alan Milburn led to a different approach to the NHS being taken.

The publication of the NHS Plan (Secretary of State for Health, 2000) came with a commitment to increased funding for the NHS, but not without significant reform. A performance management system was introduced and, working alongside new quasi-autonomous organisations that acted as a healthcare inspectorate (the Healthcare Commission) and a treatment approval body (NICE), led to an increased centralisation of healthcare and a far greater sense of the NHS being a 'national' organisation. However, during its second term in office, central government appeared to believe that it had run up against the limits of centralised performance management, and a third stage of reform began in which markets were reintroduced into healthcare on the grounds of making health services more responsive to individual patients (Greener, 2004c).

Labour's new marketplace for care is different from the Conservative internal market of the 1990s in that it makes use of private and not-for-profit providers to introduce competitive forces into the NHS. A second important difference is that the Conservatives put in place what was, for the time, radical legislation to introduce the purchaser-provider split that faced considerable medical opposition, but which was implemented in a very cautious way that resulted in very few market mechanisms. Labour, in contrast, has introduced its reforms on a far more piecemeal basis; it has not faced concerted medical opposition, but has been extremely radical in the implementation of the reforms, even effectively subsidising non-public entrants into the health marketplace in order to make sure that competitive forces become more widespread. Labour's 'continuous revolution' in policy making has led to NHS institutions being introduced, disbanded and renamed at a remarkable rate, and wave after wave of reforms and changes to performance management systems.

A sympathetic interpretation of Labour's approach is that it has come to represent a process of creative destruction in which the government has realised that the only way to reform an organisation such as the NHS is continually to change its structures and systems. A more critical reading would suggest that, although the reforms tend to combine a strong central performance management system with the increased use of market mechanisms, the contradictions and tensions that arise from this approach threaten to overwhelm health provision, which only survives because of the goodwill and hard work of those working within the NHS.

Thatcherism was summarised by political scientist Andrew Gamble's phrase 'the free economy and the strong state' (Gamble, 1987); in the NHS Labour appears to be taking a leaf out of Thatcher's book, with its approach to reform introducing market mechanisms into healthcare on a wider basis than has ever been the case before, but also making sure that a strong, centralised performance management system is in place. The NHS is increasingly resembling a combination of a regulated economy and a performance–managed state.

From a managerial state to a regulatory state?

Labour's changes to the NHS can be summarised as representing a shift from running a managerial state (pre-2000) to a regulatory state (post-2000), with the government beginning to withdraw from its commitment to provision, and instead trying to lever improvements in healthcare by creating market-type mechanisms, by setting an overall performance framework within which health services must work and by reserving direct intervention for when political problems appear. Labour's NHS is an attempt to force systematic reform through market mechanisms, an acknowledgement that there is only so much that management can achieve in terms of driving any greater performance from the existing NHS systems (Barber, 2007). Labour's return to markets mechanisms, after labelling them as inefficient in 1997 because of the red tape necessary for contracting arrangements, appears at times to resemble an article of faith (Greener, 2004c; Clarke et al, 2007).

When things go wrong, however, the government is increasingly blaming those working within the NHS, especially managers in Foundation Trusts or Primary Care Trusts. When circumstances become politically sensitive, such as when drug assessments or treatment refusals are taken up by the media, managers are held to blame for financial problems rather than the government, which still decides pay awards, sets the overall policy context requiring PFI for capital expenditure,and enforces participation in the new mixed economy of care by incentivising new entrants from the private and not-for-profit sectors. The new marketplace for care also introduces a real danger that the NHS will be left holding the bill for services that the private sector regards as too expensive to provide, and that medical (and even nurse) training will be fragmented or disappear in some specialisms in some areas.

If creative destruction was the goal of health reform, Labour policy is becoming increasingly successful – the double-bed has been reformulated, and the tripartite split faces a new solution through the increased use of market forces. The general taxation method of funding remains, propped up by private finance in order to achieve long-overdue infrastructure investment, but which imposes significant capital charges on public healthcare providers in the long term. Forcing organisations to deal with contradictions does not have to be a destructive process – contradictions are a part of everyday life. However, the heavy-handed and overbearing manner with which blame is often allocated by the government, and the characterisation of anyone caring to suggest alternatives to the reform agenda as being stuck in the past, have hardly created a positive environment for the discussion of what kind of healthcare system the NHS should be in the future. It is to the future that the next chapter looks.

Note
[1] My thanks to Matthias Beck for telling me about the early history of PFI.

TEN

Conclusion

Introduction

This final chapter of the book has two parts. The first part reviews the book's argument with the aim of exploring what the NHS is like today, summarising the previous chapters' analysis in the process. The second part considers how health services may be reformed to deal with the problems identified in the first part of the chapter. It presents the author's view of what the NHS should become.

Part One: what the NHS is like today

This book began by claiming that the creation of the NHS in 1948 put in place key organisational features that, to varying extents, are still present 60 years later. These features have persisted by various means, putting in place mechanisms for their self-reproduction and resisting attempts at change through waves of health reform.

Organisational features

Tripartism

The tripartite relationship between the three areas of NHS provision – GPs, consultants, and health services run by local authorities – remains remarkably in place 60 years after the NHS was founded. Depending on which of the tripartite elements employs a particular member of staff, differences in pay and conditions still exist, even for those working in what appear to be similar jobs. The 1970s saw attempts to work across common boundaries in the first NHS reorganisation, alongside new discourses of community care and primary care leading to a greater emphasis on the provision of local services. Policy confusion in the 1980s resulted in an explosive growth of private residential care for older people and for home visiting, and eventually local authority care managers and social care. Social care is technically outside the scope of the NHS, but lies along the boundaries of health services, and in the eyes of influential commentator (and also recent governmental health policy adviser) Julian Le Grand, presents a template for the way in which health services may be organised more competitively in the future. Hospital services remain dominant in the NHS, but are increasingly under threat as the budget for services is devolved to Primary Care Trusts and GPs, and a greater emphasis on delivering health services in the community emerges. Hospitals also face a number of potential problems in the future because of their difficulties in competing in a healthcare marketplace where they have disadvantages in terms of both higher overheads and providing a comprehensive range of services at a time when specialist, small-scale providers are competing with them.

Primary care has undergone a period of increased attention and development since the 1970s, with GPs being encouraged to drive reform and increase the NHS's responsiveness by their purchasing of care and by providing more community-based services themselves. On returning to office in 1997, Labour abolished GP purchasing (fundholding) and attempted to form partnerships between GPs, hospitals and community health services to overcome the boundary problems between health services, but the new partnership organisations often struggled to make much headway because of their long history of independence from one another. Labour's policy then became rather circular, as it first created Primary Care Groups as both purchasers and providers of care, then tried to achieve better coordination between health and community care in the creation of Primary Care Trusts and finally reintroduced GP purchasing (this time as practice-based commissioning). Meanwhile, Primary Care Trusts have taken increased responsibility for both providing and contracting for community services, but have run into considerably difficulties, underwent a period of disruptive mergers in 2006 and were graded as the lowest-performing organisations in the NHS in both 2006 and 2007 (Healthcare Commission, 2006b).

The present means of attempting to navigate through the tripartite split comes with the mixed economy of care, with GPs potentially able to commission services, in their new roles as practice-based commissioners (DH, 2004), from a remarkable range of community providers (Secretary of State for Health, 2006), but without the scope, yet, to commission social care services as well (Le Grand, 2007). The relationship between health and community health services remains contingent, with GPs positioned as care entrepreneurs in offering new services, and managers responsible for commissioning them into coherent care pathways.

General practitioners, then, are increasingly requested to occupy entrepreneurial roles, providing new services to allow Primary Care Trusts to move care from secondary into primary settings, managing their own budgets as practice-based commissioners, and attempting to get the best possible deals for their patients in local health economies, even though it is unclear whether GPs or patients are meant to be making the choice of secondary care. Equally, GPs must manage the tensions between responding to patient wishes and prescribing the latest treatments demanded by articulate patients with good access to the Internet or, at the other extreme, work out whether they should offer treatments such as homeopathy, when their practice is meant to be as 'evidence based' as possible. Consultants are also being encouraged to take on entrepreneurial roles, moving their services out of their locations in general hospitals because of the high overheads they may carry with them, and into community settings, where their service may become a 'social enterprise' provider, organisationally outside of the public sector.

The relationship between GPs and consultants has undergone another change as the result of the introduction of payment by results, which means that money, for the first time in the NHS, now notionally follows individual patients through the healthcare system, funding those who actually provide care. General practitioenrs, as practice-based commissioners, now carry the powers of the fundholders of the 1990s, and so consultants may have to foster rather closer relationships with their clinical colleagues, especially in the new mixed economy of care where there is greater scope for competition. As relationships become more necessary, and hospitals become more exposed to the rigours of contracting from the private sector, the not-for-profit sector and entrepreneurial GPs establishing services in primary care, the balance of power may shift back in favour of GPs again.

The double-bed

The double-bed relationship between the state and the medical profession survives in the present day, but has gradually been moved on to different terms. State–medical relationships at the creation of the NHS were based on the principle of mutual dependence, but from the 1980s onwards the state has increasingly imposed policy rather than consulting with the doctors, and the medical profession has found itself excluded particularly from the policy formulation process. However, the ability of the doctors effectively to veto the implementation of policy through their professional autonomy and by operating in a professional rather than managerial hierarchy means that their independence persists in most healthcare organisations to a remarkable degree, despite repeated attempts by the state to gain greater control.

It is hard for managers to either challenge or control doctors. The state has found ways of reducing its dependence on doctors working within the public sector and increasing the capacity of health services available through the creation of the mixed economy of care, but well-qualified doctors remain a scarce resource on which the state depends to deliver its care whether they are working for the public or private sector. New employment contracts have meant that doctors have found themselves increasingly treated as employees of health organisations and the state now expects health managers to measure the performance of clinicians in order to monitor their productivity and efficiency. However, doctors remain archetypal professionals, with their relationships with patients confidential and their accountability still often primarily to their peers rather than to managers. The power of the state in the double-bed has certainly increased, but doctors remain, compared with the fate of other professionals in the public and private sectors, remarkably in control of their own destinies.

The double-bed relationship has remained in place because both the state and the medical profession still need the relationship between the two groups to work out, even if they find themselves increasingly estranged. Labour is certainly continuing the trend of pushing the boundaries of the relationship further in the state's favour, and unless the medical profession manages to begin to organise some sustained resistance, it may well find the remaining bastions of its power under siege from the increased use of management controls and through challenges to autonomy in medical regulation (Greener, 2006). The relationship between the medical profession and the state has become more and more contingent, and less and less necessary, as time has gone on, and increasingly incompatible, creating the potential for conflict. Ways have to be found of re-engaging both parties in a more constructive relationship.

Health service funding

The NHS still provides care that is free at the point of use, financed primarily from general taxation. This claim was first partially compromised through the introduction of the prescription charge, but with so many exemptions applied that its effect on vulnerable groups was very limited. In today's NHS, increased managerialism means that charging at every opportunity seems to be becoming the norm, with attempts to find ways of getting patients to pay for the non-clinical aspects of their care particularly apparent. In hospitals, patients find environments where a host of optional extras exists from the use of private telephones and televisions through to a chance to visit the miniature shopping malls now present in many entrance foyers. Visitors are expected to pay 'market-based' fees for car parking, and to be offered numerous opportunities to buy flowers and gifts on their way to seeing their family and friends. Health managers are expected to find every possible income source to help cover the substantial capital costs involved in running a hospital (especially a PFI hospital), seeking out opportunities to subcontract services in return for new income streams, or offering NHS services to the private as well as public market.

The first mechanism for the preservation of the NHS remaining free at the point of care is that it would be politically extremely damaging for the government to introduce more widespread charges – it would be seen as an attack on Britain's most popular welfare institution (Klein, 1993). Charges have yet to be introduced for patients who do not turn up for GP appointments, and it seems unlikely that charges for doctor consultations will be introduced in the immediate future. It would require a brave politician to risk going down in history as the one who introduced routine charges for access to care in the NHS. Prescription charges, however, are very much in place, and continue to rise at a rate above inflation, compromising the claim that the NHS is entirely free in its care, even if substantial exemptions from them continue to exist.

The second mechanism for preserving the NHS's funding mechanism from general taxation is its fairness. This is emphasised in both the NHS Plan (Secretary of State for Health, 2000) and the Wanless Report into healthcare financing (Wanless, 2002), and, despite the cynical view that politicians are not overly concerned with fairness, it does seem valid to suggest that it is a concern for them. However, politicians also stand to gain a great deal from funding healthcare from general taxation, as it gives them a considerable degree of control over the NHS budget. This ability to control health budgets gives the Treasury, normally recognised to be the most powerful government department, a strong reason not to want to change the way the NHS is funded. NHS funding is supply-led, the government deciding the budget available for healthcare, rather than being demand-led, which would be the case if an insurance-based system were adopted instead. A combination of an insurance-based system and a mixed economy of care could be particularly inflationary of health budgets, as new providers could enter, additional capacity for care could be provided, and waiting lists almost completely removed. However, the state would have to meet the bill for all the extra healthcare capacity offered. This would potentially require an open-ended commitment from the state immediately to fund anyone needing treatment who met insurance-funding criteria.

The government, although it has dramatically increased the funds available to the NHS in the period since 2000, still does not allocate the same level of funding for healthcare as the other leading economies of the world, so there is still scope for a considerable growth in expenditure. Funding health services from general taxation keeps a limit on this growth, with the state deciding the total fund available rather than allowing the demand for services to dictate the level of funding for healthcare. Funding healthcare from a fixed budget, however, leaves it to local doctors and managers to decide who gets treated within the available funds, a role they may be increasingly reluctant to take if the state continues to criticise the decisions they make.

The other area of healthcare financing that must be considered in any account of recent NHS policy is the PFI. The PFI has, by some measures, been a remarkable success. Not since the Hospital Plan of the 1960s has there been so much capital investment in NHS infrastructure, with significant building taking place across the country. It is hard to dispute that hospitals have been built that would otherwise still be the subject of discussions over financing and planning, and investment in healthcare facilities has occurred on a level that would not otherwise have been the case. This is the upside of PFI. However, persistent concerns remain on a number of fronts. The question as to whether the PFI represents good value for money for the public sector remains a controversial one. If private organisations are making above-market returns for building or maintenance contracts, this needs to be examined urgently to see if the price of the PFI is too great. There were rumours of a moratorium on the PFI during 2006 (Talbot-Smith and Pollock, 2006), but this seems to have been overcome, with new awards being given during 2007 that were among the largest so far. The Hospital Plan of the 1960s was successful in improving NHS infrastructure, but created budgetary problems in the 1970s, as the running costs of the new builds were far greater than the buildings they replaced. The PFI has a similar problem built into it – as the capital costs of new buildings have to be paid for, the costs of running health organisations increases dramatically, and the long-term financial commitment that PFI buildings carry with them means that these increased costs will be incurred for a long time to come.

NHS principles

The NHS remains universal in that it provides care for all UK citizens, as it has always done. However, there have always been compromises in its universality, and a further erosion is now becoming apparent. In line with the discourse of the new public health, there is increasingly a sense of the deserving and undeserving sick, with those in the latter category, such as the obese or those who have abused drugs or engaged in self-harm, expected to meet additional criteria before they receive treatment from the health service. Drug abusers may have to demonstrate their commitment to giving up before they receive care, and self-harmers may expect to be treated begrudgingly in hospital facilities (Cresswell, 2005, 2007). There is a logic to care being limited by the available budget, as not everyone can receive it at once. The difficulty is that it is doctors who are left to decide who receives care and when, rather than this being the result of an explicit and rational debate either nationally from policy makers or locally from Primary Care Trusts. The NHS has always implicitly delayed care through requiring patients to wait, sometimes for years, for treatment. This waiting is now supplemented by increased opportunities for doctors to make value judgements, deciding the order in which patients should be treated according to lifestyle factors.

The comprehensiveness of the NHS has always been overstated (Powell, 1997). A range of treatments are in place that aim to provide care for every illness, but the NHS does not provide every possible treatment – this would not be possible on the grounds of cost. Comprehensiveness is an important principle of care as it guarantees at least some kind of care to be available, but that care increasingly does not have to be provided by the public sector. The increased use of not-for-profit and private organisations in the mixed economy of care leads to care contracts passing out of public provision. In theory, this doesn't really matter – patients do not mind who treats them as long as they are well looked after. What does matter is if clinical training opportunities disappear from particular specialisms as a result of care moving into the private sector, or if the provision of care can no longer be guaranteed because it has moved entirely out of public hands. Comprehensiveness may exist both locally and nationally, but it will take considerable coordination from strategic health authorities and Primary Care Trusts to make sure that this is the case. Public organisations that attempt to continue to provide comprehensive care may have additional overheads from providing medical training, and from the extensive estate required to offer a comprehensive range of services. This puts them at a disadvantage in the mixed economy of care, as private sector institutions may be operating on much smaller scales, with far lower costs.

The NHS of today, then, remains a service that is free at the point of delivery, but with a range of additional services available for a fee, as well as ample shopping opportunities, and with visitors expected to help fund the NHS through car parking charges. Equally, those paying prescription charges on a regular basis may wonder exactly whether they are receiving NHS care for free. The NHS is comprehensive in that it continues to provide some kind of treatment for the public for their illnesses and injuries, although the care offered may not be exactly what patients, increasingly cast as consumers, might have chosen, and may not be provided by public organisations, leaving open the possibility of service gaps appearing in the future should private and not-for-profit providers exit from the mixed economy of care. The NHS continues to be funded primarily from general taxation, but with that taxation being used to fund a range of non-public providers, and with health managers being encouraged to find as many additional funding sources as they possibly can. The NHS is national in the sense that there are national standards for care and only limited space for local variations, although a rhetoric of decentralisation is used to justify market-based reforms and blame managers for problems when they occur. This leads to issues of paternalism and accountability moving centre-stage.

Paternalism and accountability

The NHS, at its founding, was a healthcare organisation categorised as being one where politicians were accountable for the NHS through the parliamentary process (with all the possible failings of that system), but with considerable local autonomy for doctors, who were expected to make operational decisions on how care should be delivered. Doctors rationed care within the budget available to healthcare by GP surgeries acting as gatekeepers to care, deciding who should be treated and who not, and by consultants managing waiting lists.

The relationship between the state and the doctors at the time of the NHS's founding therefore amounted to a system of national accountability, with politicians being responsible for the running of the NHS through the parliamentary process, and local paternalism, with the doctors effectively running the NHS at the local level on behalf of the government. This could be seen as a remarkably conducive system of relationships for the doctors, who apparently held most of the power in the day-to-day running of the health service, but with politicians taking the blame when things went wrong. However, the government made decisions about the overall sum available for care within the NHS, and despite setting up an independent panel to decide doctor pay (the Whitley Council), it also had the final say on medical pay, and certainly set the budget for capital investment. Compared with most advanced economies, the growth of doctors' pay in the NHS during its first decades was remarkably restrained, and doctors have often been required to work in very poor facilities, a symptom of poor levels of both resource inheritance and investment.

In contrast to the situation at the time of the NHS's founding, the direction of reforms now is to create a situation of national paternalism, whereby the centre sets the policy framework and intervenes when it thinks things are going wrong, and local accountability, whereby semi-autonomous national organisations such as NICE (Walshe, 2003b) and local health organisations such as Foundation Trusts and Primary Care Trusts are blamed when concerns about unfair outcomes or budget deficits arise. Local organisations have been given the responsibility of running healthcare, but without the authority to fulfil that responsibility (Paton, 2005). This is a direct inversion of the situation at the founding of the NHS – accountability has moved away from the government, which is now happy to blame others when things go wrong, with managers to blame for deficits, NICE to blame when particular medicines are not approved for use in the NHS and Primary Care Trusts to blame when funds are not available for particular treatments. The local paternalism present at the founding of the NHS, based on medical professionalism and autonomy, has moved to the centre as the government has achieved stronger control over local health organisations through the use of techniques such as performance management. The government is also able to make well-publicised interventions to correct politically sensitive failings of local and health organisations, where drugs are not prescribed for patients, or where media pressure creates situations where politicians sense that they may be held to blame.

Managers

The changes described above have had an odd effect on the role of local health managers in the NHS. Increasingly, they find themselves cast in the extreme roles of heroes or villains, with managers of organisations ranked as being high performing being held up as exemplars of what it takes to lead the NHS in the 21st century, and those with budget deficits and clinical governance failings castigated by politicians and the media alike. Primary Care Trust managers are required to be entrepreneurs, commissioning services that appear seamless to patients from the increasing range of care providers, while at the same time attempting to be strategic in trying to find innovative new ways of providing care, and moving treatments from secondary (hospital) to primary (community) settings, in order to both make them more accessible to patients and reduce costs.

Primary Care Trust managers face a dilemma with respect to consumerism: should they commission services in line with patient demand, and so increasingly fund services without an evidence base, such as homeopathy, which are clearly popular with patients in an age when alternative therapies are a huge growth area, or should they only commission services that evidence suggests are best for them? Equally, Primary Care Trusts are left with the dilemma of having to work out locally how individual demands for the latest treatments square with the collective needs of their local communities to receive care, and with the problem of trying to achieve responsiveness to local demand on the one hand, but public accountability of transparency of expenditure and fairness for everyone on the other. They have to navigate their way between national guidelines for care and local responsiveness in care commissioning.

Hospital managers are left to compete in the health marketplace on often unfair terms, as they must provide comprehensive care, providing the full range of services, and carry the overhead of clinical training, while their private and not-for-profit competitors are often much smaller in size, specialist in their focus (in the sense of providing only one treatment) and have lower overheads as a result. Hospital managers have found themselves hamstrung in the mixed economy of care even where they have been able to persuade clinicians to offer additional capacity, as Primary Care Trusts have often been unable to provide the funding for the additional treatments they can offer. This problem, well known within the NHS but illustrated vividly in a BBC2 (2007) investigation by businessman Gerry Robinson into the NHS, is clearly madness. Salaried, public employees are finding ways of being more productive, but their ideas and more-efficient practices are blocked because they cannot be paid for by another public organisation, when the NHS as a whole must meet these salary costs anyway.

Patients

Patients too are being given new roles. They are expected to challenge GPs and consultants as informed consumers, choosing their GP with care and conducting research into which secondary provider would be best for them. However, patients still do not appear to have the appetite or capacity to seek out health organisation performance information to form the basis of their choices, and may not even want increased choice at all (Fotaki et al, 2005). Patients are meant to be using 'choice' rather than 'voice' to drive the new mixed economy of care (Minister of State for Department of Health et al, 2005), but are struggling in this role. This is not to suggest that patients are fools, or passive participants in their healthcare. They do know when they are being treated with dignity and respect, but it is hard to see how they can make this count within the mixed economy of care as it is presently configured. Patients are being actively encouraged to use choice mechanisms as an 'exit' strategy from poor service providers, but are often reluctant to change GP because their choice is usually linked to the proximity of the practice to their home (Greener, 2003a) and the very episodic nature of the relationship with hospital medicine is likely to mean that the choice to avoid a particular service in the future as the result of a bad experience might prove to be irrelevant. Encouraging a discourse of health consumerism runs the very real risk of patients raising their expectations of care to unrealistically high levels from which they can only be disappointed, a symptom of the 'consumer society' more generally (Bauman, 2007) that has the potential to be brought into healthcare. Equally, patients appear to be unwilling to travel very far for non-tertiary (regional specialist) care, and this has to impose a limit on the potential for increasing patient choice (but see Propper et al, 2006, for a different interpretation of the data on this point).

Summary of the NHS's problems

The new mixed economy of care, according to policy makers, is a source of innovation, creating the potential for entrepreneurial behaviour from managers and doctors. It is also meant to cause disruption to the delivery of health services in a way that causes 'creative destruction', in that old, outdated practices are driven out and a new responsive NHS is created. All this change and dynamism means that the planning of local services is made extremely difficult as new providers enter and exit markets, and hospitals find themselves having to work extremely hard to continue to operate as comprehensive providers of care. Equally, allowing greater health consumerism risks raising the expectations of the public to unrealistic levels, so causing disaffection with a public service that has, despite its many failings, remained remarkably popular throughout its history. Patients in desperate need of expensive new drugs find themselves having to fight for them as individual consumers, while

Primary Care Trusts struggle to consider the implications of funding new treatments within limited budgets, at the same time holding a responsibility for commissioning care for the rest of their community. At the same time, local and national media, sometimes alongside politicians, accuse managers of making heartless and insensitive decisions that, in practice, they may have little control over.

The new mixed economy of care decentralises blame, has an unrealistic notion of the role of the patient in improving care standards, distracts clinicians from medicine by encouraging them to be entrepreneurs instead, and puts managers into roles where they must meet centrally imposed targets or face losing their jobs, while at the same time being expected to act according to longstanding principles of high public standards. Labour is to be congratulated for its increased investment in the NHS, but criticised for the cumbersome, contradictory (Harrison and McDonald, 2008) and inconsistent way in which it has implemented reform since 2000. Table 10.1 summarises the NHS's problems at the end of 2007.

Part Two: the future of the NHS. What should be done?

If the NHS is ridden with tensions, and the government's approach to reform is struggling to find answers and is proving destructive, what should be done instead? What follows is a pragmatic attempt, based on the analysis of the preceding chapters, to take the best from the health service's history to combine what seems to have worked best with the understanding that any changes must start, not with a blank slate, but with the inheritance of 60 years of policy.

The role of professions in the policy process

First of all, the medical profession must be brought back into policy making in recognition that its role is crucial if the health service is to improve. To be sure, the doctors have not always been the most cooperative of partners in the past, but the relationship between the government and the doctors has to be a two-way street rather than the government attempting to simply impose policy from the centre through the increased use of managerial technologies and market forces. Doctors deserve a say in policy. But equally, nurses must also have a place at the table. Despite the lack of nursing will to put forward its interests as assertively as the doctors through routes such as industrial action, it is surely time to recognise the centrality of nursing to the NHS,

Table 10.1: The NHS's problems at the end of 2007

Problem	Description
Creative destruction from wave after wave of reform	NHS managers experience reforms as 'redisorganisation' (Smith et al, 2001) and cynicism about reforms increases from profession
Mixed economy of care makes planning extremely difficult	Market reforms mean that planning of services becomes extremely problematic because of lack of predictability and stability
Difficulty in guaranteeing comprehensiveness of service	Market dynamic means that public provision may no longer guarantee the local provision of particular services
Public expectations of service based on consumerism grow too high	Even with improvement, health services can never meet the increasingly raised expectations of service of the public, whose expectations are forced higher still through choice agendas
Patients experience financial decentralisation as a barrier to getting care	Primary Care Trusts are blamed for rationing healthcare, having to take responsibility for the commissioning of care for their community within nationally set guidelines
Clinicians encouraged to become entrepreneurs	Clinicians are increasingly distracted from clinical roles and engage in providing new services
Managers blamed for problems	Politicians decentralise blame – national paternalism, but local accountability

and to allow nurse leaders a voice in deciding what direction health policy should take. At present, the government appears to be bent on spending vast sums on special advisers and management consultants when the NHS already employs vast numbers of experts who need to be better incorporated into the policy-making process.

There has been much debate over an 'independent board' to run the NHS 'free from politics'. This seems a rather naive dream. Choices over the direction of health policy are inherently ideological – judgements about the use of markets and the role of doctors in health service administration are not technical judgements, but carry a great deal of ideological baggage. It has been possible to pass control of interest rate policy to the Bank of England since 1997 because it involves making a single technical decision, so a range of different expertise and beliefs can be combined to form a judgement as to whether action is necessary.

Health policy, in contrast, involves a bewildering range of variables and entirely unforeseeable events. There will always be a role for politics in healthcare, as the principles of the political party in place have a role to play in deciding what policy should consider from the almost endless lists of things that could be done. But politicians must work closely with health professionals to decide what direction future policy should take, and health professionals, in turn, must accept that if given a seat in policy making, they have a duty to contribute constructively to debates and to take responsibility for making collectively made decisions work on the ground.

A national health service or a local health service?

The centralisation of health policy and organisation that has been particularly clear from 2000 onwards has meant that the NHS has become a 'national' health service more than ever before. But as this has occurred, policy makers have utilised market mechanisms to a far greater extent than ever before and tried to blame local health managers for the problems that have emerged as a result. Labour appears to regard the tension between a national performance system and local markets as a creative one, but there is little evidence to support this view.

One alternative to the combination of a centralised performance management system and a decentralised market is to try to make health services genuinely national, with the same treatments available everywhere. This approach carries with it a logic of central government accountability, with management and doctors primarily in an implementation role. There seems to be little space for markets in this model, as markets in healthcare are about creating greater local responsiveness for services (as in present policy), and this runs directly against the grain of centrally specified services, which are about standardisation. Attempting to balance the two, as Labour is presently trying to achieve, gives policy makers an almost irresistible urge to interfere in local decisions they do not like, invalidating their reasons for setting up the market in the first place. Policy makers often characterise the NHS's organisation between 1948 and 1989 as being one of command and control, as a performance management system would entail, but the analysis in this book suggests that NHS organisation during this period time was very far from centrally run.

However, a centrally run performance management system is probably near impossible to achieve in practice. Central government lacks the capacity to run the NHS on a day-to-day basis with any degree of consistency, with the critiques of government overload being particularly apposite (Le Grand, 1991). The performance management system presently in the NHS involves a huge amount of data of very mixed quality being collected, summarised and reported, but still the government probably has very little idea of what goes on in hospitals, Primary Care Trusts, GP surgeries and other NHS organisations on an everyday level.

There is merit in trying to secure a standardisation of services and treatments across the country, but this seems to be an unrealistic dream that stifles the ability of local managers to be responsive to the needs of the communities they serve. This ties in Fox and Miller's (1995) criticisms of accountability measures of public organisations designed around systems that rely on politicians and periodic elections, where they suggest that the 'democratic loop' has never really functioned as most people do not even know who their elected officials are, never mind how they can influence the running of public services through them.

Instead of a national health service, it is time we treated seriously the idea of a local health service instead. Within such a service it would still be the role of the government to set policy, but local organisations would be allowed far greater discretion in how it was carried out. In return for this increased local discretion and authority, those running local health services would have to accept the responsibility for meeting the standards required by the government. This is different from the way that local health services are presently run because of the overbearing and interfering practices central government adopts to get its way in local health economies. It has been recognised since the early 1980s, and the Griffiths Management Inquiry, that this has to stop, but the government has lacked the political will to grasp the nettle and allow it to happen.

This is not to say that the government does not have a role in setting minimum standards of care and deciding, at the highest level, what the priorities for health expenditure should be. But systemic improvement does not come from remote politicians trying to squeeze more and more from the system using top-down performance management, something even the head of the Prime Minister's Delivery Unit appears to have come to believe towards the end of his time in office (Barber, 2007).

The logic of this argument leads to the conclusion that health services should be allowed to offer locally different services, with experiments in local democracy carried out to make sure that they are also accountable for these differences. It has been a long-running theme of NHS organisation that the obvious site for achieving greater local involvement in healthcare is local government. The decline of local authorities over the past 30 years has been sad to watch, as they have been stripped of authority and resources, and the resulting decline in involvement from local people in local politics is hardly surprising (Jenkins, 2006). To make local government a vibrant and dynamic site from which health services might be run, two changes need to take place. First, local people must believe that local politics matter, and that the decisions being taking are important. Putting local health organisations under the control of local authorities would mean that the decisions taken there would matter to local people – health services remain among the highest profile of all those in the public sector. There would therefore be an incentive for local people to be involved in local politics to a far greater extent. Second, mechanisms would have to be established to show that their involvement paid off, and that local people had a genuine role in deciding the future of their health services once involved. Greater local participation in health services will only be secured if the decisions given to local people are important, and if their views are taken seriously.

A greater use of local democratic mechanisms does not remove the need for planning in health services; there is a need to ensure adequate provision in each area, and this should become the job of strategic health authorities, with Primary Care Trusts then expected to find ways of locally conforming to the regional plans. Again, though, there is a key role for local government in working with these bodies to make sure that the needs of local people are being met, and for far greater local involvement in decision-making processes within them.

National Institute for Health and Clinical Excellence (NICE) should continue to make recommendations on the care to be funded within the NHS, but politicians should be kept out of its decision making. If NICE has demonstrated a clear criteria for making decisions as to whether NHS care is funded or not, those decisions should be respected. Treatments that do not meet public standards of demonstrating clinical efficacy should not be funded through the NHS. If patients want to consume services with no evidence base, they should do so with their own funds, but NICE must also be funded so that it is able to perform analyses of newly available treatments quickly and effectively.

The tripartite split

The tripartite split between health services has been a central organisational problem since the creation of the NHS in 1948. Putting healthcare in the hands of local authorities would allow both social care and healthcare to be overseen by the same government organisations, and for the leaders of local authorities to be accountable to a local electorate for their ability to run them.

The role of clinicians within the NHS should be to make sure they are up to date in their practice, providing high standards of care and treating patients with respect and dignity. Patients should be able to challenge doctors where necessary, but they also have to understand that there are collective limits to what can be funded within health services, and that they cannot have every possible service or treatment. Where a low standard of service is being received, or where patients have been treated discourteously or without respect, they have a right to complain, and to have those complaints treated seriously. The right to greater local involvement in the running of the NHS through the mechanisms of local government carries with it a duty for the public to participate in the decisions made available to them. If particular members of the public choose not to get involved in debates about what services should or should not be funded, and later demand funding for services that become important to them, their complaints will fall not on deaf ears, but on less sympathetic ones than had the complainants participated when less directly or personally interested.

Within hospitals the role of consultants should be focused on providing excellent services rather than trying to behave as entrepreneurs finding new locations to deliver care with lower overheads. Consultants must be more accountable for their work and actions; their inspection bodies must be simplified and accountability achieved where mistakes can be a source of learning rather than of legal action. Clinical governance has had some success in this area, by encouraging hospital doctors to learn from errors in the past, and to account for the success (or otherwise) of their medical and surgical practice.

Consultants, in line with many public professionals, have not always been held accountable for their decisions (Marquand, 2004). This does not mean, however, that the government must step in. Doctors can be held to account by their peers, and it is right that they are made accountable for the resource implications of their decisions. The regulatory mechanisms of the GMC must be overhauled to make decisions and processes more transparent than at present, and more lay involvement in key decision-making panels in order that clinicians are forced to be more accountable to those outside of their profession. Their processes must also be streamlined dramatically, as health organisations are presently often put in the invidious position of having to suspend doctors on full pay and begin their own investigations of doctors' performances, while at the same time having to wait for GMC hearings to be conducted before they are able to decide whether any charges brought against doctors are valid or not. In the end, the issue of doctor competence can only be decided by other doctors, but if self-regulation is to be preserved, the GMC has to become far more responsive and consistent in its decision-making processes.

The role of GPs should remain the likely first port of call into the NHS for patients, with GPs and patients making referrals within the framework of contracts put in place by the Primary Care Trusts for the location where secondary or tertiary care (where necessary) takes place. General practitioners are increasingly the lead figures in primary care teams rather than individuals working with other doctors alone, and their key role, which is providing the majority of frontline healthcare in the NHS, has to be recognised and celebrated. There are areas of GP practice where improvements need to be made, however.

The patient choice process must take place within the GP surgery, rather than the job being delegated to telephone call centres. General practitioners should work with patients through additional appointments, or by referring them to specialist choice advisers. The information systems underpinning patient choice and contracting must be substantially overhauled from their present state. It seems odd that the government continues to reify the efficiency of the private sector when at the same time it has failed so badly, so frequently, to provide the public sector with adequate information technology. Primary Care Trusts must become more locally engaged, and work more closely with GPs to address the difficulties of the gatekeeper function. General practitioners should be held to account for their prescribing and referral patterns in a similar way to consultants being required to explain the average length of patients' hospital stays and treatment patterns. However, they should not be constrained by individual budgets, as the evidence of the 1990s suggests that the savings that can be generated are not significant (Baines et al, 1997) and that GP budget holding does not necessarily lead to an increase in patient satisfaction (Dusheiko et al, 2004b).

Nursing

In line with nursing being a graduate profession, it is time that nurses were treated with greater respect. Matron roles have placed nurses in important liaison roles between hospital boards and wards and clinics, giving them key middle management positions as well as responsibilities for areas such as infection control and cleanliness. Nurses are renegotiating their roles with doctors and taking on more and more responsibilities, but it is important that they are rewarded adequately rather than being viewed as a way of delivering health services more cheaply.

Pay settlements with doctors in the 2000s have not been ungenerous, but they started from a low base. The budgetary implications of giving the pay rises now necessary to nurses are considerable, but worthwhile, for the NHS depends almost entirely on graduate nurses and nursing assistants for the routine delivery of care. It is no mystery why there are continuing shortages of nurses in many areas of the country. Until the profession is treated as an important partner in healthcare and paid accordingly, nursing seems set to remain positioned on the sidelines of NHS organisation.

The healthcare market

The main mechanism for the allocation of care at the secondary level is becoming the mixed economy of care. This presents a particular challenge. It may be illegal under international treaties to reduce the role of non-public sectors once they have been introduced into public service provision (Pollock, 2004), so a way must be found of making this increased capacity available from the new entrants into the NHS work with the grain of the service, rather than against it.

One answer would be a reversion to the logic applied by Labour in 1997 on resuming office, and placing new entrants not in competitive relationships with one another and with public providers, but as part of a network of collaborative provision. If the government is correct and extra capacity is needed in order to bring and hold down waiting times, achieving this goal through competition appears wasteful (in terms of potential duplication, not to mention the possible need to advertise services within health economies) as well as unfair to public provision, which, as suggested above, may not be competing on equal terms because of the increased cost base comprehensive provision carries with it.

Putting local economies of care on a collaborative basis also allows Primary Care Trusts and strategic health authorities to plan, ensuring that public provision is available in each area as a back-up should non-public providers decide that they wish to leave the marketplace, as well as to continue to provide training opportunities for the clinicians of the future. Where vital training work is taking place in public facilities, those providers need to receive a clear premium in their staffing establishment payments for this work – public providers should not be put at a disadvantage for carrying out crucial work. Primary Care

Trust should have a statutory duty to continue training in their local areas at a level prescribed by the strategic health authority.

Contracts in the mixed economy of care should be made longer term, as Labour attempted to do in 1997, with poor providers warned that, should their service standards fall, they risked losing their contracts for care. Where new entrants are necessary to make good the shortfalls resulting from planned withdrawals of contracts, they should be given contracts on a planned basis in line with forecasted need rather than entering health economies on a competitive basis. Keeping the size of services at a planned level should bring and hold down waiting times through the strategic health authority planning service need in advance, and awarding extra contracts where unexpected additional need appears. Services would therefore be supply-organised (in terms of having a fixed establishment of staff, which could be compared with other health economies to make sure it is working at an appropriate level given the case mix it has before it) but demand-led, with Primary Care Trusts having a duty to meet clinical need and keep waiting times down. Because of the increased ability to forecast the incidence of illness in localities, Primary Care Trusts should receive greater funding where it is likely to be necessary. Rather than relying on historical data, the possibilities of predictive modelling offer the opportunity to fund health services more in line with contemporary need than historical illness.

Strategic health authorities and Primary Care Trusts must make sure that general hospitals are supported in order to ensure that they remain comprehensive providers of care. Where hospitals are failing to provide care at the appropriate level, there may well be a case for the present combination of managers and clinicians being removed in order for the service to start afresh, but the wholesale removing of services from public provision is not sensible. Public provision must remain the cornerstone of the NHS, not only because it is where training takes place, but also because it remains the provider of last resort. Non-public providers cannot be made to enter the mixed economy of care to fill gaps, but public provision allows services to be guaranteed, and they should be.

The Private Finance Initiative

The PFI needs to be urgently reviewed. Difficulties in evaluating the cost-effectiveness of the policy have sometimes been prevented because of claims that information about contracts is 'commercially sensitive' (Monbiot, 2001). This should not be allowed to happen – if private firms wish to contract for public money, the processes need to be fully transparent. A commission needs urgently to review existing PFI projects to establish whether they have represented a good return for the state, and to make recommendations for how the mechanism can be improved for the future. PFI contracts need to be both transparent and accountable. Equally, there needs to be a review to examine whether existing PFI builds have reached the required standard, or whether, as has been alleged by some leading architects, the builds are not really fit for purpose (Liddle, 2006).

There is an upside to PFI in terms of the increased range of capital projects it has put in place, but where grave concerns exist about the long-term value for money that they offer, an urgent review is surely required before the financial commitment it represents is extended further. Equally, it seems odd for a government that claims to embrace market forces to offer only one scheme for capital projects to be funded within the whole of the healthcare system. The PFI is the 'only game in town', and it does not seem to be entirely sensible or fair that the NHS's crumbling infrastructure is being updated with no alternative means of attracting funding available.

The role of the public in health services

Consumers or customers?

The role of the user in health services should not be that of the consumer, but instead that of the customer. This may seem to be splitting hairs, but there is a key difference. Consumers are assumed to be empowered individuals, capable of driving reform through their choices and of making informed decisions. This isn't quite right in the case of healthcare; patients often make choices about health services based on their closeness to home rather than their clinical performance, and may not be able to differentiate between good and bad care before they experience it. The public taking a customer role, in contrast, would mean that they would be routinely asked whether they have been treated fairly and with dignity, and whether their condition is improving, but would carry with it an acknowledgement that patients generally lack the clinical knowledge to be the judge of whether they are receiving the right treatment or not, and whether it is being given to them competently – this is the job of inspection regimes and of doctors' peers.

Patients positioned as customers must clearly have a voice, but primarily on the grounds of whether they are being treated fairly and with dignity. Complaints within this framework become extremely important because they combine individual dissatisfaction with the potential for systemic change. Complaints procedures must be overhauled, with mixed panels of patient representatives and clinical representatives examining cases. Patients who make serial complaints without grounding need to be reminded of their public responsibilities, and doctors who receive justifiable complaints need to change their practices.

Citizens

In terms of the public's citizen role, the greater involvement of the public in local authority decision making as a result of them being given control over health services would hopefully create far more opportunities for meaningful public service. As well as this, Foundation Trusts need to continue down the line of democratic experimentation, with this being part of accepting that services become more localised. One of the key areas where local people should be given more input, in consultation with doctors and managers from health organisations, is in considering the range of treatments to be provided within their area. It is surely sensible to allow some localisation of care, as long as basic comprehensive services and standards are kept in place. People are used to finding whether other local facilities are in place when they move house, and there is no reason why the range of health services provided in a particular area should not be taken into account as well.

If an area with a large number of older people wishes to provide an enhanced range of services for that group, local NHS services should be flexible enough to cope with that. Local plans based on population need should be agreed. This creates the chance to link health services more explicitly with local government, with a 'top-up' for locally distinct health services appearing through Council Tax payments, and a duty for local government to consult with respect to options for health service expenditure. As Mohan (2002, p 220) puts it in terms of hospitals, 'Participation and community support would be best assured through local government control'.

The obvious criticisms of such a system would be that it creates a 'postcode lottery' of care, and that it leaves health services open to politicisation at the local level. The media have become fond of creating publicity where they find some treatments available in some areas, but not in others. However, if these decisions were made in a transparent and open manner, with both public and clinical involvement, the sense of such decisions being a 'lottery' would no longer be a valid criticism. A free press cannot be made to behave responsibly, but it can be shown that decisions about which care should be funded are made in an open and democratic way.

The criticism of health services potentially becoming more politicised as a result of greater local involvement is harder to answer, as it could genuinely result, in extreme cases, in treatments that are popular becoming funded at the expense of treatments that actually work. The Oregon experiment of the 1980s asked the public to rank treatments in the order in which they believed they should be funded, with odd outcomes such as orthodontic work to straighten teeth coming higher than tried-and-tested, but less glamorous health interventions, such as smoking cessation (Halliday, 1995).

However, securing greater local involvement in NHS decisions does not mean that local people are given a free reign over policy making, it means that they must work with professional groups and managers to come to difficult decisions about how their local health services should be run. The public would be a part of decision making, but would not have the final say, in the same way that local managers or local clinicians would not. As important as the final decisions are, is the way that they are reached, through deliberation and consideration and respect, with Fox and Miller (1995, Chapter 5) suggesting practical ways of attempting to achieve sincere, honest and genuine communication in public forums.

Health service managers

The role of the manager within the NHS should be to make sure that standards of clinical care (judged by medical peers as well as others) are kept high; that patients are treated with respect and dignity; that the public are involved in the decision making of their organisation; and that resources are used wisely. Managers are collectively responsible in local heath economies for removing nonsensical situations where, for example, operating theatres are lying unused, there are long waiting lists for particular conditions and consultants who could be working on them appear to be underemployed. Managers should be ensuring that health services provide public value (Moore, 1997), searching not for new ways of extracting money from the general public through increased opportunities for charging, but for ways of ensuring that the public routinely receive high levels of service.

Those responsible for planning in hospitals and Primary Care Trusts should work with public health observatories to make sure that sufficient capacity is available in local health economies, and that contracts for care are issued for them, as well as to lobby for increased funding where capacity is not sufficient. The government should work with local planners to put in place more of a bottom-up system for the planning of health need. Remarkable steps forward have been made in predictive modelling of care, and it seems ridiculous to blame local health managers for running up deficits for funding care the need for which was predicted the previous year. The argument that there is infinite demand for healthcare (economists argue that any service with a 'price' of zero will have infinite demand) needs to be treated with a pinch of salt – would most people really like to spend more time at the doctor's?

A greater use of local democratic mechanisms to underpin the accountability of health services may also mean greater involvement in planning processes, not only extending the citizen role of the public (see above), but also leading to the potential for public decisions to make a real difference to their local health services, and so breaking the deadlock of apathy that tends to exist in local democratic elections. Health services can be instrumental in creating a 'politics for amateurs' (Stoker, 2006), in which greater local participation and involvement can lead to a virtuous circle of improved political engagement.

Inspection

Central inspection is a controversial element within the NHS, but clearly has an important role to play. All NHS providers should have to meet defined standards to remain in the mixed economy of care, with new opportunities for entry offered to either existing or new providers where these standards are not met. The inspection process, however, needs central government intervention in order to rationalise it. At present, government and accreditation bodies bombard health providers with requests for information, often in different formats, despite, one presumes, trying to achieve much the same end of ensuring a high-quality, safe service for patients.

Accreditation bodies and health service inspectorate organisations must work far more closely together to relieve the often ridiculous burden placed on health service workers at present, while at the same time assuring the goals of inspection are met. Doctors' treatment decisions must be regularly examined by other doctors, with a substantial overhaul of peer review complementing a streamlined and simplified external inspection system. Comparisons of clinical practice are now possible across a range of indicators, but this should be treated as an opportunity for doctors to learn from one another's practice rather than being used as a stick with which to beat the medical profession.

Doctors must be more accountable for their practice, based on the assumption that the vast majority of them are doing a good job rather than the presumption that they need to be bullied and cajoled into doing the right thing (Klein, 2005). Clinical governance has meant that doctors have become used to justifying their decisions to their peers, but also to managers. This must be encouraged as a means of improving practice and identifying further training needs, as well as finding inadequate and outdated practice.

Conclusion

The NHS is a remarkable institution. It is undergoing a period of unprecedented change. But it is time to question the direction of that change and to look to alternative futures where the pressures to deliver better services are combined with organisational forms that go with the grain of how health services were delivered in the UK in 1948, rather than working so much against them. Reforms that recognise the history of the NHS surely stand a better chance of working than those that appear to want to erase the past. We should be celebrating the achievements of health services in the UK, and looking forward to their improvement in the future rather than risk losing what makes the NHS special through unrealistic, badly thought-out, market-based reforms.

References

6, P. (2003) 'Giving consumers of British public services more choice: what can be learned from recent history?', *Journal of Social Policy*, 32(2), 239-70.

Abel-Smith, B. (1975) *A History of the Nursing Profession*, London: Heinemann.

Abel-Smith, B. and Titmuss, R. (1956) *The Cost of the National Health Service*, Cambridge: Cambridge University Press.

Acheson, D. (1981) *A Survey of Primary Care in London*, Occasional Paper 16, London: Royal College of General Practitioners.

Acheson, D. (1988) *Public Health in England: The Report of the Committee of Inquiry into the Future Development of the Public Health Function*, London: Department of Health.

Addison, P. (1975) *The Road to 1945*, London: Cape.

Aldcroft, D. (2001) *The European Economy 1914-2000*, London: Routledge.

Alford, R. (1972) 'The political economy of health care: dynamics without change', *Politics and Society*, 12, 127-64.

Alford, R. (1975) *Health Care Politics*, Chicago, IL: University of Chicago Press.

Allen, I. (1988) *Any Room at the Top? A Study of Doctors and their Careers*, London: Policy Studies Institute.

Allen, I. (1997) *Committed by Critical: An Examination of Young Doctors' Views of their Core Values*, London: British Medical Association.

Allender, P. (2001) 'What's new about "New Labour"?', *Politics*, 21(1), 56-62.

Allsop, J. (1995) *Health Policy and the NHS: Towards 2000*, London: Longman.

Allsop, J. and Jones, K. (2008) 'Withering the citizen, managing the consumer: complaints in healthcare settings', *Social Policy and Society*, 7(2), 233-43.

Allsop, J., Baggott, R. and Jones, K. (2002) 'Health consumer groups and the national policy process', in S. Henderson and A. Peterson (eds) *Consuming Health*, London: Routledge, pp 48-65.

Allsop, J., Jones, K. and Baggott, R. (2004) 'Health consumer groups in the UK: a new social movement?', *Sociology of Health and Illness*, 26(6), 737-56.

Andalo, D. (2004) 'Hospitals charged high premiums for PFI projects', http://society.guardian.co.uk/privatefinance/story/0,8150,1358757,00.html

Archer, M. (1995) *Realist Social Theory: The Morphogenetic Approach*, Cambridge: Cambridge University Press.

Archer, M. (1996) *Culture and Agency: The Place of Culture in Social Theory*, Cambridge: Cambridge University Press.

Archer, M. (2000) *Being Human: The Problem of Agency*, Cambridge: Cambridge University Press.

Archer, M., Bhaskar, R., Collier, A., Lawson, T. and Norrie, A. (eds) (1998) *Critical Realism: Essential Readings*, London: Routledge.

Asenova, D. and Beck, M. (2003) 'The UK financial sector and risk management in PFI projects: a survey', *Public Money and Management*, 23(3), 195-202.

Audit Commission (2003) *Waiting List Accuracy: Assessing the Accuracy of Waiting List Information in NHS Hospitals in England*, London: Audit Commission.

Audit Commission (2006) *Learning the Lessons from Financial Failure in the NHS*, London: Audit Commission.

Bacon, R. and Eltis, W. (1978) *Britain's Economic Problem: Too Few Providers*, London: Macmillan.

Baggott, R. (1994) 'Getting politics out of health? Ministers, managers and the market', *Public Policy and Administration*, 9(3), 33-51.

Baggott, R. (2004) *Health and Health Care in Britain*, Basingstoke: Palgrave.

Baggott, R. (2005) 'A funny thing happened on the way to the forum? Reforming patient and public involvement in the NHS in England', *Public Administration*, 83(3), 533-51.

Baggott, R., Allsop, J. and Jones, K. (2004) 'Representing the repressed? Health consumer groups and the national policy process', *Policy & Politics*, 32(3), 317-31.

Baines, D., Tolley, K. and Whynes, D. (1997) *Prescribing, Budgets and Fundholding in General Practice*, London: Office of Health Economics.

Baker, R. (1992) 'The inevitability of rationing: a case study of rationing in the British National Health Service', in M. Strosberg (ed) *Rationing America's Health Care*, Washington, DC: Brookings Institute.

Balint, E. and Norell, J. (1973) *Six Minutes for the Patient: Interactions in General Consultation*, London: Tavistock Institute.

Balint, M. (1957) *The Doctor, his Patient and the Illness*, London: Pitman.

Barber, M. (2007) *Instruction to Deliver: Tony Blair, the Public Services and the Challenge of Achieving Targets*, London: Portoco's Publishing.

Bauman, Z. (2007) *Consuming Life*, Cambridge: Polity Press.

BBC2 (2007) 'Can Gerry Robinson fix the NHS? – One year on', 12 December.

BBC News (1999) 'Health managers rebuked over £115m hospital overspend', http://news.bbc.co.uk/1/hi/health/436046.stm

BBC News (2001) '£30m to improve "dirty" hospitals', http://news.bbc.co.uk/1/hi/health/1121300.stm

BBC News (2004) 'Doctors fear recruitment crisis', http://news.bbc.co.uk/1/hi/england/leicestershire/3082242.stm

BBC News (2006a) 'NHS deficit doubles to over £500m', http://news.bbc.co.uk/1/hi/health/5055602.stm

BBC News (2006b) 'Judge me on NHS finances – Hewitt', http://news.bbc.co.uk/1/hi/health/4785032.stm

BBC News (2006c) 'PFI schemes "to cost NHS £53bn"', http://news.bbc.co.uk/1/hi/health/6089122.stm

BBC News (2006d) '"Meddling" to blame for NHS deficits', http://news.bbc.co.uk/1/hi/health/5052976.stm

BBC News (2007) 'PFI "forcing public service cuts"', http://news.bbc.co.uk/1/hi/uk_politics/7113770.stm

Beardwood, B., Walters, V., Eyles, J. and French, S. (1999) 'Complaints against nurses: a reflection of "the new managerialism" and consumerism in health care?', *Social Science and Medicine*, 48, 363–74.

Beck, U. (1992) *Risk Society: Towards a New Modernity*, London: Sage Publications.

Berridge, V. (1996) *AIDS in the UK: The Making of Policy 1981-1994*, Oxford: Oxford University Press.

Berridge, V. (1999) *Health and Society in Britain since 1939*, Cambridge: Cambridge University Press.

Beveridge, W. (1942) *Social Insurance and Allied Services*, London: HMSO.

Birchall, J. (2003) 'Mutualism and the governance of foundation trusts', Paper presented at the Manchester Centre for Healthcare Management Conference, Manchester, 13 June.

Bloomfield, B. (1991) 'The role of information systems in the NHS: action at a distance and the fetish of calculation', *Social Studies of Science*, 21, 701–34.

Bloomfield, B. and Best, A. (1992) 'Management consultants: systems development, power and the translation of problems', *Sociological Review*, 40, 533–60.

Bolton, S. (2001) 'Changing faces: nurses as emotional jugglers', *Sociology of Health and Illness*, 23(1), 85–100.

Bolton, S. (2002) 'Consumer as king in the NHS', *International Journal of Public Sector Management*, 15(2), 129-39.

Boseley, S. (2003) 'Babies at risk from midwife shortage', http://society.guardian.co.uk/NHSstaff/story/0,7991,1040428,00.html

Bowling, A. (1981) *Delegation in General Practice: A Study of Doctors and Nurses*, London: Tavistock.

Boyne, G. (2002) 'Public and private management: what's the difference?', *Journal of Management Studies*, 39(1), 97-122.

Brandt, A. and Gardner, M. (2003) 'The golden age of medicine?', in Cooter, R. and Pickstone, J. (eds) *Companion to Medicine in the Twentieth Century*, London: Routledge, pp 21-37.

Brazier, J., Hutton, J. and Jeavons, R. (1990) 'Evaluating the reform of the NHS', in A. Culyer, A. Maynard and J. Posnett (eds) *Competition in Health Care: Reforming the NHS*, London: Macmillan,

Brewis, J. (1999) 'How does it feel? Women, managers, embodiment and changing public-sector cultures', in S. Whitehead and R. Moodley (eds) *Transforming Managers: Gendering Change in the Public Sector*, London: UCL Press, pp 84-106.

British Medical Journal (1942) 'Editorial', *British Medical Journal*, 26 September.

British Medical Journal (1950) 'Editorial', *British Medical Journal*, 2 December.

Brown, A. (1992) 'Managing change in the NHS: the resource management initiative', *Leadership and Organization Development Journal*, 13(6), 13-17.

Brown, R. and Stones, R. (1973) *The Male Nurse*, London: Bell.

Burt, R. (1993) 'The social structure of competition', in R. Swedburg (ed) *Explorations in Economic Sociology*, New York, NY: Russell Sage Foundation, pp 65-103.

Burt, R. (2000) 'The network entrepreneur', in R. Swedburg (ed) *Entrepreneurship: The Social Science View*, Oxford: Oxford University Press.

Butler, J. (1992) *Patients, Policies and Politics*, Buckingham: Open University Press.

Buxton, M. and Packwood, T. (1991) *Hospitals in Transition: The Resource Management Initiative*, Buckingham: Open University Press.

Calnan, M. and Gabe, J. (1991) 'Recent developments in general practice: a sociological analysis', in J. Gabe, M. Calnan and M. Bury, (eds) *The Sociology of the Health Service*, London: Routledge.

Cameron, J. (1965) *A Charter for the Family Doctor Service*, London: British Medical Association.

Carrier, J. and Kendall, I. (1986) 'NHS management and the Griffiths Report', in M. Brenton and C. Ungerson (eds) *The Year Book of Social Policy in Britain*, London: Routledge.

Carvel, J. (2004) 'NHS "relies too heavily on foreign nurses"', *The Guardian*, http://society.guardian.co.uk/NHSstaff/story/0,7991,1340529,00. html

Central Health Services Council Standing Medical Advisory Committee (1963) *The Field and Work of the Family Doctor* (Gillie Report), London: HMSO.

Clarke, A. (1999) *The Tories: Conservatives and the Nation State: 1922-1997*, London: Phoenix.

Clarke, J. (2004) *Changing Welfare, Changing Welfare States*, London: Sage Publications.

Clarke, J. and Newman, J. (1997) *The Managerial State*, London: Sage Publications.

Clarke, J., Cochrane, A. and Smart, C. (1992) *Ideologies of Welfare: From Dreams to Disillusion*, London: Routledge.

Clarke, J., Gewirtz, S. and McLaughlin, E. (2000) 'Reinventing the welfare state', in J. Clarke, S. Gewirtz and E. McLaughlin (eds) *New Managerialism: New Welfare?*, Buckingham: Open University Press, pp 1-26.

Clarke, J., Newman, J., Smith, N., Vidler, E. and Westmarland, L. (2007) *Creating Citizen-Consumers: Changing Publics and Changing Public Services*, London: Paul Chapman Publishing.

Cohen, H. (1943) 'A comprehensive health service', *Agenda*, 1-20.

Collings, J. (1950) 'General practice in England today: a reconnaissance', *Lancet*, 555-85.

Commission for Health Improvement (2001) *A Guide for Clinical Governance Reviews in NHS Trusts*, London: Commission for Health Improvement.

Committee of Inquiry into Normansfield Hospital (1978) *Report*, London: HMSO.

Conger, J. and Kanungo, R. (1998) *Charismatic Leadership in Organizations*, New York, NY: Sage Publications.

Coulter, A. (1995) 'Evaluating general practice fundholding in the UK', *European Journal of Public Health*, 5, 233-9.

Cox, D. (1991) 'Health service management – a sociological view: Griffiths and the non-negotiated order of the hospital', in J. Gabe, M. Clanan and M. Bury (eds) *The Sociology of the Health Service*, London: Routledge.

Cresswell, M. (2005) 'Self-harm "survivors" and psychiatry and England, 1988-1996', *Social Theory and Health*, 3, 259-85.

Cresswell, M. (2007) 'Self-harm and the politics of experience', *Journal of Critical Psychology*, 7(1), 9–17.

Crinson, I. (1998) 'Putting patients first: the continuity of the consumerism discourse in health policy', *Critical Social Policy*, 55, 227–39.

Crossman, R. (1969) *Paying for the Social Services*, London: Fabian Society.

Daly, M. and Rake, K. (2003) *Gender and the Welfare State*, Cambridge: Polity Press.

Davies, A. (2000) 'Don't trust me, I'm a doctor: medical regulation and the 1999 NHS reforms', *Oxford Journal of Legal Studies*, 20(3), 437–56.

Davies, A. and Thomas, R. (2002) 'Gendering and gender in public service organizations: changing professional identities under New Public Management', *Public Management Review*, 4(4), 461–84.

Davies, C. (1995) *Gender and the Professional Predicament in Nursing*, Buckingham: Open University Press.

Davis, F. and Olesen, V. (1963) 'Initiation into the women's profession: identity problems in the status transition of coed to student nurse', *Sociometry*, 26, 89–101.

Dawson, S. and Dargie, C. (2002) 'New Public Management: a discussion with special reference to UK health', in K. McLaughlin, S. Osborne and E. Ferlie (eds) *New Public Management: Current Trends and Future Prospects*, London: Routledge, pp 34–56.

Day, P. and Klein, R. (1992) 'Constitutional and distributional conflict in British medical politics: the case of general practice, 1911–1991', *Political Studies*, 40(3), 462–78.

Deacon, A. and Mann, K. (1999) 'Agency, modernity and social policy', *Journal of Social Policy*, 28(3), 413–35.

Deakin, N. (2001) *In Search of Civil Society*, London: Palgrave.

DH (Department of Health) (1989), *Caring for People: Community Care in the Next Decade and Beyond*, Cm 849, London: HMSO.

DH (1991) *The Patient's Charter*, London: DH.

DH (1999) *Supporting Doctors, Protecting Patients*, London: DH.

DH (2001a) *Extending Choice for Patients*, London: DH.

DH (2001b) *NHS Performance Ratings: Acute Trusts 2000/2001*, London: DH.

DH (2001c) *The Expert Patient: A New Approach to Chronic Disease Management for the 21st Century*, London: DH.

DH (2002a) *Learning from Bristol: The Department of Health's Response to the Report of the Public Inquiry into Children's Heart Surgery at the Bristol Royal Infirmary 1984-1995*, London: HMSO.

DH (2002b) *Reforming NHS Financial Flows: Introducing Payment by Results*, London: DH.

DH (2002c) *Shifting the Balance of Power within the NHS: Securing Delivery*, London: DH.

DH (2004) *Practice Based Commissioning – Engaging Practices in Commissioning*, London: DH.

DH (2006a) 'Good doctors, safer patients', London: DH.

DH (2006b) *Our Health, Our Care, Our Say*, Cm 6737, London: HMSO.

DH (2006c) *Patient Choice Becomes a Reality Across the NHS*, London: DH.

DH and OPCS (Office of Population Censuses and Surveys) (1994) *Departmental Report*, London: HMSO.

DHSS (Department of Health and Social Security) (1968) *Report of the Committee on Local Authority and Allied Personal Social Services*, London: HMSO.

DHSS (1970) *National Health Service: The Future Structure of the National Health Service*, London: HMSO.

DHSS (1971) *National Health Service Reorganisation: Consultative Document*, London: HMSO.

DHSS (1975) *The Separation of Private Practice from National Health Service Hospitals: A Consultative Document*, London: DHSS.

DHSS (1976) *Regional Chairman's Enquiry into the Working of the DHSS in Relation to Regional Health Authorities*, London: DHSS.

DHSS (1983) *NHS Management Inquiry*, London: HMSO.

Digby, A. (1999) *The Evolution of General Practice 1850-1948*, Oxford: Oxford University Press.

Dingwall, R., Rafferty, M. and Webster, C. (1988) *An Introduction to the Social History of Nursing*, London: Routledge.

Dopson, S. and Stewart, R. (1990) 'Public and private sector management: the case for wider debate', *Public Money and Management*, 10(1), 37-40.

Dowling, B. (2000) *GPs and Purchasing in the NHS*, Aldershot: Ashgate.

Doyal, L. (1979) *The Political Economy of Health*, London: Pluto Press.

Du Gay, P. (2000) *In Praise of Bureaucracy: Weber, Organization, Ethics*. London: Sage Publications.

Dunleavy, P. and Hood, C. (1994) 'From old public administration to New Public Management', *Public Money & Management*, 14(3), 9-16.

Dusheiko, M., Gravelle, H. and Jacobs, R. (2004a) 'The effects of practice budgets on waiting times: allowing for selection bias', *Health Economics*, 13, 941-58.

Dusheiko, M., Gravelle, H. and Jacobs, R. (2004b) 'The impact of budgets for gatekeeping physicians on patient satisfaction: evidence from fundholding', Technical Paper No 30, York: Department of Economics, University of York.

Easington Primary Care Trust (2006) *Choosing your Hospital*, Peterlee: Easington Primary Care Trust.

Eckstein, H. (1958) *The English Health Service*, Cambridge, MA: Harvard University Press.

Edwards, B. and Fall, M. (2005) *The Executive Years of the NHS: The England Account 1985-2003*, Oxford: Radcliffe Publishing.

Ehrenreich, J. (1978) *The Cultural Crisis of Modern Medicine*, Boston, MA: Monthly Review Press.

Enthoven, A. (1985) *Reflections on the Management of the National Health Service: An American Looks at Incentives to Efficiency in Health Service Management in the UK*, London: Nuffield Provincial Hospitals Trust.

Enthoven, A. (2000) 'In pursuit of an improving National Health Service', *Health Affairs*, 19, 102-19.

Evidence-Based Medicine Working Group (1992) 'Evidence-based medicine: a new approach to the practice of medicine', *Journal of the American Medical Association*, 268, 2420-5.

Exworthy, M. and Peckham, S. (2006) 'Access, choice and travel: implications for health policy', *Social Policy and Administration*, 40(3), 267-87.

Ferlie, E. and Pettigrew, A. (1996) 'Managing through networks: some issues and implications for the NHS', *British Journal of Management*, 7(Special Issue), S81-S99.

Firth-Cozens, J. (1990) 'Sources of stress in women junior house officers', *British Medical Journal*, 301, 89-91.

Flynn, R. (2004) '"Soft bureaucracy", governmentality and clinical governance: theoretical approaches to emergent policy', in A. Gray and S. Harrison (eds) *Governing Medicine,* Maidenhead: Open University Press, pp 11-26.

Forbes, I. (1986) *Market Socialism: Whose Choice?*, London: Fabian Society.

Fotaki, M., Boyd, A., Smith, L., McDonald, R., Roland, M., Sheaff, R., Edwards, A. and Elwyn, G. (2005) 'Patient choice and the organization and delivery of health services: scoping review', London: National Co-ordinating Centre for Service Delivery and Organisation.

Fox, C. and Miller, H. (1995) *Post-Modern Public Administration: Towards Discourse*, London: Sage Publications.

Fox, N. (1993) *Postmodernism, Sociology and Health*, Buckingham: Open University Press.

Gaffney, D., Pollock, A., Price, D. and Shaoul, J. (1999) 'The politics of the Private Finance Initiative and the new NHS', *British Medical Journal*, 319, 252.

Gamarnikow, E. (1991) 'Nurse or woman: gender and professionalism in reformed nursing 1860-1923', in P. Holden and J. Littlewood (eds) *Anthropology and Nursing*, London: Routledge, pp 110-29.

Gamble, A. (1987) *The Free Economy and the Strong State*, London: Macmillan.

General Medical Services Committee (1962) *A Review of the Medical Services of Great Britain: Report of the Medical Services Review Committee*, London: Social Assay.

Gherardi, S. (1995) *Gender, Symbolism and Organisational Culture*, London: Sage Publications.

Giddens, A. (2002) *What Now for New Labour?*, Cambridge: Polity Press.

Gillespie, R. (1997) 'Managers and professionals', in N. North and Y. Bradshaw (eds) *Perspectives in Health Care*, Basingstoke: Macmillan, pp 84-109.

Glasby, J. (2007) *Understanding Health and Social Care*, Bristol: The Policy Press.

Glasby, J. and Peck, E. (2003) *Care Trusts: Partnership Working in Action*, Abingdon: Radcliffe Medical Press.

Glendinning, C., Halliwell, S., Jacobs, S., Rummery, K. and Tryer, J. (2000) 'Bridging the gap: using direct payments to purchase integrated care', *Health and Social Care in the Community*, 8(3), 192-200.

Glendinning, C., Dowling, B. and Powell, M. (2005) 'Partnerships between health and social care under "New Labour": smoke without fire? A review of policy and evidence', *Evidence & Policy: A Journal of Research, Debate and Practice*, 1(3), 365-82.

Glennerster, H. (1995) *British Social Policy since 1945*, Oxford: Blackwell.

Glennerster, H. (2000) *British Social Policy since 1945* (2nd edn), Oxford: Blackwell.

Godber, G. (1975) *The National Health Service: Past, Present and Future*, London: The Athlone Press.

Goldman, P. and Macleod, I. (1958) *The Future of the Welfare State*, London: Conservative Political Centre.

Goss, E. (1963) 'Patterns of bureaucracy among hospital staff physicians', in E. Frieson (ed) *The Hospital in Modern Society*, New York, NY: Free Press, pp 170-94.

Graham, H. (1979) 'Prevention and health: every mothers' business', in C. Harris (ed) *The Sociology of the Family*, Keele: Keele University, pp 160-85.

Granovetter, M. (1973) 'The strength of weak ties', *American Journal of Sociology*, 78(6), 1360-80.

Grant, C. (1973) *Hospital Management*, London: Churchill Livingstone.

Greener, I. (2001) '"The ghost of health services past" revisited: comparing British health policy of the 1950s with the 1980s and 1990s', *International Journal of Health Services*, 31(3), 635-46.

Greener, I. (2002a) 'Understanding NHS reform: the policy-transfer, social learning, and path-dependency perspectives', *Governance*, 15(2), 161-84.

Greener, I. (2002b) 'Agency, social theory and social policy', *Critical Social Policy*, 22(73), 688-706.

Greener, I. (2003a) 'Patient choice in the NHS: the view from economic sociology', *Social Theory and Health*, 1(1), 72-89.

Greener, I. (2003b) 'Performance in the NHS: insistence of measurement and confusion of content', *Public Performance and Management Review*, 26(3), 237-50.

Greener, I. (2003c) 'Who choosing what? The evolution of "choice" in the NHS, and its implications for New Labour', in C. Bochel, N. Ellison and M. Powell (eds) *Social Policy Review 15*, Bristol: The Policy Press, pp 49-68.

Greener, I. (2004a) 'Health service organisation in the UK: a political economy approach', *Public Administration*, 82(3), 657-76.

Greener, I. (2004b) 'The drama of health management', in M. Learmonth and N. Harding (ed) *Unmaking Health*, New York, NY: Nova Science, pp 143-55.

Greener, I. (2004c) 'The three moments of New Labour's health policy discourse', *Policy & Politics*, 32(3), 303-16.

Greener, I. (2005a) 'The potential of path dependence in political studies', *Politics*, 25(1), 62-72.

Greener, I. (2005b) 'The role of the patient in healthcare reform: customer, consumer or creator?', in S. Dawson and C. Sausmann (eds) *Future Health Organisations and Systems*, Basingstoke: Palgrave, pp 227-45.

Greener, I. (2005c) 'Health management as strategic behaviour: managing medics and performance in the NHS', *Public Management Review*, 7(1), 95-110.

Greener, I. (2005d) 'Talking to health managers about change: heroes, villains and simplification', *Journal of Health Organisation and Management*, 18(5), 321-35.

Greener, I. (2006) 'Where are the medical voices raised in protest?', *British Medical Journal*, 330, 660.

Greener, I. (2007) 'The politics of gender in the NHS: impression management and "getting things done"', *Gender, Work and Organization*, 14(3), 281-99.

Greener, I. (2008a) 'Decision making in a time of significant reform: managing in the NHS', *Administration and Society*, 40(2), 194-210.

Greener, I. (2008b) 'Markets in the public sector: when do they work, and what do we do when they don't?', *Policy & Politics*, 36(1), 93-108.

Greener, I. and Mannion, R. (2006) 'Does practice-based commissioning avoid the problems of fundholding?', *British Medical Journal*, 333, 1168-70.

Greener, I. and Powell, M. (2008) 'The changing governance of the NHS; reform in a post-Keynesian health service', *Human Relations*, 61(5), 617-636.

Greener, I. and Powell, M. (2009: forthcoming) 'The evolution of choice policies in UK housing, education and health policy', *Journal of Social Policy*.

Hadfield, S. (1953) 'Field survey of general practice 1951-52', *British Medical Journal*, 683-706.

Halcrow, M. (1989) *Keith Joseph: A Single Mind*, London: Macmillan.

Hall, P. (1993) 'Policy paradigms, social learning and the state', *Comparative Politics*, 25, 275-96.

Hallam, J. (2000) *Nursing the Image: Media Culture and Professional Identity*, London: Routledge.

Halliday, I. (1995) *The NHS Transformed*, Manchester: Baseline Books.

Ham, C. (1980) 'Approaches to the study of social policy making', *Policy & Politics*, 8(1), 55-71.

Ham, C. (2000) *The Politics of NHS Reform 1988-97: Metaphor or Reality*, London: King's Fund.

Ham, C. (2004) *Health Policy in Britain: The Politics and Organisation of the NHS*, London: Palgrave.

Harris, B. (2004) *The Origins of the British Welfare State*, Basingstoke: Palgrave Macmillan.

Harrison, S. (1988a) *Managing the National Health Service: Shifting the Frontier?*, London: Chapman and Hall.

Harrison, S. (2002) 'New Labour, modernisation and the medical labour process', *Journal of Social Policy*, 31(3), 465–85.

Harrison, S. (2004) 'Medicine and management: autonomy and authority in the National Health Service', in A. Gray and S. Harrison (eds) *Governing Medicine*, Maidenhead: Open University Press, pp 51–9.

Harrison, S. and McDonald, R. (2008) *The Politics of Healthcare in Britain*, London: Sage Publications.

Harrison, S. and Pollitt, C. (1994) *Controlling Health Professionals: The Future of Work and Organization in the National Health Service*, Buckingham: Open University Press.

Harrison, S. and Wistow, G. (1993) 'Managing health care: balancing interests and influence', in B. Davey and J. Popay (eds) *Dilemmas in Health Care*, Buckingham: Open University Press, pp 12–26.

Harrison, S., Hunter, D. and Pollitt, C. (1990) *The Dynamics of British Health Policy*, London: Unwin Hyman.

Harrison, S., Hunter, D., Marnoch, G. and Pollitt, C. (1992) *Just Managing: Power and Culture in the NHS*, London: Macmillan.

Hart, C. (1994) *Behind the Mask: Nurses, their Unions and Nursing Policy*, London: Baillière Tindall.

Hart, L. (1991) 'A ward of my own: social organization and identity amongst hospital domestics', in P. Holden and J. Littlewood (eds) *Anthropology and Nursing*, London: Routledge, pp 84–109.

Haug, M. and Sussman, M. (1969) 'Professional autonomy and the revolt of the client', *Social Problems*, 17(2), 153–61.

Healey, D. (1993) *The Time of My Life*, Harmondsworth: Penguin.

Health Policy and Economic Research Unit (2006) *Survey of GP Practice Premises: Report*, London: British Medical Association.

Healthcare Commission (2005) *The Healthcare Commission's View of NHS Foundation Trusts*, London: Healthcare Commission.

Healthcare Commission (2006a) *Results of the Annual Health Check 2005/2006*, London: Healthcare Commission.

Healthcare Commission (2006b) *Annual Health Check Press Release*, London: Healthcare Commission.

Hennessy, P. (1994) *Never Again: Britain 1945-1951*, London: Pantheon Books.

Hill, M. (1993) *The Welfare State in Britain: A Political History since 1945*, London: Edward Elgar.

Hirschman, A. (1970) *Exit, Voice and Loyalty: Responses to Decline in Firms, Organizations and States*, London: Harvard University Press.

Hofling, C., Brozman, E., Dalyrymple, N. and Pierce, C. (1966) 'An experimental study in nurse–physician relationships', *Journal of Nervous and Mental Disease*, 143, 171–80.

Honigsbaum, F. (1979) *The Division in British Medicine: A History of the Separation of General Practice from Hospital Care 1911-1968*, New York, NY: St Martin's Press.

Honigsbaum, F. (1989) *Health, Happiness and Security: The Creation of the National Health Service*, London: Routledge.

Hood, C. (1991) 'A public management for all seasons?', *Public Administration*, 69, 3–19.

Hoque, K., Davis, S. and Humphreys, M. (2004) 'Freedom to do what you are told: senior management team autonomy in an NHS acute trust', *Public Administration*, 82(2), 355–76.

Howe, G. (1994) *Conflict of Loyalty*, London: Macmillan.

Hughes, D. (1988) 'When nurse knows best: some aspects of nurse/doctor interaction in a casualty department', *Sociology of Health and Illness*, 10(1), 1–22.

Hunter, D. (1986) *Managing the Health Service in Scotland: Review and Assessment of Research Needs*, Edinburgh: Scottish Home and Health Department.

Hunter, D. (1992) 'Doctors as managers: poachers turned gamekeepers?', *Social Science and Medicine*, 35(4), 557–66.

Hunter, D. (1993a) 'Care in the community: rhetoric or reality?', in B. Davey and J. Popay (eds) *Dilemmas in Health Care*, Buckingham: Open University Press, pp 121–42.

Hunter, D. (1993b) 'The internal market: the shifting agenda', in I. Tilley (ed) *Managing the Internal Market*, London: Paul Chapman Publishing, pp 31–43.

Hunter, D. (1994a) 'From tribalism to corporatism: the managerial challenge to medical dominance', in J. Gabe, D. Kelleher and G. Williams (ed) *Challenging Medicine*, London: Routledge, pp 1–22.

Hunter, D. (1994b) 'Managing medicine: a response to the "crisis"', *Social Science and Medicine*, 32(4), 441–9.

Hunter, D. (1997) *Desperately Seeking Solutions: Rationing Health Care*, Harlow: Addison Wesley Longman.

Hutton, J. (2003) Speech to the Royal College of Nursing Annual Congress, Harrogate, 30 April.

Illich, I. (1977) *Limits to Medicine*, Harmondsworth: Penguin.

Jenkins, S. (2006) *Thatcher and Sons: A Revolution in Three Acts*, London: Allen Lane.

Johnson, J. (2005) *Funding Matters, Workbook 4*, Milton Keynes: Open University.

Jones, H. (1994) *Health and Society in Twentieth Century Britain*, London: Longman.

Jones, K. (1954) 'Problems with mental after-care in Lancashire', *Sociological Review*, 2, 34–56.

Kanter, R. (1977) *Men and Women of the Corporation*, New York, NY: Anchor Press.

Kavanagh, D. (1985) 'Whatever happened to consensus politics?', *Political Studies*, XXII, 529–46.

Kavanagh, D. and Morris, P. (1991) *Consensus Politics from Attlee to Major*, Oxford: Blackwell.

Keegan, W. (2003) *The Prudence of Mr. Gordon Brown*, London: John Wiley and Sons.

Kelleher, D. (1994) 'Self-help groups and their relationship to medicine', in J. Gabe, D. Kelleher and G. Williams (eds) *Challenging Medicine*, London: Routledge, pp 104–17.

Kelleher, D., Gabe, J. and Williams, G. (1994) 'Understanding medical dominance in the modern world', in J. Gabe, D. Kelleher and G. Williams (eds) *Challenging Medicine*, London: Routledge, pp xi–xxix.

Keynes, J. (1997) *The General Theory of Employment, Interest and Money*, New York, NY: Prometheus Books.

King's Fund (2006) *NHS Reform: Getting Back on Track*, London: King's Fund.

King's Fund and *The Sunday Times* (2005) *An Independent Audit of the NHS under Labour (1997-2005)*, London: King's Fund.

King's Fund Institute (1988) *Health Care Finance: Assessing the Options*, London: King's Fund Institute.

Kitchener, M. (2000) 'The "bureaucratization" of professional roles: the case of clinical directors in UK hospitals', *Organization*, 7(1), 129–54.

Klein, R. (1979) 'Ideology, class and the National Health Service', *Journal of Health Politics, Policy and Law*, 4(3), 464–90.

Klein, R. (1983) 'The politics of ideology vs. the reality of politics', *Milbank Quarterly*, 62(1), 82–109.

Klein, R. (1986) 'Why Britain's Conservatives support a socialist health care system', *Health Affairs*, 4(1), 41–58.

Klein, R. (1990) 'The state and the profession: the politics of the double-bed', *British Medical Journal*, 301, 700-2.

Klein, R. (1993) 'The goals of health policy: church or garage?', in King's Fund (ed) *Health Care UK 1992/3*, London: King's Fund, pp 136–38.

Klein, R. (1997) 'Learning from others: shall the last be the first?', *Journal of Health Politics, Policy and Law*, 33(5), 1267-78.

Klein, R. (1998) 'Why Britain is reorganizing its National Health Service – yet again', *Health Affairs*, 17(4), 111-25.

Klein, R. (2001) *The New Politics of the NHS*, Harlow: Longman.

Klein, R. (2003) 'Governance for NHS foundation trusts', *British Medical Journal*, 326, 174-5.

Klein, R. (2005) 'The great transformation', *Journal of Health Economics, Policy and Law*, 1(1), 91-8.

Klein, R. (2006) *The New Politics of the NHS: From Creation to Reinvention*, Abingdon: Radcliffe Publishing.

Klein, R. and Lewis, J. (1976) *The Politics of Consumer Representation: A Study of Community Health Councils*, London: Centre for Studies in Social Policy.

Klein, R., Day, P. and Redmayne, S. (1995) 'Rationing in the NHS: the dance of the seven veils – in reverse', *British Medical Bulletin*, 51, 769-80.

Labour Party (1997) *New Labour Because Britain Deserves Better*, London: Labour Party.

Land, H. (1991) 'The confused boundaries of community care', in J. Gabe, M. Calnan and M. Bury (eds) *The Sociology of the Health Service*, London: Routledge, pp 203-21.

Lawson, N. (1991) *The View from No. 11*, London: Corgi.

Le Fanu, J. (1999) *The Rise and Fall of Modern Medicine*, London: Abacus.

Le Grand, J. (1991) 'The theory of government failure', *British Journal of Political Science*, 21, 423-42.

Le Grand, J. (1997) 'Knights, knaves or pawns? Human behaviour and social policy', *Journal of Social Policy*, 26(2), 149-69.

Le Grand, J. (1999) 'Competition, cooperation or control? Tales from the British Health Service', *Health Affairs*, 18(3), 27-44.

Le Grand, J. (2003) *Motivation, Agency and Public Policy: Of Knights, Knaves, Pawns and Queens*, Oxford: Oxford University Press.

Le Grand, J. (2007) *The Other Invisible Hand*, Woodstock, NJ: Princeton University Press.

Le Grand, J., Mays, N. and Dixon, J. (1998a) 'The reforms: success or failure or neither?', in J. Le Grand, N. Mays and J. Mulligan (eds) *Learning from the NHS Internal Market*, London: King's Fund, pp 117-43.

Le Grand, J., Mays, N. and Mulligan, J. (1998b) *Learning from the NHS Internal Market*, London: King's Fund.

Le Grand, J., Winter, D. and Woolley, F. (1991) 'The National Health Services: safe in whose hands?', in J. Hills (ed) *The State of Welfare: The Welfare State in Britain since 1974*, Oxford: Clarendon Press, pp 88-134.

Learmonth, M. (2001) 'NHS Trust chief executives as heroes?', *Health Care Analysis*, 9(4), 417-36.

Leathard, A. (1990) *Healthcare Provision, Past, Present and Future*, London: Chapman and Hall.

Lee, P. and Raban, C. (1988) *Welfare Theory and Social Policy: Reform or Revolution?*, London: Sage Publications.

Lee Potter, J. (1998) *A Damn Bad Business*, London: Orion.

Levitt, R. (1976) *The Reorganised National Health Service*, London: Croom Helm.

Levitt, R. (1980) 'The illusion of change in the National Health Service', *Policy & Politics*, 8(2), 205-16.

Lewis, J. (1990) 'Mothers and maternity policies in the twentieth century', in J. Garcia, R. Kilpatrick and M. Richards (eds) *The Politics of Maternity Care: Services for Childbearing Women in Twentieth Century Britain*, Oxford: Oxford University Press, pp 15-29.

Lewis, J. (1992) 'Providers, "consumers", the state and the delivery of health services in twentieth century Britain', in A. Wear (ed) *Medicine in Society*, Cambridge: Cambridge University Press, pp 317-45.

Lewis, J. (1999) 'The concepts of community care and primary care in the UK: the late 1960s to the 1990s', *Health and Social Care in the Community*, 7(5), 333-41.

Leys, C. (2003) *Market-Driven Politics: Neoliberal Democracy and the Public Interest*, London: Verso.

Liddle, C. (2006) 'Quality design through PFI', *Hospital Development*, www.hdmagazine.co.uk/story.asp?storyCode=2040650

Ling, T. (1998) *The British State since 1945: An Introduction*, Cambridge: Polity Press.

Lowe, R. (1989) 'Resignation at the Treasury: the Social Services Committee and the failure to reform the welfare state, 1955-1957', *Journal of Social Policy*, 18(4), 505-26.

Lowe, R. (1990) 'The Second World War, consensus and the foundation of the welfare state', *Twentieth Century British History*, 1(2), 152-82.

Lowe, R. (1993) *The Welfare State in Britain since 1945*, London: Macmillan.

Maddock, S. (2002) 'Making modernisation work: new narratives, change strategies and people management in the public sector', *International Journal of Public Sector Management*, 15(1), 13-43.

Mannion, R. and Goddard, M. (2002) 'Performance measurement and improvement in health care', *Applied Health Economics and Health Policy*, 1(1), 13-24.

Mannion, R., Goddard, M., Kuhn, M. and Bate, A. (2003) 'Earned autonomy in the NHS: a report for the Department of Health', London: Department of Health.

Mannion, R., Davies, H. and Marshall, M. (2004) *Cultures for Performance in Health Care*, Buckingham: Open University Press.

Mannion, R., Davies, H. and Marshall, M. (2005) 'Impact of star performance ratings in NHS Acute Trusts', *Journal of Health Services Research and Policy*, 10(1), 18-24.

Marinker, M. (1998) '"What is wrong" and "how we know it": changing concepts of illness in general practice', in I. Loudon, J. Horder and C. Webster (eds) *General Practice under the National Health Service 1948-1997*, London: Clarendon Press, pp 65-91.

Mark, A. and Scott, H. (1992) 'Management in the National Health Service', in L. Willcocks and J. Harrow (eds) *Rediscovering Public Services Management*, London: McGraw-Hill, pp 197-234.

Marquand, D. (2004) *Decline of the Public*, Cambridge: Polity.

Marshall, J. (1984) *Women Managers: Travellers in a Male World*, London: John Wiley.

Marshall, T.H. (1950) *Citizenship and Social Class*, Cambridge: Cambridge University Press.

Maynard, A. (1993) *Creating Competition in the NHS: Is it Possible? Will it Work?*, London: Paul Chapman Publishing, pp 58-68.

Maynard, A. (2001) 'Izzy whizzy, let's get busy! Is Sooty alive and well in the NHS?', *British Journal of Health Care Management*, 8(10), 422.

Maynard, A. (2006) 'On restructuring and redundancy', *Health Service Journal*, 16 March, p 16.

McDonald, R., Waring, J. and Harrison, S. (2005) 'Balancing risk, that is my life: the politics of risk in a hospital operating theatre', *Health, Risk and Society*, 7(4), 397-411.

McKeown, T. (1962) 'Reasons for the decline of mortality in England and Wales in the nineteenth century', *Population Studies*, 16, 94-122.

McKeown, T. (1976) *The Role of Medicine: Dream, Mirage or Nemesis?*, New York, NY: Academic Press.

McLachlan, G. (1971) *In Low Gear?*, Oxford: Oxford University Press.

Means, R. and Smith, R. (1994) *Community Care: Policy and Practice*, Basingstoke: Macmillan.

Means, R., Morbey, H. and Smith, R. (2002) *From Community Care to Market Care?: The Development of Welfare Services for Older People*, Bristol: The Policy Press.

Means, R., Richards, S. and Smith, R. (2003) *Community Care: Policy and Practice*, London: Palgrave.

Merrison, A. (1979) *Royal Commission on the National Health Service: Report*, Cmnd 7615, London: HMSO.

Milburn, A. (2002) 'Diversity and choice within the NHS', Speech to the NHS Confederation, 24 May.

Miles, A. (1991) *Women, Health and Medicine*, Buckingham: Open University Press.

Minford, P. (1991) *The Supply-Side Revolution in Britain*, London: Edward Elgar.

Minister of Health (1962) 'A Hospital Plan for England and Wales', London: HMSO.

Minister of State for Department of Health, Minister of State for Local and Regional Government and Minister of State for School Standards (2005) *The Case for User Choice in Public Services*, London: Public Administration Select Committee into Choice, Voice and Public Services.

Ministry of Health (1944) *A National Health Service*, London: HMSO.

Ministry of Health (1950) *Circular ECL 98/50*, London: Ministry of Health.

Ministry of Health (1953) *Annual Report*, London: Department of Health.

Ministry of Health (1956) *Committee of Enquiry into the Cost of the National Health Service*, London: HMSO.

Ministry of Health (1968) *National Health Service: The Administrative Structure of the Medical and Related Services in England and Wales*, London: HMSO.

Mitchell, A. and Wienir, D. (1997) *Last Time: Labour's Lessons from the Sixties*, London: Bellew Publishing.

Mohan, J. (2002) *Planning, Markets and Hospitals*, London: Routledge.

Monbiot, G. (2001) *Captive State: The Corporate Takeover of Britain*, London: Pan.

Monitor (2006) 'NHS foundation trusts – preliminary results for year ended 31 March 2006', London: Monitor.

Mooney, G. (2003) *Economics, Medicine and Healthcare*, London: FT Prentice Hall.

Moore, G. (1990) 'Doctors as managers: frustrating tensions', in D. Costain (ed) *The Future of Acute Services: Doctors as Managers*, London: King's Fund.

Moore, M. (1997) *Creating Public Value: Strategic Management in Government*, Cambridge, MA: Harvard University Press.

Moran, M. (1995) 'Explaining change in the National Health Service: corporatism, closure and democratic capitalism', *Public Policy and Administration*, 10(2), 21-33.

Moran, M. (1999) *Governing the Healthcare State: A Comparative Study of the United Kingdom, the United States and Germany*, Manchester: Manchester University Press.

Morgan, K. (1990) *The People's Peace*, Oxford: Oxford University Press.

Morrell, D. (1998) 'Introduction and overview', in I. Loudon, J. Horder, and C. Webster (eds) *General Practice under the National Health Service 1948-1997*, London: Clarendon Press, pp 1-19.

Morrell, K. (2006) 'Policy as narrative: New Labour's reform of the National Health Service', *Public Administration*, 84(2), 367-85.

Muir Gray, J. (1996) *Evidence-Based Health Care*, New York, NY: Churchill Livingstone.

Multiple Sclerosis Society (2003) *Measuring Up: Experiences of People with MS of Health Services*, London: MORI/Multiple Sclerosis Society.

NAO (National Audit Office) (2007) *Pay Modernisation: A New Contract for NHS Consultants in England*, London: The Stationery Office.

NAO (2008) *Making Changes in Operational PFI Projects*, London: HMSO.

National Association for Mental Health (1961) *Emerging Patterns of the Mental Health Services*, London: National Association for Mental Health.

Nettleton, S. (2006) *The Sociology of Health and Illness*, Cambridge: Polity Press.

Nettleton, S. and Burrows, R. (2003) 'E-scaped medicine? Information, reflexivity and health', *Critical Social Policy*, 23(2), 173-93.

Newman, J. (2002) 'The New Public Management, modernization and institutional change', in K. McLaughlin, S. Osborne and E. Ferlie (eds) *New Public Management: Current Trends and Future Prospects*, London: Routledge, pp 77-91.

Newman, J. and Vidler, E. (2006) 'Discriminating customers, responsible patients, empowered users: consumerism and the modernisation of health care', *Journal of Social Policy*, 35(2), 193-209.

NHS Executive (1994) *Hospital and Ambulance Services: Comparative Performance Guide 1993-1994*, London: Department of Health.

Nuffield Trust for Research and Policy Studies in Health Services (1953) *The Work of Nurses on Hospital Wards: Report of Job Analysis*, London: Nuffield Provincial Hospitals Trust.

O'Conner, J. (1973) *The Fiscal Crisis of the State*, London: Macmillan.

O'Dowd, A. (2005) 'New medical contracts hamper trusts' financial performance', *British Medical Journal*, 331, 251.

O'Reilly, D., Steele, K., Patterson, C., Milsom, P. and Harte, P. (2006) 'Might how you look influence how well you are looked after? A study which demonstrates that GPs perceive socio-economic gradients in attractiveness', *Journal of Health Services Research and Policy*, 11(4), 231-4.

Oakley, A. (1984) *The Captured Womb: A History of the Medical Care of Pregnant Women*, Oxford: Basil Blackwell.

Offer, A. (2006) *The Challenge of Affluence*, Oxford: Oxford University Press.

Oliver, M. (1996) 'Social learning and macroeconomic policy in the UK since 1979', *Essays in Economic Business History*, 14, 117-31.

Oliver, M. (1997) *Whatever Happened to Monetarism? Economic Planning and Social Learning in the United Kingdom since 1979*, Aldershot: Ashgate.

Osborne, S. and McLaughlin, K. (2002) 'The New Public Management in context', in K. McLaughlin, S. Osborne and E. Ferlie, E. (eds) *The New Public Management: Current Trends and Future Prospects*, London: Routledge, pp 7-14.

Pater, J. (1981) *The Making of the National Health Service*, London: King's Fund.

Paton, C. (1998) *Competition and Planning in the NHS*, Cheltenham: Nelson Thornes.

Paton, C. (2005) 'The state of the healthcare system in England', in Dawson, S. and Sausman, C. (eds) *Future health organisations and systems*, Basingstoke: Palgrave Macmillan, pp 57-79.

Paton, C. (2007) 'Visible hand or invisible fist? The new market and choice in the English NHS', *Health Economics, Policy and Law*, 2(3), 317-26.

Payer, L. (1996) *Medicine and Culture*, New York, NY: Henry Holt.

Peckham, S. (2006) 'The changing context of primary care', *Public Finance and Management*, 6(4), 504-38.

Peckham, S. and Exworthy, M. (2003) *Primary Care in the UK: Policy, Organisation and Management*, Basingstoke: Palgrave.

Peckham, S., Exworthy, M., Greener, I. and Powell, M. (2005a) 'Decentralisation as an organisational model in England', London: National Co-ordinating Centre for Service Delivery and Organisation.

Peckham, S., Exworthy, M., Greener, I. and Powell, M. (2005b) 'Decentralizing health services: more local accountability or just more central control?', *Public Money & Management*, 25(4), 221-8.

Pemberton, H. (2000) 'Policy networks and policy learning: UK economic policy in the 1960s and 1970s', *Public Administration*, 78(4), 771-92.

Petchey, R. (1986) 'The Griffiths reorganisation of the National Health Service', *Critical Social Policy*, 17(2), 87-101.

Petchey, R. (1995) 'General practitioner fundholding: weighing the evidence', *The Lancet*, 346, 1139-42.

Peters, J. and Waterman, R. (1982) *In Search of Excellence: Lessons from America's Best Run Companies*, London: HarperCollins.

Peterson, A. and Lupton, D. (1996) *The New Public Health: Health and Self in the Age of Risk*, London: Sage Publications.

Pettigrew, A., Ferlie, E. and McKee, L. (1992) *Shaping Strategic Change*, London: Sage Publications.

Pierson, C. (1998) *Beyond the Welfare State: The New Political Economy of Welfare*, Cambridge: Polity Press.

Pollitt, C. (1985) 'Measuring performance: a new system for the National Health Service', *Policy & Politics*, 13(1), 1-15.

Pollitt, C., Harrison, S., Hunter, D. and Marnoch, G. (1988) 'The reluctant manager: clinicians and budgets in the NHS', *Financial Accountability and Management*, 4(3), 213-33.

Pollock, A. (1995) 'The politics of destruction: rationing in the UK health care market', *Health Care Analysis*, 3(4), 299-308.

Pollock, A. (2004) *NHS Plc: The Privatisation of our Health Care*, London: Verso.

Poole, L. (2000) 'Health care: New Labour's NHS', in J. Clarke, S. Gewirtz and E. McLaughlin (eds) *New Managerialism: New Welfare?*, Buckingham: Open University Press, pp 102-21.

Pope, C., Roberts, J. and Black, N. (1991) 'Dissecting a waiting list', *Health Service Management Research*, 4(2), 112-19.

Powell, J.E. (1972) 'Foreword', in D. Davies (ed) *Health or Health Service?*, London: Charles Knight and Co Ltd.

Powell, J.E. (1966) *Medicine and Politics*, London: Pitman Medical.

Powell, M. (1994) 'The forgotten anniversary? An examination of the 1944 White Paper', *Social Policy and Administration*, 28(4), 333-47.

Powell, M. (1996) 'The ghost of health services past: comparing health policy of the 1930s with the 1980s and 1990s', *International Journal of Health Services*, 26(2), 253–68.

Powell, M. (1997) *Evaluating the National Health Service*, Buckingham: Open University Press.

Powell, M. (1998) 'New Labour and the "new" UK NHS', *Critical Public Health*, 8(2), 167–73.

Prime Minister (1991) *The Citizen's Charter*, London: HMSO.

Pringle, R. (1998) *Sex and Medicine*, Cambridge: Cambridge University Press.

Propper, C., Croxson, B. and Shearer, A. (2002) 'Waiting times for hospital admissions: the impact of GP fundholding', *Journal of Health Economics*, 21, 227–52.

Propper, C., Wilson, D. and Burgess, S. (2006) 'Extending choice in English health care: the implications of the economic evidence', *Journal of Social Policy*, 35(4), 537–57.

Public Finance (2007) 'PFI hospitals "costing NHS extra £480m a year"', www.cipfa.org.uk/publicfinance/news_details.cfm?News_id=30216

Public Records Office (1953) 'Butler to Macleod', 94501/9/1, London: Department of Health.

Public Records Office (1955) 'Treasury Social Services Division file on the Guillebaud Report', Ref T.227.424

Public Records Office (1957) 'CC (57) 5th meeting', CAB 128.31

Richmond, C. (1996) 'NHS waiting lists have been a boon for private medicine in the UK', *Canadian Medical Association Journal*, 154, 378–81.

Rintala, M. (2003) *Creating the National Health Service: Bevan and the Medical Lords*, London: Frank Cass Publishers.

Rivett, G. (1998) *From Cradle to Grave: Fifty Years of the NHS*, London: King's Fund.

Robb, B. (ed) (1967) *Sans Everything: A Case to Answer*, London: Trevor Nelson and Sons.

Roberts, A. (2003) *Hitler and Churchill: Secrets of Leadership*, London: Phoenix.

Ross, J. (1952) *The National Health Service in Great Britain*, Oxford: Oxford University Press.

Royal College of General Practitioners (1972) *The Future General Practitioner: Teaching and Learning*, London: Royal College of General Practitioners.

RCN (Royal College of Nursing) (1974) *The State of Nursing: Submission to the Secretary of State for Social Services*, London: RCN.

Royal Commission on Doctors' and Dentists' Remuneration (1960) *Royal Commission on Doctors' and Dentists' Remuneration 1957-1960* (Pilkington Report), London: HMSO.

Royal Commission on Long-Term Care (1999) *With Respect to Old Age: Long Term Care – Rights and Responsibilities*, London: HMSO.

Ruggie, M. (1996) *Realignments in the Welfare State: Health Policy in the United States, Britain and Canada*, New York, NY: Columbia University Press.

Sackett, D., Richardson, W., Rosenberg, W. and Haynes, R. (1997) *Evidence-Based Medicine: How to Practice and Teach EBM*, London: Churchill Livingstone.

Saks, M. (1994) 'The alternatives to medicine', in J. Gabe, D. Kelleher, and G. Williams (eds) *Challenging Medicine*, London: Routledge, pp 84-103.

Salter, B. (1993) 'The politics of purchasing in the National Health Service', *Policy & Politics*, 21(3), 171-84.

Salter, B. (2004) *The New Politics of Medicine*, London: Palgrave.

Salvage, J. (1982) 'Angles, not angels', *Health Service Journal*, 3(9), 12-13.

Salvage, J. (1985) *The Politics of Nursing*, London: Heinemann.

Sang, B. (2004) 'Choice, participation and accountability: assessing the potential impact of legislation promoting patient and public involvement in health in the UK', *Health Expectations*, 7, 187-90.

Savage, W. (1986) *A Savage Enquiry*, London: Virago.

Schofield, J. (2001) 'The old ways are the best? The durability and usefulness of bureaucracy in public sector management', *Organization*, 8(1), 77-96.

Schulman, S. (1958) 'Basic functional roles in nursing: mother surrogate and healer', in E. Jaco (ed) *Patients, Physicians and Illnesses*, Glencoe, IL: Free Press, pp 528-37.

Schwartz, B. (2004) *The Paradox of Choice: Why Less is More*, New York, NY: HarperCollins.

Scottish Home and Health Department (1966) *Administrative Practice of Hospital Boards in Scotland: Report of the Scottish Health Services Council*, London: HMSO.

Secretary of State for Health (1989) *Working for Patients*, London: HMSO.

Secretary of State for Health (1992) *The Health of the Nation: A Strategy for Health in England*, London: HMSO.

Secretary of State for Health (1996) *The NHS: A Service with Ambitions*, London: HMSO.

Secretary of State for Health (1997) *The New NHS: Modern, Dependable*, London: HMSO.

Secretary of State for Health (1998) *A First Class Service: Quality in the New NHS*, London: Department of Health.

Secretary of State for Health (1999) *Long-Term Care: The Government's Response to the Health Committee's Report on Long-Term Care*, London: HMSO.

Secretary of State for Health (2000) *The NHS Plan: A Plan for Investment, A Plan for Reform*, London: HMSO.

Secretary of State for Health (2002) *Delivering the NHS Plan: Next Steps on Investment and Reform*, London: HMSO.

Secretary of State for Health (2006) *Our Health, Our Care, Our Say: A New Direction for Community Services*, London: HMSO.

Secretary of State for Health and Social Services (1972) *The National Health Service Reorganisation: England*, London: HMSO.

Sethi, S. and Dimmock, S. (1982) *Industrial Relations and Health Services*, London: Croom Helm.

Sheldon, T. (1990) 'When it makes sense to mince your words', *Health Service Journal*, 121, 16 August.

Simmons, R., Birchall, J., Doheny, S. and Powell, M. (2007) '"Citizen governance": opportunities for inclusivity in policy and policy making?', *Policy & Politics*, 35(3), 457-78.

Smee, C. (2005) *Speaking Truth to Power: Two Decades of Analysis in the Department of Health*, Oxford: Radcliffe Publishing/The Nuffield Trust.

Smith, J. (2002) *The Shipman Inquiry: First Report, Volume One: Death Disguised*, London: HMSO.

Smith, J., Walshe, K. and Hunter, D. (2001) 'The "redisorganisation" of the NHS: another reorganisation leaving unhappy managers can only worsen the service', *British Medical Journal*, 323, 1262-3.

Smith, M. (1993) *Pressure, Power and Policy*, London: Harvester Wheatsheaf.

Smith, P. (2002) 'Performance management in British health care: will it deliver?', *Health Affairs*, 21(3), 103-15.

Stacey, M. (1998) 'The health service consumer: a sociological misconception', in Mackay, L., Soothill, K. and Melia, K. (eds) *Classic Texts in Health Care*, Oxford: Butterworth-Heinemann, pp 54-9.

Stark Murray, D. (1971) *Why a National Health Service?*, London: Pemberton Books.

Stewart, J. and Walsh, K. (1992) 'Change in the management of public services', *Public Administration*, 70, 499-518.

Stocking, B. (1985) *Initiative and Inertia: Case Studies in the NHS*, London: Nuffield Provincial Hospitals Trust.

Stoker, G. (2006) *Why Politics Matters: Making Democracy Work*, London: Palgrave.

Strauss, A., Schatzman, L., Ehrlich, D., Bucher, R. and Sabsin, M. (1963) 'The hospital and its negotiated order', in E. Frieson (ed) *The Hospital in Modern Society*, New York, NY: Free Press, pp 147-69.

Street, A. (2000) 'Confident about efficiency measurement in the NHS?', *Health Care UK*, 47-52.

Strong, P. and Robinson, J. (1988) *New Model Management: Griffiths and the NHS*, Warwick: Nursing Policy Studies Centre.

Talbot-Smith, A. and Pollock, A. (2006) *The New NHS: A Guide*, London: Routledge.

Tallis, R. (2005) *Hippocratic Oaths: Medicine and its Discontents*, London: Atlantic Books.

Taylor, F. (2006) 'Terms and conditions', *Community Care*, 12-18 January, pp 38-39.

Taylor, S. (1954) *Good General Practice*, London: Oxford University Press.

Taylor-Gooby, P. and Lawson, R. (eds) (1993) *Markets and Managers*, Buckingham: Open University Press.

Thatcher, M. (1993) *The Downing Street Years*, London: HarperCollins.

Timmins, N. (1995a) *The Five Giants*, London: Fontana.

Timmins, N. (1995b) 'How three top managers nearly sank the reforms', *Health Service Journal*, 29 June, pp 11-13.

Timmins, N. (2002) 'A time for change in the British NHS: an interview with Alan Milburn', *Health Affairs*, 21(3), 129-35.

Titmuss, R. (1950) *Problems of Social Policy*, London: HMSO.

Titmuss, R. (1958) *Essays on the Welfare State*, London: Allen and Unwin.

Titmuss, R. (1961) *Daily Herald*, 2 February.

Toynbee, P. (2008) 'Quackery and superstition: available soon on the NHS', *The Guardian*, www.guardian.co.uk/Columnists/Column/0,2236974,00.html

Tudor-Hart, J. (1971) 'The inverse care law', *Lancet*, 1, 405-12.

Tudor-Hart, J. (1988) *A New Kind of Doctor*, London: Merlin Press.

Turner, B. (1987) *Medical Power and Social Knowledge*, London: Sage Publications.

Wainwright, D. (1998) 'Disenchantment, ambivalence and the precautionary principle: the becalming of British health policy', *International Journal of Health Services*, 28(3), 407-26.

Walmsley, J. (2006) 'Organisations, structures and community care, 1971-2001: from care to citizenship?', in J. Welshman and J. Walmsley, (eds) *Community Care in Perspective: Care, Control and Citizenship*, Basingstoke: Palgrave Macmillan, pp 77-96.

Walshe, K. (2003a) 'Foundation hospitals: a new direction for NHS reform?', *Journal of the Royal Society of Medicine*, 96, 106-10.

Walshe, K. (2003b) *Regulating Health Care: A Prescription for Improvement?*, Maidenhead: Open University Press.

Walshe, K. and Smith, J. (eds) (2006) *Healthcare Management*, Buckingham: Open University Press.

Wanless, D. (2002) *Securing our Future Health: Taking A Long Term View – Final Report*, London: HM Treasury.

Watkin, B. (1978) *The National Health Service: The First Phase*, Old Woking: Unwin.

Watkins, S. (2004) 'Medicine and government: partnership spurned?', in A. Gray and S. Harrison (eds) *Governing Medicine*, Maidenhead: Open University Press, pp 37-50.

Webster, C. (1988) *The Health Services since the War, Vol 1, Problems of Health Care: The National Health Services before 1957*, London: HMSO.

Webster, C. (1994) 'Conservatives and consensus: the politics of the National Health Service 1951-64', in A. Oakley and S. Williams (eds) *The Politics of the Welfare State*, London: University College Press.

Webster, C. (1996) *The Health Services since the War, Vol 2, Government and Health Care: The British National Health Service 1958-1970*, London: HMSO.

Webster, C. (1998a) *The National Health Service: A Political History*, Oxford: Oxford University Press.

Webster, C. (1998b) 'The politics of general practice', in I. Loudon, J. Horder and C. Webster (eds) *General Practice Under the National Health Service 1948-1997*, London: Clarendon Press, pp 20-44.

Welshman, J. (2006a) 'Ideology, ideas and care in the community, 1948-71', in J. Welshman and J. Walmsley (eds) *Community Care in Perspective: Care, Control and Citizenship*, Basingtoke: Palgrave Macmillan, pp 17-37.

Welshman, J. (2006b) 'Organisations, structures and community care, 1948-71: from control to care?', in J. Welshman and J. Walmsley (eds) *Community Care in Perspective: Care, Control and Citizenship*, Basingstoke: Palgrave Macmillan, pp 59-76.

West, P. (1998) 'Market – what market? A review of health authority purchasing in the NHS internal market', *Health Policy*, 44, 167-83.

White, R. (1985) 'Political regulators in British nursing', in R. White (ed) *Political Issues in Nursing: Past, Present and Future, Vol 1*, Chichester: John Wiley and Sons.

Whiteside, N. (1996) 'Creating the welfare state in Britain 1945-1960', *Journal of Social Policy*, 25(1), 83–103.

Wicks, D. (1993) *Nurses and Doctors at Work: Theorising the Sexual Division of Labour*, Newcastle, New South Wales: University of Newcastle.

Wilmot, S. (2004) 'Foundation trusts and the problem of legitimacy', *Health Care Analysis*, 12(2), 157–69.

Wilson, P. (2001) 'A policy analysis of the expert patient in the United Kingdom: self-care as an expression of pastoral power?', *Health and Social Care in the Community*, 9(3), 134–42.

Witness Seminar (2006) *Consumerism and Choice in the Conservative Internal Market 1987-1992 (draft transcript)*, London: Institute for Historical Research, University of London.

Witz, A. (1994) 'The challenge of nursing', in J. Gabe, D. Kelleher, and G. Williams (eds) *Challenging Medicine*, London: Routledge, pp 23-45.

World Health Organization (2000) *The World Health Report 2000: Health Systems Improving Performance*, Geneva: World Health Organization.

Wright, K., Haycox, A. and Leedham, I. (1994) *Evaluating Community Care*, Buckingham: Open University Press.

Index

1940s
  funding 116–17
  NHS 39–49
  nursing 163–7
1940s and 1950s
  GPs 43–8
  Local authority health services 49
1950s
  double-bed relationship 81–3
  funding 117–20
  NHS 39–49
  nursing 165–9
1960s
  double-bed relationship 84–8
  funding 120–3
  General Practitioners 53–6
  local authority care 56–7
  mental health services 51–3
  NHS 50–8
  nursing 167–72
  public role in health policy 188–92
  tripartite healthcare 57–8
1970s
  1974 reorganisation 141–2
  double-bed relationship 88–92
  economic problems 125–6
  funding 124–7
  Keynesianism 125–6
  NHS 58–60
  nursing 172–4
  public health 59
  public role in health policy 188–92
1974 reorganisation 141–2
  double-bed relationship 89tab
1980s
  community care 61–2
  double-bed relationship 93–101
  funding 127–9
  General Practitioners 61
  Hospitals 60–1
  NHS 60–3
  nursing 174–7
  public health 62
  public role health policy 192–6
1980s and 1990s: criticisms of care 193
1990s
  double-bed relationship 101–6
  NHS 63–6
  nursing 177–81
  public health 65
  public role in health policy 192–6
2000s
  consultants 71tab

double-bed relationship 106–11
General Practitioners 71tab
NHS 66–71
nursing 177–81
public role in health policy 197–204
social care 71tab
6, P. 197

A

Abel-Smith, B. 117, 171
accountability
  doctors 108–9
  managers 160
  and paternalism 238–9
Acheson, D. 61
Acheson Report 62
Addison, P. 41
administration: early NHS 138–40
Alford, R. 60, 81, 94, 144, 158, 163
Allen, I. 70
Allender, P. 131
Allsop, J. 22, 189, 196, 214
alternative therapies 193
ambulance workers' strike 90
ancillary services 148
Andalo, D. 134
Archer, M. 11, 77
Asenova, D. 133, 218

B

Bacon, R. 93, 124
Baggott, R.
  health policy under Labour 212, 216
  management 150
  nursing 180
  public role in health policy 191, 203
  tripartite split 63
Baines, D. 210, 248
Balint, M. 55
Barber, M. 68, 153, 220, 223, 228, 245
Bauman, Z. 198, 241
Beardwood, B. 178–9
Beck, M. 133, 218
Beck, U. 65
Berridge, V.
  double-bed relationship 93
  health policy under Labour 211
  management 150
  nursing 168, 171, 176
  public role in health policy 193, 200
  tripartite split 56, 62
Best, A. 94
Bevan, Aneurin 17, 25–9, 82

concessions to medical profession
30*tab*
Beveridge Report 9, 21–2
Birchall, J. 68, 203
Blair, Tony 106, 131–2
Bloomfield, B. 94, 104
BMA
  creation of NHS 22, 23, 26–7
  'double-bed' relationship 77, 84, 85,
    89–90, 95, 99
  health policy under Labour 224, 225,
    226
  and internal market 99
  tripartite split 43, 48, 53, 54, 70
Bolton, S. 178–9, 201
Boseley, S. 178
Bowling, A. 55
Boyne, G. 159
Brandt, A. 41
Brazier, J. 77
Bretton Woods 125, 216
Brewis, J. 158
Bristol Royal Infirmary 105
Brown, Gordon 214, 217
Brown, R. 170
budget deficits 134–5, 154, 224–5
bureaucracy 139, 210–11
Burrows, R. 199
Burt, R. 159
Butler, J. 130
Buxton, M. 128, 145

C

Calnan, M. 44, 55, 70
Cameron, J. 54, 85–6
capital building plan: 1960s 84–5
capital expenditure 121–2, 123*tab*,
  216–19
care, criticisms of 188–9, 193
Care Trusts 215–16
Carrier, J. 141
Carvel, J. 178
Castle, Barbara 91–2, 173
charges 117–19, 234–5
Charter for the Family Doctor Service
  54, 85
childbirth 53
choice 191–2, 197, 222–3, 248
'Choose and Book' 222
citizenship
  creation of NHS 187–8
  future of NHS 252–3
  health 203–4
Clarke, A. 126
Clarke, J.
  creation of NHS 24
  health policy under Labour 211, 221
  management 146–7, 148

public role in health policy 188
  tripartite split 63
Clarke, Kenneth 94–5, 98–100, 101–2,
  149
clinical audit 104, 105–6
clinical budgeting 128
'Cogwheel' system 85
Cohen, H. 19
Collings, J. 45
Commission for Health Improvement
  106, 211
community care 59–60, 61–2, 211
  mental health services 51–52
1990 Community Care Act 62–3
Community Health Councils (CHCs)
  189–91, 214
community health services 27, 29–30
community medicine 59
complementary therapies 193
comprehensive care 17, 22, 36–7, 237
compulsory competitive tendering
  127–8, 147–8, 176–7
Confederation of Health Service
  Employees (COHSE) 169–70,
  172–3, 174–5, 177
Conservatives
  1950s 117–20
  1980s 127–31
  1980s and 1990s 93–104
consultants
  contracts 99
  image 184
  and GP's 20, 43, 44*tab*, 46, 64, 212,
    223, 233
  and NHS 27–8, 31–2, 71*tab*, 233, 247
  and patients 186–7
  pay 89–90
  and pay-beds 91–2
  public and private practise 114, 115
  rationing care 115
consumerism 197–9, 241
  and funding 201–3
    future of NHS 251–2
  and nurses 178–9
  problems with 201–3
consumers contracts
  consultants 99
  General Practitioners 99
  internal market 129–30
contributory system 83, 118–19, 120
cost of NHS: 1948-51 116*tab*
Coulter, A. 64
Cox, D. 141, 146
Crossman, R. 123*tab*
customers
  future of NHS 251–2
  patients as 206–7

D

Danckwerts award 47, 82
Dargie, C. 152, 159, 224
Davies, A. 106, 163, 166
Dawson, S. 152, 159, 224
Deakin, N. 204
deficits 134–5, 154
demand 113, 115
Department for Health and Social
    Services 98
Digby, A. 19
Dimmock, S. 171
Dingwall, R. 2, 53, 164, 166, 171
direct payments 221
Directors of Public Health 62
disability rights campaigners 188
District General Hospital 50–1
doctors
  accountability 108–9, 148–9
  future of NHS 247–8
  and management 83, 145, 150–1
  relationship with patients 193–6,
      199–200
Dopson, S. 152
double-bed relationship 75–112, 76*tab*
  1950s 81–3
  1960s 84–8
  1970s 88–92
  1980s 92–101, 148–9
  1990s 101–6
  2000s 106–11
  2008 233–4
  creation of NHS 9, 14*tab*, 15, 33–4
  and internal market 101*tab*
  under Labour 111*tab*, 224
  logics of 78*tab*
Dowling, B. 45
Doyal, L. 9, 114, 174
Du Gay, P. 158
Dusheiko, M. 65, 194, 210, 248

E

Eckstein, H. 20, 26, 44, 46, 138
economic problems: 1970s 89, 125–6
Edwards, B. 68, 100, 102, 146, 209, 211
Eltis, W. 93, 124
Ely Hospital: 1960s 52
Emergency Medical Service (EMS) 21
enrolled nurses 169, 171, 173, 176
Enthoven, Alain 98, 150
entrepreneurship
  consultants 247
  doctors 223
  General Practitioners 53, 72, 232
  managers 156, 157, 159, 239
evidence-based medicine 109
expenditure

1940s 116*tab*
1950s 118
Expert Patient 201
Exworthy, M. 61, 130, 134

F

Fall, M. 68, 100, 102, 146, 209, 211
Farquharson Lang Report 139
feminism 52–3, 188, 193
finance *see* funding
Firth-Cozens, J. 178
fiscal crisis 124–5
Forbes, I. 42
Fotaki, M. 156, 198, 205, 241
Foundation Trusts 67–8, 107, 213–15
Fowler, Norman 94–5
Fox, N. 184–95, 245, 253
free care 34–5
fundholders, GP 194–5, 210
funding 59, 106–7, 113–35, 234–6 *see*
    also Private Finance Initiative (PFI)
  1940s 116–17
  1950s 117–20
  1960s 120–3
  1970s 124–7
  1980s 127–9
  2008 234–6
  and consumerism 201–3
  general taxation 14*tab*, 15–16, 34, 83,
      113
  health insurance 16, 83, 118, 235–6
  Labour 1997 onwards 131–5
  problems 114
  problems with 121–2
The Future General Practitioner (Royal
    College of General Practitioners)
    55
future of NHS 242–55
  citizenship 252–3
  consultants 247
  customers 251–2
  doctors 247–8
  healthcare market 249–50
  inspection 254–5
  local authorities 245–7
  managers 253–4
  National Institute for Health and
      Clinical Excellence (NICE) 246
  nursing 248–9
  public role in health services 251–3
  tripartite split 246–8

G

Gabe, J. 44, 55, 70
Gaffney, D. 218
Gamarnikow, E. 164–5, 169
Gardner, M. 41
gatekeeping 75–6, 115

gender
  medical profession 69–70
  in NHS development 9
  nursing 164–5, 170, 178
general managers 60, 143–4
General Medical Council (GMC) 105,
  107, 149, 247–8
General Practitioners 28–9, 32–3, 63–5,
  98–9, 132, 210
  1940s 41, 47*tab*
  1940s and 1950s 43–8
  1960s 53–6
  1980s 61
  2000s 71*tab*
  2008 232–3
  and consultants 20, 43, 44*tab*, 46, 64,
    212, 223, 233
  contracts 72, 99
  at creation of NHS 183–4
  fundholding 66
  future of NHS 248
  as gatekeepers 75–6, 115
  image 184
  and NHS 75–6
  and patients 183–4, 185–6, 193–6,
    197
  pay 44–5, 47, 53, 54, 82, 83, 85–6,
    89–90
  practice-based commissioning 221–2
  pre-NHS 20
  prescribing 75–6
Gherardi, S. 166
Giddens, A. 212
Gillespie, R. 77, 145–6
Gillie Report 54
Glasby, J. 69, 216
Glendinning, C. 69, 221
Glennerster, H. 21, 26, 141, 174
  double-bed 86, 87
  tripartite split 50, 62, 63
Godber, G. 44, 138
Goddard, M. 153
'golden age' of welfare 7–8
Goss, E. 140
GP fundholders 63–5, 98–9, 132, 210,
  221–2
GPs *see* General Practioners
Graham, H. 62
Granovetter, M. 159
Grant, C. 140
Greener, I. 8
  creation of NHS 30–1
  double-bed 77, 80, 99, 109
  funding 128
  health policy under Labour 215, 219,
    221, 223, 226, 227
  management 137, 143, 153, 155, 157
  NHS 2008 234, 241

public role in health policy 183, 206
  tripartite split 67, 72
Griffiths, Roy 63, 94, 143–4, 176, 192
Guillebaud Report 82–3, 84, 95

H

Hadfield, S. 45
Hall, P. 172
Hallam, J. 165, 166, 173
Halliday, I. 253
Ham, C. 57, 61, 77, 99–100, 103, 209
Harris, B. 19
Harrison, S. 5–6, 6–7, 242
  double-bed 96, 102, 109
  management 143, 146, 158
Hart, C. 170, 173, 175, 182
Hart, L. 176–7
Haug, M. 158
health and social care 215–16
health centres 49
health citizenship 203–4
health consumerism 197–9, 201–3
health economics 211–12
health information 199–201
The Health of the Nation (Secretary of
  State for Health) 65
health policy 4–9
  1992-1997 209–10
  1997 213
  development 4–9
  under Labour 1997 onwards 209–29
  public role in 183–207
  role of professional in 242–4
  shared version 5–7
health services: local authority provision
  244–6
health user groups 188–9, 191, 199,
  200
healthcare assistants 176
Healthcare Commission 211, 215, 220
healthcare market: future of NHS
  249–50
healthcare: pre-NHS 18–25
Hennessy, P. 116
Hercepton 110
Hewitt, Patricia 154
Hill, M. 7
Hirschman, A. 84, 147
Honigsbaum, F. 41, 116
  creation of NHS 14, 20, 21, 22, 23,
    26, 28
Hoque, K. 68, 153, 213, 215
Hospital Activity Analysis 85
Hospital Management Committees 40
Hospital Plan 50–1, 84–5, 121–2,
  216–17
hospitals
  1940s and 1950s 40–3

1980s 60–1
choice of 197
competition problems 156, 232, 249
at creation of NHS 31–2
managers 240
nationalisation 25–6
performance management system 213
pre-NHS 19–20
and wartime 41
Howe, Geoffrey 52
Hughes, D. 176
Hunter, D. 10, 62, 103, 149, 150
Hutton, J. 214

I

Illich, I. 58, 189
industrial action
and compulsory competitive
tendering 148
nurses 172–4, 177
inflation: 1970s 125–6
inspection: future of NHS 254–5
insurance system 16, 63, 118, 235–6
internal market 149–50, 152, 193–6,
209–10
and double-bed relationship 98–100,
101*tab*, 104
funding 129–31
tripartite split 61, 64*tab*
International Monetary Fund (IMF)
126
Internet 199–201

J

Jenkins, S. 131, 214, 246
Johnson, J. 61, 223
Jones, H. 28, 33, 193
Jones, K. 49, 163, 196
Jones, Sir Cyril 82
Joseph, Keith 87–8

K

Kanter, R. 169
Kavanagh, D. 7
Keegan, W. 212
Kelleher, D. 151, 179, 193
Kendall, I. 141
Keynes, J. 21
Keynesianism 79, 125–6
Kitchener, M. 108
Klein, R. 2, 3, 7, 9, 235, 255
creation of NHS 15, 24, 26–7, 28
the double-bed relationship 75, 76,
77, 80, 81, 82, 85, 87, 90, 95, 97, 99,
110
funding 113, 115, 117, 120, 121, 129,
135
health policy under Labour 209, 215

management 138, 139, 142, 146, 150
public role in health policy 186, 189,
190, 203
tripartite split 61, 65, 68, 70

L

Labour
1997 onwards 104–11
and double-bed relationship 110–12
funding, 1997 onwards 131–5
health management 152–61
health policy under, 1997 onwards
209–29
Hospital Plan 121–2, 123
NHS reforms, 1997 onwards 227–9
post war 25–9
public participation in health 204
tripartite split under 71*tab*
Land, H. 49
Lawson, N. 127
Lawson, R. 129
Le Fanu, J. 24, 25, 37, 41, 58, 193
Le Grand, J. 221, 231–2, 244–5
double-bed relationship 77, 93, 100
funding 125
public role in health policy 185, 195,
202
tripartite split 64, 69
leadership 159
Learmouth, M. 137
Leathard, A. 20–1
Lee, P. 126
Lee Potter, J. 128
Levitt, R. 190
Lewis, J.
funding 115
nursing 163, 164
public role in health policy 190
tripartite split 57, 59, 60
Leys, C. 105, 218
Liddle, C. 250
lifestyle and health 68, 193, 205
limited list prescribing 61, 94–5
local accountability and national
paternalism 109–10
local authorities
care: 1960s 56–7
future of NHS 245–7
health services 49, 72–3
pre-NHS 19
local health services 244–6
Local Involvement Networks (LINks)
203
local paternalism and national
accountability 80, 81*tab*
London: internal market problems 130
Lowe, R. 8, 20, 21, 119
Lupton, D. 65, 68, 205

M

McDonald, R. 226, 242
McKeown, T. 58
McKinsey's 141
McLachlan, G. 85
McLaughlin, K. 21
Maddock, S. 157
Major, John 196
malpractice 105–6
management 137–61
  1980s 94
  administration 138–40
  budget deficits 224–5
  doctors in 83
  failures 142
  Griffths Report 143–4
  managerialism 140–2
  under New Labour 152–60, 161*tab*
  nurses in 174, 176
  prescribing decisions 225–6
  problems 151, 219–20
  review 1983 93–4
  Thatcher government 145–6
managers
  future of NHS 253–4
  hospitals 240
  NHS 2008 239–40
  numbers of 151
  problems of 153, 154, 155–8
  roles 161*tab*
Mannion, R.
  health policy under Labour 213, 219, 221
  management 153
  tripartite split 67, 68, 72
Marinker, M. 55, 56
Mark, A. 143
Marquand, D. 247
Marshall, T. H. 187
maternity services: 1960s and 1970s 188
matrons 165, 166, 168, 179
Maynard, A. 108, 194
Means, R. 14, 62
Medical Act (1858) 19
medical audit 150
Medical Officers of Health (MOH's) 39, 49, 59
Medical Practitioners' Union 90
medical profession
  gender 69–70
  militancy 84
  and the NHS 2, 6
  and patients 192
  pay 77
  and state 9, 148–9, 226, *see also* double-bed relationship

medical regulation 105–6
medicine
  history of 19–20
  hospital 40–1
  pre-NHS 24–5
mental health services: 1960s 51–3
Merrison, A. 127
midwives 163–4, 178
Milburn, Alan 211, 212, 213, 214, 227
Miles, A. 157
Miller, H. 245, 253
Minford, P. 103
Minister of Health, role of 80
Ministry of Health 22
Mitchell, A. 121
mixed economy of care 66–7, 155–8, 220–4
  future of NHS 249–50
  private sector 221
Mohan, J. 14, 121, 133, 203, 252
Monbiot, G. 250
Monitor 110
Mooney, G. 63, 96
Moore, M. 253
Moran, M. 48, 77, 81, 120, 148–9
Morgan, K. 25, 118
Morrell, D. 43, 215
Morris, P. 7
Morrison, Herbert 26–7, 28*tab*
municipal health services: pre-NHS 19–20
mutual governance 214–15

N

national accountability and local paternalism 80, 81*tab*
National Health Insurance (NHI) 20
The National Health Service Reorganisation (Secretary of State for Health and Social Services) 191–2
National Institute for Health and Clinical Excellence (NICE) 106, 201–3, 211–12, 225–6, 246
1911 National Insurance Act 18, 19–20
national insurance: NHS funding 118
national paternalism and local accountability 109–10
National Service Frameworks 109
National Union of Public Employees (NUPE) 169–70, 172–3
nationalisation 41–2, 93
Nettleton, S. 188, 199
New Labour: health management 152–8
The New NHS: Modern, Dependable (Secretary of State for Health) 210–11
New Public Management 146–51

and the NHS 147–9
Newman, J. 8, 63, 146–7, 148, 153, 204
NHS
  1940s and 1950s 39–49
  1960s 50–8, 86–7
  1970s 58–60
  1980s 60–3
  1990s 63–6
  1997-2000 210–13
  2000s 66–71
  cost of: 1948-51 116*tab*
  creation of 13–37, 21–5, 27*tab*
  criticisms of: 1960s and 1970s 188–9
  effect on nursing 163–4
  funding 113–35, 119*tab*
  future 242–55
  management 137–61
  managers 2008 239–40
  nature of 1–2
  organisational features 13–17
  principles 16*tab*, 17, 34–7, 237–8
  problems 241–2
  public role in creation 183–5
  reorganisation 122–3
  review: 1989 98–100
  today 231–41
  tripartism 2008 231–3
NHS Management Inquiry 143–4, 192
NHS Plan 106–7, 132, 152, 213–26,
  227–9, 235
NHS 'stamp' 118
Norell, J. 55
Normansfield Hospital 142
not-for-profit providers 221
nurse practitioner 177
nursing 163–82
  1940s and 1950s 163–7
  1960s 167–72
  1970s 172–4
  1980s 174–7
  1990s and 2000s 177–81
  2000s 177–81
  conservatism in 182
  effect of NHS on 163–4
  future of NHS 248–9
  gender 170, 178, 181
  industrial action 172–4, 177
  management 174, 176
  minority ethnic workers 173–4
  pay 171–3, 174–5, 180–1
  professionalism 176–7
  recruitment problems 165, 168, 178
  relationship with medical profession
    163–4
  role 179–80
  sexism in 181
  splits within 169–71
  stereotypes 166–7, 173

  training 165, 176–7
  vocationalism 167, 168–9, 181
nursing auxiliaries 171, 177

O

Oakley, A. 164
O'Connor, J. 124
Offer, A. 193
Oliver, M. 89, 125
Oregon experiment 253
Osborne, S 21
Our Bodies, Ourselves (Boston Women's
  Health Collective) 193
overspending: 1940s 116–17

P

Packwood, T. 128, 145
Pater, J. 29
paternalism and accountability 238–9
Patient Advice Liaison Services (PALS)
  203
Patient Forums 214
patients
  care 188–9
  choice 66–7, 197–9, 205, 222–3, 248
  and consultants 186–7
  as consumers 197–9, 251–2
  as customers 179, 196, 206–7, 251–2
  and doctors 192, 199–200
  and General Practitioners 183–4,
    185–6, 193–6, 197
  NHS 2008 240–1
  roles of 206*tab*
Patient's Charter (DH) 196
Paton, C. 139, 150–1, 156, 211, 239
pay
  disputes 85–6, 88–91
  and funding 114
  General Practitioners 82, 83, 85–6,
    89–90
  medical profession 77
  nursing 171–3, 174–5, 180–1
pay body 83
pay-beds 91–2, 115
Payer, L. 45, 193, 203, 205
Peck, E. 216
Peckham, S.
  'double-bed' relationship 93
  funding 130, 134
  health policy under Labour 213
  management 144
  public role in health policy 193
  tripartite split 61
Pemberton, H. 45, 121, 125
Performance Assessment Framework
  153
performance indicators 95–7, 145–6

performance management 152–4, 213,
  219–20
performance measurement 107, 143–4
Petchey, R. 143, 176, 194, 210
Peters, J. 148
Peterson, A. 65, 68, 205
Pettigrew, A. 150
Pierson, C. 8, 89, 126
policy *see* health policy
politics 2–3, 109–10, 239
  2000s 224–6
  and charging 235
  and expenditure 121–2
  future of NHS 252–3
  and treatment provision 202
Pollitt, C. 95, 96, 144, 145, 146
Pollock, A. 236, 249
  double-bed relationship 107
  funding 115, 133, 134
  health policy under Labour 223
  management 154
Poole, L. 211
Pope, C. 115
Porritt Report 50
postcode lottery 35, 103, 201, 225–6
Potter, Lee 112
Powell, Enoch 50–1, 52, 53, 189
Powell, M. 212, 237
  creation of NHS 17, 20, 23
  double-bed relationship 78, 80, 87,
    104
  management 145, 152
  nursing 183
  tripartite split 66
practice-based commissioning 107,
  132, 221–2, 223, 232
prescriptions
  charges 82, 117–18, 120–1, 128
  decisions 225–6
  limited list 94–5
Primary Care Groups 104–5, 211
Primary Care Trusts 232, 239–40
  funding 132
  future of NHS 249–50
  health policy under Labour 211,
    225–6
  management 157
  public role in health policy 201–2,
    204
principals and agents 192, 197, 203, 206
Pringle, R. 70, 157
private care 114
Private Finance Initiative (PFI) 67, 107,
  133–4, 154–5, 217–19
  arguments for and against 134*tab*
  future of NHS 250–1
  problems with 218–19, 236
private sector 93, 192, 194–5

funded by NHS 107
and mixed economy of care 221
and NHS 112, 128–9
professionalism: nursing 176–7
Propper, C. 194, 210
public
  relationship with GP's 183–4
  role in health policy 183–207
  role in health services 251–3
  role of at creation of NHS 187–8
public health
  1970s 59
  1980s 62
  1990s 65
public organisations: competition
  problems 237–8
public role in health policy 183–207
  1950s 183–8
  1960s and 1970s 188–92
  1980s and 1990s 192–6
  1990s 192–6
  2000s 197–204
  creation of NHS 183–8

R

Raban, C. 126
rating systems 213
rationing care 75–6, 103, 115, 120, 128,
  201–2
RAWP (resource allocation working
  party) 130
Raynor 'scrutinies' 143
RCN 169–70, 172–3, 174–5, 177, 182
recruitment problems: nursing 168, 178
Regional Hospital Boards (RHBs) 40
registered nurses 169, 171, 177
reorganisation: 1960s and 1970s 86–7,
  122–3
Resource Management Initiative 96,
  128, 145
restructuring 93–4
revenue expenditure 123*tab*
Richmond, C. 115
Rintala, M. 27, 98, 138
Rivett, G.
  creation of NHS 24, 25
  double-bed relationship 85
  nursing 165, 168, 172
  tripartite split 46, 48, 54, 59
Robb, B. 51
Robinson, Gerry 240
Robinson, J. 176
Robinson, Kenneth 85–6
Royal College of Nursing (RCN)
  169–70, 174–5, 176, 177, 182
Royal Colleges
  creation of NHS 14, 28, 31

double-bed relationship 77, 90, 95,
 97, 105
health policy under Labour 226
management 149
tripartite split 70
Royal Commission on Doctors' and
 Dentists' Renumeration 48, 83
Royal Commission on the National
 Health Service 92
Ruggie, M. 14 (M)

S

Saks, M. 193
Salmon Report 168
Salter, B. 105, 108, 109, 130
Salvage, J. 173, 178
Sang, B. 198
Savage, J. 178
Savage, Wendy 193
Schofield, J. 159
Schwartz, B. 205, 223
Scott, H. 143
secondary care: choosing 197, 202, 205,
 222, 233
Secretary of State for Health 9
Seebohm Report 59, 87
Sethi, S. 171
sexism: in nursing 181
Shaoul, Jean 218
Sheldon, T. 100, 209
Simmons, R. 215
situational logics 11
Smee, C. 80
Smith, J. 33, 220
Smith, M. 77
Smith, R. 62
social capital 124, 204
social care 68–9, 71*tab*, 221
social expenses 124
social rights 187
socialism 79
Stacey, M. 188
staff costs 114
Standing Medical Advisory Committee
 53–4
Stark Murray, D. 86
The State of Nursing 173
state: relationship with medical
 profession *see* double-bed
 relationship
stereotypes: nursing 173
Stewart, J. 187
Stewart, R. 152
Stocking, B. 146
Stones, R. 170
Strauss, A. 140
strikes: nurses 177
Strong, P. 176

Supporting Doctors, Protecting Patients
 (DH) 105
surgery 41
Sussman, M. 158

T

Talbot-Smith, A. 223, 236
Tallis, R. 186
tariffs 155–6
taxation, general 14*tab*, 15–16, 34, 83,
 113, 235
 and capital expenditure 216–17
 redistributionary effect 113, 114, 115,
 117–18
Taylor, F. 68
Taylor, S. 45, 55
Taylor-Gooby, P. 129
Thatcher, Margaret 129, 149
Thatcher government: NHS
 management 93–100, 143–6
'Third Way' 131
Thomas, R. 166
Thorneycroft, Peter 118–19
Timmins, N. 99–100, 211, 212
Titmuss, R.
 creation of NHS 21, 26
 double-bed relationship 83
 funding 117, 119
 public role in health policy 184, 189
 tripartite split 45, 58
Toynbee, P. 68
training: nursing 165, 176–7
tripartite split 14–15, 29–33, 39–73,
 40*tab*
 1960s 57–8
 future of NHS 246–8
 and internal market 64*tab*
 under Labour 71*tab*
 NHS 2008 231–3
Tudor-Hart, J. 55–6
Turner, B. 58, 169, 181

U

universal care 17, 22, 35–6, 237

V

Vidler, E. 8
vocationalism: nursing 167, 168–9, 181
voluntary hospitals: pre-NHS 19–20
volunteerism 191, 204

W

Wainwright, D. 103, 209
waiting lists 114
Waldegrave, William 99–100
Walmsley, J. 61, 63
Walshe, K. 110, 187, 215, 239
Wanless, Derek 132, 235

wartime: creation of the NHS 21–5, 41
Waterman, R. 148
Watkin, B. 50, 133, 139, 189
Watkins, S. 109
Webster, C.
    creation of NHS 14, 20, 21, 22, 25–6
    double-bed relationship 83, 85
    funding 113, 118, 119–20
    public role in health policy 183
    tripartite split 42, 47
Welshman, J. 49, 52, 56, 188
West, P. 100, 130, 155, 210
White, R. 165
White Paper 1944 22–3
Whiteside, N. 119
Whitley Council 171, 172, 174, 175
Wicks, D. 70
Wiener, D. 121
Wilmot, S. 215
Wilson, P. 201
'winter of discontent' 90, 173
Wistow, G. 102
Witness Seminar 129, 149
Witz, A. 179
women 157–8
    and nursing 181
    role of 164–5
Wood Report 165
Working for Patients (Secretary of State
    for Health) 98–100
Wright, K. 59